Introduction to Sensory Processes

A Series of Books in Psychology

Editors: Jonathan Freedman
Gardner Lindzey
Richard F. Thompson

Introduction to
Sensory Processes

Jacqueline Ludel

GUILFORD COLLEGE

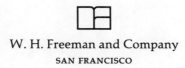

W. H. Freeman and Company
SAN FRANCISCO

Figure on page 86 after "Visual Cells" by Richard W. Young.
Copyright © 1970 by Scientific American, Inc. All rights
reserved.

Figure on page 126 after "How Cells Receive Stimuli" by
William H. Miller, Floyd Ratliff, and H. K. Hartline.
Copyright © 1961 by Scientific American, Inc. All rights
reserved.

Library of Congress Cataloging in Publication Data

Ludel, Jacqueline.
    Introduction to sensory processes.

    (A Series of books in psychology)
    Bibliography: p.
    Includes index.
    1. Senses and sensation.   2. Psychology, Physiological.
I. Title.
BF233.L8   612.8   77–16785
ISBN 0–7167–0032–8
ISBN 0–7167–0031–X pbk.

Printed in the United States of America

1 2 3 4 5 6 7 8 9

Contents

Preface

This book is intended for students who are just beginning their study of the senses. It does not assume any prior knowledge of sensory anatomy and physiology or of perception. It does explore topics in depth, but the material is gradually developed, beginning at an introductory level. The book would be most appropriate as a primary text for sensory-systems courses—whether offered by a psychology department (often under the title "Sensation and Perception") or by a biology department—and as a supplemental text for courses in physiological psychology (psychobiology), experimental psychology, and human physiology.

The first three chapters contain background information in neuro-anatomy and neurophysiology. The treatment is simplified and abbreviated, but it provides an adequate basis for understanding the remainder of the book. Even students who have had prior training in these areas should be encouraged to read the material; it will provide a review and a means of becoming acquainted with the style and terminology used throughout the book.

The next twelve chapters treat each sensory system in detail. They are best read in the order presented because succeeding chapters often build upon information given in earlier chapters. The final chapter summarizes some of the general issues and themes developed throughout the book.

This book differs markedly in style from most college texts. The tone is conversational; there are mnemonic and pronunciation aids; figures and tables are placed directly within the text; analogies appear often; there are questions and imaginary experiments; instead of reference citations, there are recommended readings for each chapter; each chapter ends with a summary that stresses key concepts and words, and that contains explicit directions to the reader; there is a brief treatment of metric measurements in an appendix; there is a glossary with page references to more complete definitions in the text, as well as an index with a more complete listing of page references. In short, I've tried to write for and to students, and to provide the reader with the same information, cues, hints, and prompts that I give my own students in lectures and discussions. I hope the result is a book that will prove more satisfactory, enjoyable, and challenging to students than traditional texts.

Several individuals reviewed the text during its development. The comments, criticisms, and questions provided by William D. Kalberer, Lester A. Lefton, Conrad G. Mueller, and Richard F. Thompson were enormously helpful. Claire K. Morse not only critically read the text and explored various topics with me, she also provided a great deal of very welcome enthusiasm. W. Hayward Rogers, Larry McCombs, and the staff at W. H. Freeman and Company have been as supportive as an author could want. To all of them, my thanks. And to all of those from whom I've learned—especially Robert E. Lana, Conrad G. Mueller, and Jesse Smith—my continuing gratitude and affection.

JACQUELINE LUDEL
September 1977

Introduction

The sensory systems are complicated. Their complexity is worth unraveling, if for no other reason than the fact that whatever we know about the world is based on what we find out through the senses. The senses impose limits on what we know, and they bias our understanding of the world. The limits and biases will become obvious as we go along. But you might, right now, think about how different our understanding of the world would be if we had the eyes of animals such as bulls. (Bulls don't see in color. Their visual world is made up of shades of gray, and they will charge a waving flag no matter what color it is.) Try to imagine what changes we might make in our dress, food, advertising, electrical wiring, photography, painting, poetry, language, and so on, if we couldn't see in color.

Receptors (such as the eyes and ears) are fantastic pieces of equipment. They collect energy in the form of light or sound or temperature or some other stimulus. But, most importantly, they convert that energy into a code the nervous system can use. The conversion is crucial, and it is not entirely understood. We know a great deal about how the various types of receptors collect energy and about the code used in the nervous system. The step in between, that most vital step, is largely a mystery. It's a problem, but it's a problem we seem to live with fairly comfortably in other situations. Consider what you know about pianos or cars or antibiotics or light switches. For the most part, you know how to use these things (the input side) and the results of using them (the output). But most of us don't really know much about what goes on in between.

One tricky aspect of understanding the senses is realizing that the receptors are not the only important structures; the nervous system also analyzes, changes, and abstracts the sensory information. The nervous system too imposes limits on what we know. Consider, for example, what our world would look like if our brains were not able to handle information about color. We could have the same eyes we now have but, if the brain weren't organized to analyze color information, we'd still see in shades of gray.

Because we will need to consider the nervous system, no matter which sensory system we're discussing, we'll begin with some material on the nervous system. Then we'll move on to discuss the sensory systems in detail.

The next three chapters are concerned with the way the nervous system functions. If you already have a good working knowledge of the nervous system, the material will be a review for you. If you don't know much about the way the nervous system functions, the next three chapters will give you enough information to understand the later parts of the book.

Before you begin, let me tell you a bit about the style of this book. Its tone is conversational. Often you'll find suggestions, such as mnemonic devices, that are aimed at helping you remember the material. Sometimes there are questions for you to ponder. There are aids to help you learn how to pronounce new terms. There is a glossary at the back of the book containing definitions of all the important terms; if you discover that you're having trouble recalling the meaning of a term, you can use the glossary to jog your memory. The glossary also gives references to the pages in the text where terms are introduced and explained in detail. The index gives a more complete listing of references to various subjects in the book. All the figures are simple and straightforward. They are placed right in the text so you won't have to search around for them. Sometimes there are instructions that will tell you how to go about experiencing various kinds of sensations.

You are often asked to use your imagination. At the end of each chapter, there is a summary and there are suggested readings. All of this has one aim: to make it easier for you to be an active reader who gets involved in the material, rather than a passive reader who just watches the material go by. I've tried to write this book as if I were talking to you, telling you about the senses, and inviting you to get excited about their marvels. Now it's up to you to be alert and alive, to question, to wonder, and to participate in your own learning process.

This book isn't terribly long. It is concise, and you should not try to read a large number of pages all at once. Read slowly and thoughtfully. And please don't just read on if you feel you don't understand something. Go back and carefully reread the section that's giving you trouble. After each section, pause long enough to think about what you've just read. The senses are fantastic, difficult, exciting things. Allow yourself time to experience how incredible they are; allow yourself time to enjoy your own senses.

1

Neurons

The vertebrate nervous system contains two major portions: the *central nervous system* (abbreviated *CNS*) includes the brain and spinal cord; the *peripheral nervous system* includes all the nerve cells that carry information into or out of the CNS. The entire nervous system is made up of nerve cells called *neurons*. Each neuron has a *cell body* (or *soma*). Extending out from the soma are many small filaments and one large filament. The single large filament is called an *axon*. The small, many-branched filaments are called *dendrites*. (The study of trees is called dendrology. The dendrites are so-named because they do look vaguely like little trees.) Each neuron is specialized to carry information from the dendrites to the soma and on to the axon.

Each neuron is a cell, complete with cell nucleus (located inside the soma), mitochondria (the energy suppliers), and a variety of other organelles (small internal structures). Typical neurons are quite small: somas range in diameter from just a few micrometers to 100 micrometers. (One micrometer is one ten-thousandth of a centimeter. If you are unfamiliar with metric units of measurement, please take a look at the appendix on Measurement Units following Chapter 16.) However, the axons of some neurons are very long. In the giraffe, for example, there are neurons whose cell bodies are located near the base of the tail and whose axons extend all the way to the brain. In an adult giraffe, that may be a distance of three meters (more than seven feet).

Although neurons differ in their details, we can sketch a "typical" neuron.

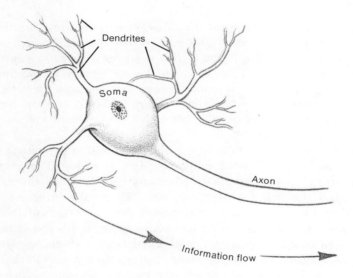

This sketch is just a two-dimensional view of a neuron. Neurons do have depth and you should try to picture the axon as a thick, soft straw coming out of a large central mass (the soma). The dendrites would be thinner, branching straws.

The Nerve Impulse

Suppose we could take just a piece of an axon and keep it alive for a while. Then suppose we could take a meter (similar to what you use to test a battery or electrical circuit) and put one of its probes inside the axon.

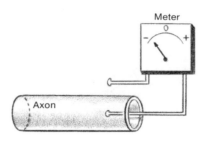

If the inside and outside of the axon are electrically equal, the meter will read zero. If the inside is more positive than the outside, we'll get a positive reading. If the inside is less positive, we'll get a negative reading. In fact, when the measurement is actually made, the reading is always negative. The very small probes that are used in such an experiment are called *microelectrodes* ("tiny probes"), and the meter needle swings to approximately -90 millivolts (a millivolt, mV, is one one-thousandth of a volt).

Two questions arise: first, why is the inside less positive than the outside and, second, what difference does it make? The second question can be answered briefly: when axons are disturbed, the inside and outside become approximately equal electrically. After a short time, the inside becomes less positive again. And that's really all that an axon does: it goes from having its interior some 90 mV less positive than its exterior, to having the interior and exterior about equal, and then back again. The "information" that an axon transmits is this change from inequality to equality and back to inequality. When we hear sounds, see sights, think thoughts, move muscles, write poems, sing, love, laugh or cry, some of our axons are going from their resting state (inequality) to their active state (equality) and then back to their resting state.

The first question requires a lengthier answer. But if you're going to understand the way the nervous system works, it's an important question and a crucial answer. Therefore, please read the following section slowly and thoughtfully.

Neurons are bathed in a fluid that closely resembles blood plasma. The fluid contains quite a few chemicals but we will be concentrating on just four: protein molecules, chloride ions, sodium ions, and potassium ions (ions are atoms that carry a positive or negative charge).

Imagine that we could take just the membrane (the "skin") of an axon, with its contents cleaned out, and place it in pure water.

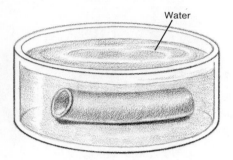

Suppose we throw in some potassium ions. They are positively charged. Within a brief time, the potassium ions (abbreviated K+) will become equally distributed inside and outside the axon.

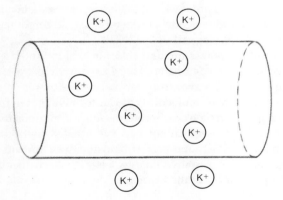

There are two reasons for the equal distribution. First, the ions will "spread out" because their positive charges repel each other. (When the ions have become equally distributed, they are said to be in *electrical equilibrium*.) Second, the ions will "spread out" so that the interior and exterior of the axon will have essentially equal concentrations of the ions. (That is, diffusion of the ions will create what's called *osmotic equilibrium*.)

If we now add some chloride ions (abbreviated Cl−), which are negatively charged, they too will become equally distributed inside and outside. Again, this is due to an attempt to reach electrical equilibrium (in this case, the negatively charged chloride ions are both repelled by each other and attracted by the positively charged potassium ions) and osmotic equilibrium (equal concentrations of chloride ions inside and outside).

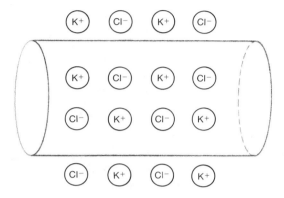

Notice that, if at this point we put one microelectrode inside the axon and one microelectrode outside, our meter will read zero: the inside and outside are electrically equal.

When we put the potassium and chloride ions in the water, some of them moved to the inside of the axon. In the normal state, chemicals move in and out of the axon through very small pores in the axon's membrane. If an atom or molecule is too large, it will not fit through the pores. This appears to be true of protein, which is manufactured by the neuron. Thus, the protein cannot become equally distributed on the inside and outside; it is found primarily inside the axon and it behaves as if it had a double negative charge. Let's go back to our original condition but let's include the protein.

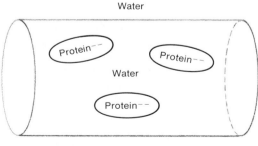

Now let's add the potassium and chloride ions.

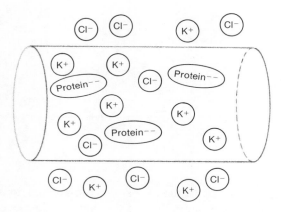

Because the protein behaves as if it had a double negative charge and because it cannot escape from the axon's interior, positive charges (K+) will be attracted to the axon's interior and negative charges (Cl−) will be repelled. We will find more potassium ions inside than outside, and more chloride ions outside than inside. If we put one microelectrode inside and one microelectrode outside, the meter will read close to zero. The inside and outside are close to electrical equilibrium. (In the figure, the net charge inside is −2; the net charge outside is −3.) But the inside and outside are not in osmotic equilibrium—that is, none of the chemicals is found in equal concentrations inside and outside.

There's one more chemical to be added: the sodium ions (abbreviated Na+), which have a positive charge. Something very strange occurs when the sodium ions are added. Instead of becoming distributed inside and outside the axon, they remain outside. Sodium ions are small enough to fit through the axon's pores, but the axon has a mechanism that does not permit sodium ions to stay in the axon. The ions are forced out. It really is not clear what the mechanism is or exactly how it forces the sodium ions out. But it has been given an expressive name: the mechanism is called the *sodium pump*. And it does seem to pump out any sodium ions that get into the axon. Now we have the following situation.

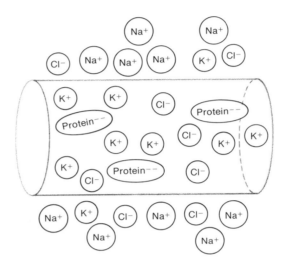

The protein is stuck inside as before; the sodium ions are kept outside by the sodium pump. Notice that most of the potassium ions are inside, attracted by the negative-acting protein and repelled by the positive sodium ions outside. However, notice that some of the chloride ions are inside and some are outside. (Of all the chemicals, the chloride ions most nearly reach electrical and osmotic equilibrium.) The tendency toward electrical balance moves the chloride ions toward the outside, while the tendency toward osmotic balance moves them back toward the inside. As it turns out, these opposing forces are just about equal for the chloride ions. The total result of the distribution of all chemicals is an imbalance in electrical charge between the inside and outside of the axon. If we now put one microelectrode inside and one microelectrode outside, the meter no longer reads close to zero. It will give a negative reading, indicating that the inside is less positive than the outside. (In the figure, the net charge inside is −3; the net charge outside is +8.)

Think back through this discussion. The protein, behaving as if it has a double negative charge, is too large to get outside. The positive sodium ions are kept outside by the sodium pump. The potassium and chloride ions are able to move through the membrane, and they become distributed both inside and outside. However, they do not reach true electrical or osmotic equilibrium, because it turns out to be impossible to reach both states of equilibrium at once. Instead, the system achieves a balance somewhere in between the two equilibrium states. The result is that the inside contains fewer net positive charges than the outside. The inside is less positive.

As long as the sodium pump keeps working, this situation will continue. If the sodium pump stops working, sodium ions will rush in (trying to achieve electrical and osmotic equilibrium). And some of the positive potassium ions will move to the exterior (also trying to achieve electrical and osmotic equilibrium). These movements result in the ion arrangement shown in the following figure.

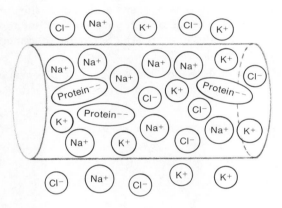

If we use our microelectrodes, we'll discover that the meter will now read very close to zero. (The net charge inside is $+3$; the net charge outside is $+2$.)

If the sodium pump comes back on again, the sodium ions will be forced out. As a result, the potassium ions will move back in. The axon gradually returns to the condition in which the interior is less positive than the exterior.

You now have the general concept of how an axon works. What you need now are some technical terms to describe the axon's activities.

1. When the axon is at rest, undisturbed, the interior is less positive than the exterior by approximately 90 mV. This is called the axon's *resting potential* (the term "potential" signifies that we're making a comparison between the inside and outside). One way to describe this inequality between the interior and exterior is to say that the axon is *polarized.*

2. When the axon is disturbed, the sodium pump briefly shuts off. This allows the sodium ions to rush in. Following the inrush, some potassium ions move out. During this period, the interior and exterior of the axon become approximately equal electrically. This is called the axon's *action potential.* The action potential is sometimes referred to as a *nerve impulse* or *spike.* One way to describe this approximate equality that occurs between the interior and exterior is to say that the axon is now *depolarized.* (The prefix "de-" signifies a reduction or removal of the polarization. Consider the word "defuse." It means to remove a fuse. Try finding one or two other words that use the prefix "de-" to mean reduction or removal. If you take the time now to find other words using "de-," it will be easier to remember the meaning of "depolarize.")

3. Following the disturbance, the sodium pump comes on again. Gradually the axon recovers and reaches its resting potential once again.

This process can be summarized in one graph.

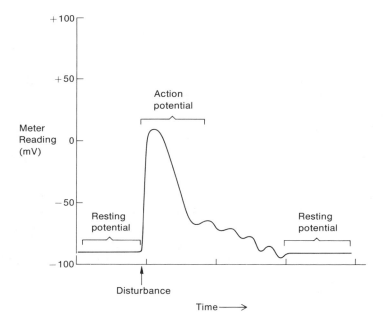

Notice that, in the graph, the meter reading is shown as slightly positive during the action potential. What this means is that the inside of the axon actually becomes a bit more positive than the outside during an action potential. The reason for this is fairly straightforward. The sodium ions rush into the axon as soon as the sodium pump shuts off. Potassium ions do not move out of the axon until many sodium ions have entered. During the short interval between the inrush of the sodium ions and the exit of potassium ions, there will be a greater concentration of positive ions inside the axon than outside. It is during this time that the meter reading will be slightly positive. As the potassium ions leave, the interior and exterior of the axon will become electrically equal; the meter reading will be zero. Therefore, if we want to be precise in our description of the action potential, we should indicate that, during this event, the interior and exterior of the axon do not simply become electrically equal; the interior actually becomes slightly more positive than the exterior for a brief period of time.

The Conduction of The Nerve Impulse

Usually information flows in a neuron from the dendrites or soma toward the axon. At the point where the axon protrudes from the soma (an area called the *axon hillock*), an action potential can be formed. Suppose we use a series of meters, each with one microelectrode inside and one outside the axon.

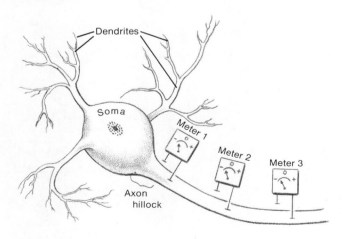

While the neuron is at rest, all the meters will read -90 mV, indicating that the axon's interior is less positive than its exterior along the axon's entire length. Now we can disturb the dendrites or the soma and see what happens. We can disturb the dendrites or soma by warming them, squeezing them, or delivering an electric shock to them. The electric-shock method is most often used because it's easy to control the precise intensity of the shock that is delivered. Suppose we deliver a fairly intense shock to the soma. Within a few milliseconds (thousandths of a second), meter 1 will read zero but meters 2 and 3 will still read -90 mV. Just a moment later, meter 1 will read -90 mV, meter 2 will read zero, and meter 3 will read -90 mV. After that, meters 1 and 2 will read -90 mV, and meter 3 will read zero. Finally, all three meters will read -90 mV.

What has happened is that an action potential was formed at the axon hillock and it traveled down the length of the axon. Each portion of the axon, in turn, shut off its sodium pump and then turned it on again. Let's take a closer look at the situation when meter 1 reads zero but the other two meters read -90 mV.

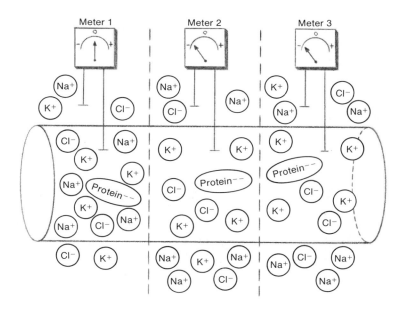

In the segment of axon under meter 1, the sodium pump has been shut off. Sodium ions have rushed in, and some potassium ions have moved to the exterior. The result is that the interior and exterior of that segment of the axon are approximately equal in electric charge. In a moment, the sodium pump will come back on and restore the resting potential. But before it does, some of the ions in the segment of axon under meter 2 are going to react to the arrangement of ions in the first segment. Notice that the exterior of the first segment contains fewer positively charged sodium ions than the exterior of the second segment. As a result, some of the sodium ions will move, along the exterior, toward the first segment. On the inside, there are more sodium ions in the first segment than in the second and some of these will move, along the interior, toward the second segment.

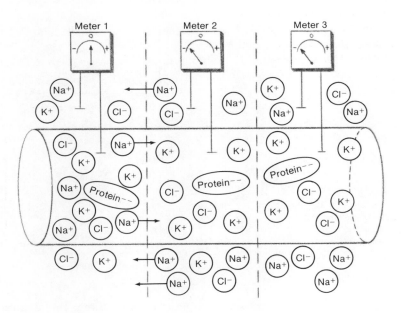

This movement of ions somehow forces the sodium pump in the second segment to shut off. Just as the first segment's sodium pump is beginning to restore the resting potential, the second segment's sodium pump is shutting off and an action potential is created in the second segment. This sequence goes on and on, down the length of the axon. The result is that an action potential moves down the length of the axon in a self-propagating fashion.

The action potential we can record from each of the meters is always the same size. The only difference is the time when the action potential occurs.

Meter 1

The action potential is seen first at meter 1.

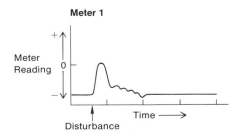

Sometime later, the action potential is seen at meter 2.

Meter 2

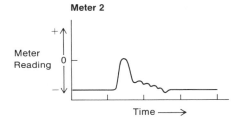

Sometime after that, the action potential is seen at meter 3.

Meter 3

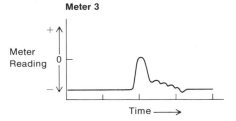

The action potential always signifies the same thing: the sodium pump in a particular segment of the axon has briefly gone off.

The fact that the action potential does not change size turns out to be rather important. It means that, no matter how long or short an axon is, the action potential will be the same size at the end as it was at the beginning. This characteristic of the action potential is called *nondecremental conduction* (which literally means that there is no decrement or reduction in the action potential's size as it is conducted along the length of the axon).

Most axons have very small branches at their ends.

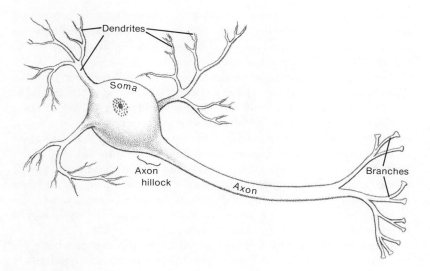

Imagine that we place a meter and microelectrodes at several of the branches. If we set off a disturbance in the dendrites or soma, we now know that (after a while) an action potential will be formed at the axon hillock. The action potential will be nondecrementally conducted down the length of the axon. The question is, what will happen when the action potential reaches the branches? What will we record with the meters? Before you answer, recall what an action potential is (the sodium pump briefly shuts off, allowing the interior and exterior of the axon to become approximately equal electrically) and what nondecremental conduction means (an action potential does not change size as it travels).

Each of the meters at each of the branches will indicate that a full-sized action potential takes place in each branch. You can think of each branch as a skinny axon. Any axon, no matter how skinny, will go from a -90 mV inequality to equality and back to inequality when it's sufficiently disturbed. Thus the action potential will be the same size in each branch as it was in the main part of the axon.

The only functional difference between skinny and thick axons (or portions of axons) is that the skinnier they are, the slower the action potential moves along. If you were designing a nervous system and wanted to send information quickly over a long distance, you would use a long, thick axon. It is not surprising that natural selection has favored the development of such axons where rapid conduction of information is advantageous to an organism.

There are many examples of thick axons. The most famous are the "giant axons" of the squid. They run from the head end of the animal to the muscles of the tail end. When the squid receives information through its eyes and chemical sensors that suggests it is in danger, messages are sent to the dendrites and somas of neurons that have giant axons. Once the disturbances reach the axon hillocks, the action potentials move speedily along, quickly reaching the ends of the giant axons and stimulating the muscles to contract. The squid then jet-propels itself away from the danger. If the axons were skinnier, the message would take longer to reach the muscles, and the squid would be exposed to danger for a longer period of time.

Remember that axons and portions of axons (no matter what their diameter) produce full-sized action potentials, and the action potentials always remain full-sized no matter how far they travel (nondecremental conduction).

Let's go back to the situation we started with. We deliver an electric shock to the dendrites or soma and then record what happens to the axon. We said earlier that one advantage of using electric shock is that the amount of shock delivered can be precisely controlled. If an extremely mild electric shock is delivered to the dendrites or soma, the axon does not produce any action potential. It does nothing. If the intensity of the shock is gradually increased, a point will be reached when the axon does produce an action potential. Therefore, we can say that the axon has a *threshold;* that is, the axon requires a certain level of disturbance before it reacts. And an axon either reacts completely by producing a full-sized action potential, or else it does nothing. An axon cannot produce a half-sized or quarter-sized action potential. Either the sodium pump shuts off or it stays on; either an action potential is produced or the resting potential is maintained. This characteristic is called the *All-or-None Principle:* either the axon reacts by doing all it can (producing an action potential) or it does nothing. If the axon is to react, the disturbance that arrives at the axon hillock must reach or exceed the axon's threshold. Anything less intense will not cause an action potential.

If we go back to the case of the squid, we can consider what the All-or-None Principle means. If the squid's eyes and chemical sensors receive only minimal danger signals, the disturbance may not be sufficient to trigger action potentials in the giant axons. If the visual and chemical signals become more intense (if, for example, a squid-eating whale swims closer and closer), the disturbance will reach or exceed the thresholds of the giant axons. Action potentials will be produced and the jet-propulsion muscles will contract. If the signals become even more intense (the whale closes in), the giant axons will produce more and more action potentials. The muscles will contract more and more rapidly, and the speed of the squid's movements will increase.

If we tested several squids, we might find that some react when the whale is at a considerable distance while others don't react until the whale is quite close. One reason for the differences in the behavior of the squids is their differing sensitivities. Suppose some squids have keener eyes and chemical sensors than others. Those with the keener sensors will detect the whale at a greater distance, and they will send information to the neurons with giant axons while the whale is still far away.

Notice that, when the danger signals become more and more intense, the giant axons produce more and more action potentials. Each action potential is the same size as every other one; there are just more of them. This is true of all axons: when a stimulus becomes increasingly intense, the axons produce more action potentials.

Stimulus Level	*Axon's Response*	
Below the axon's threshold:	nothing	⎫ All-or-None
Just at the axon's threshold:	one action potential	⎬ Principle
Above the axon's threshold:	several action potentials	

Axons differ in their thresholds. Some are quite sensitive, and they will produce an action potential in response to a relatively mild stimulus. Other axons have high thresholds and will not produce an action potential until the stimulus is fairly intense.

Imagine that you've been sitting in a darkened room for 10 or 15 minutes. Then an extremely dim light is turned on and it is gradually made brighter and brighter. The information from the eyes is sent to the brain via the optic nerves (two collections of axons). Think, step by step, about how the axons of the optic nerves will react as the light's intensity increases.

	Light	Optic-Nerve Axons	Perception
1.	Extremely dim (below the threshold of all the axons).	No response.	No light is seen.
2.	Slightly more intense (at the threshold of some axons).	Some axons are mildly stimulated and they each produce one action potential.	A dim light might be on but I'm not certain.
3.	More intense (above the threshold of some axons and at the threshold of others).	Some axons produce several action potentials. Additional axons produce one action potential each.	I see a dim light.
4.	Even more intense (above the threshold of all axons).	All axons are producing several action potentials.	I see a moderately bright light.

Notice that, as the light gets brighter, two things happen: axons with low thresholds produce more action potentials than they did before, and axons with high thresholds begin to react. Thus, we can say that axons translate the intensity of a stimulus into a number code: as the stimulus is made more intense, more axons produce more action potentials.

There is an upper limit to the number of action potentials an axon can produce in a given amount of time. This is the case because an axon requires a recovery period following each action potential before it can respond again. During the recovery period, the sodium pump is restoring the resting potential. Only when the axon is at or near its resting potential can it respond with another action potential.

There is one more point to consider when discussing axons. Most axons are covered by an insulating layer called *myelin*. Myelin is wrapped around the length of the axon. At intervals, there are breaks in the myelin called *nodes of Ranvier* (pronounced "ron'-ve-ay"). In a simplified sketch, the myelin and nodes look like this.

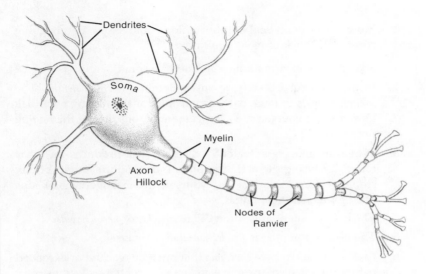

Because axons often lie close to each other, whenever an action potential occurs in one axon, action potentials might be induced in neighboring axons were it not for the myelin. Thus myelin acts in a way similar to the insulation placed around individual strands of wire in a cable.

Myelin has an important additional effect on the conduction of the action potential. Wherever myelin is found, chemicals cannot pass from the exterior of the axon to the interior or vice versa. However, at the nodes of Ranvier, myelin is not present. Thus it is only at the nodes that chemicals can pass into and out of the axon. When an action potential is produced at the axon hillock, sodium ions and potassium ions move through the axon's membrane at that location. The next place along the axon where an action potential can occur is the first node of Ranvier. In between the axon hillock and the first node, myelin prevents the passage of ions into or out of the axon. Thus the action potential does not move smoothly along the length of the axon as we previously indicated. Instead, the action potential appears first at the axon hillock, then at the first node, then the second node and so on, skipping from node to node down the length of the axon. The skipping conduction of the action potential is called *saltatory conduction* ("saltatory" comes from the Latin word *saltare*, meaning to jump or leap). Its primary effect is to speed things up: it takes less time for the action potential to be carried down the axon via saltatory conduction than for it to move smoothly along the length of the axon.

You now have a good deal of information about axons. Before going any further, take stock of what you know.

1.   Axons carry information *away* from the soma.

2.   In the undisturbed state, axons maintain a *resting potential*. The *sodium pump* is in large part responsible for the resting potential. Describe for yourself the arrangement of ions during the resting potential.

3.   When an axon is sufficiently disturbed, it produces an *action potential*. During the action potential, the sodium pump briefly stops working. Describe for yourself the arrangement of ions during the action potential.

4.   The action potential is often called a *spike*, or *nerve impulse*.

5.   The action potential is *nondecrementally conducted*.

6.   Each axon has its own *threshold* that must be reached or exceeded before the axon will produce an action potential. All axons obey the *All-or-None Principle*.

7.   As a stimulus is made more intense, more action potentials are produced; the axon translates the intensity of a stimulus into a number code.

8.   In those axons that have myelin, action potentials are conducted in a *saltatory* fashion down the length of the axons.

Dendrites and Somas

Dendrites and somas have a resting potential of approximately −90 mV, just like axons. The arrangement of protein, sodium ions, potassium ions, and chloride ions is the same as it is in axons. The activity of the sodium pump during the resting potential is the same. However, there are some critically important differences.

To begin, dendrites and somas do not obey the All-or-None Principle. Instead, dendrites and somas respond to small disturbances by making small responses, and to large disturbances by making large responses. Because the size of the response varies with the intensity of the stimulus, the response is not called an action potential. Rather, the responses of dendrites and somas are called *graded potentials*.

Imagine that we've placed some microelectrodes and meters on a dendrite.

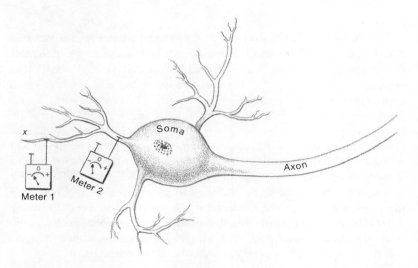

In the undisturbed state, both meters will read −90 mV, indicating that the inside of the dendrite is some 90 mV less positive than the outside. If we deliver an electric shock to the dendrite at point x, first meter 1 and then meter 2 will change from a reading of −90 mV toward zero, and then back to −90 mV. If the shock is mild, the change may be from −90 mV to −70 mV, and then back to −90 mV. If the shock is strong, the change may be from −90 mV to −50 mV, and then back to −90 mV. Because dendrites and somas react in this graded fashion to all stimuli, they are not said to have thresholds.

One way to think of graded potentials is to imagine that the sodium pump hesitates or "sputters," but does not really shut off in response to a disturbance. The greater the disturbance, the more the sodium pump hesitates. But in dendrites and somas, the sodium pump never stops completely.

When a disturbance is created at point x, the graded potential recorded at meter 1 will always be greater than the graded potential recorded at meter 2. This is completely unlike the axon, in which an action potential remains the same size as it travels. Graded potentials get smaller and smaller as they travel. This reduction in size is called *decremental conduction*. If a dendrite is long, a graded response that begins at one end may die out completely before it reaches the soma. Even if a dendrite is quite short, a mild disturbance may produce a graded response so small that, by the time it travels the length of the dendrite and soma, the graded response will not be sufficient to activate the axon.

Let's consider what this means. If, for example, you touch something that is just slightly warm, receptors in the skin may be activated. Dendrites located near the receptors are activated by them. If the receptors are only slightly activated, the dendrites will produce small graded responses. As a graded response moves toward the soma, it gets smaller and smaller. As it travels through the soma, it gets still smaller. By the time the graded responses reach the axon hillock, they may be below the axon's threshold, so that the message of "warm" is never sent to the brain. If the stimulus is more intense (if the object is warmer), a larger graded response is produced initially. It also gets smaller in size as it moves toward the soma and then to the axon hillock. However, it may still be large enough to cause the axon to produce an action potential. An even more intense stimulus would produce a larger graded potential and, by the time it arrived at the axon hillock, it might still be large enough to produce several action potentials.

Try to picture what's going on.

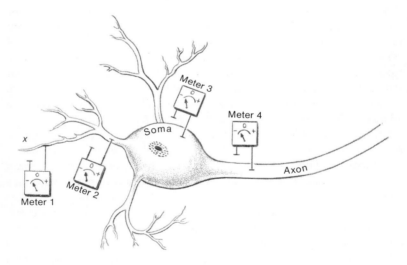

To begin with, all the meters will indicate -90 mV. If a very mild stimulus is applied at point x, we might see the following.

	Meter 1:	-90 mV to -80 mV to -90 mV.
Then,	Meter 2:	-90 mV to -82 mV to -90 mV.
Then,	Meter 3:	-90 mV to -85 mV to -90 mV.
Then,	Meter 4:	remains at -90 mV (no action potential).

If a stronger stimulus is applied at point x, the result will be quite different.

	Meter 1:	-90 mV to -60 mV to -90 mV.
Then,	Meter 2:	-90 mV to -62 mV to -90 mV.
Then,	Meter 3:	-90 mV to -65 mV to -90 mV.
Then,	Meter 4:	-90 mV to 0 to -90 mV (an action potential).

Let's represent this information in a different way.

Very Mild Stimulus   **Stronger Stimulus**

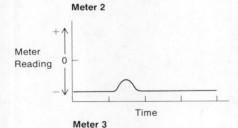

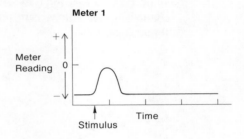

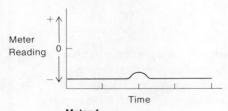

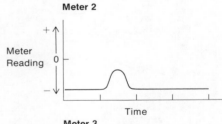

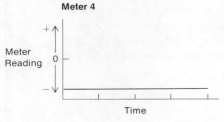

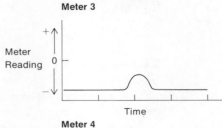

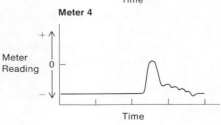

Additional Properties of Dendrites and Somas

Because dendrites and somas respond with graded potentials, they don't r ꓒ recovery periods before they can react again. In fact, dendritꓶ ꓒnd somas can add up two disturbances that occur in rapid succession. One mild disturbance at point x will produce a small graded response at meter 1. A second disturbance of the same intensity will produce a second graded response of the same size. If the second disturbance occurs very soon after the first disturbance, one larger graded response will be produced. This larger graded potential travels down the dendrite in the normal way (and, as always, it is decrementally conducted). Because the dendrite has added together two disturbances that happened at slightly different times, the dendrite is said to have performed *temporal* ("over-time") *summation.*

Dendrites and somas can also add up disturbances that occur at different locations.

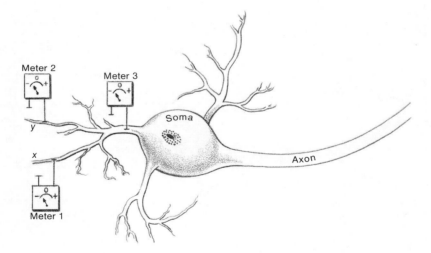

If a disturbance is produced at point x, we will see a graded potential at meter 1. Later, we will see a smaller graded potential at meter 3. Similarly, a disturbance at point y will produce a graded response at meter 2 and, sometime later, a smaller response at meter 3. If two disturbances, one at point x and one at point y, are produced simultaneously, we will see graded responses at meters 1 and 2. A bit later, we will see one graded response at meter 3 that is the combination of the two original graded responses. Let's represent this in graph form.

Stimulate Point *x* Alone

Meter 1

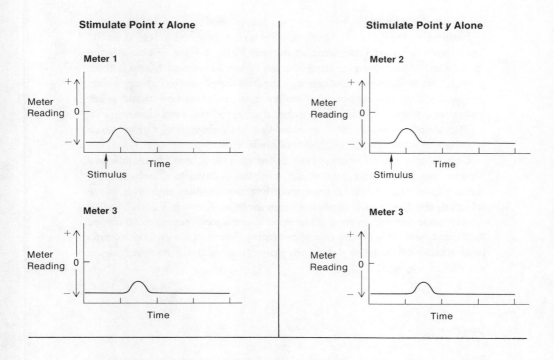

Meter 2

Meter 3

Meter 3

Stimulate Point *y* Alone

Stimulate Point *x* and Point *y* Simultaneously

Meter 1

and

Meter 2

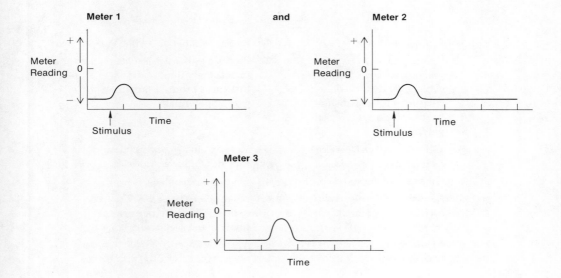

Meter 3

Notice that the graded potential at meter 3 is somewhat less than the actual sum of what was found at meters 1 and 2. This is because the graded potentials coming from the areas under meters 1 and 2 have gotten smaller (decremental conduction) as they traveled along. What is clear is that the response at meter 3 is greater when x and y are stimulated together than when either x or y is stimulated alone.

This ability of dendrites and somas to add up disturbances that occur at different locations is called *spatial summation.*

One final point of comparison between axons, and dendrites and somas: dendrites and somas do not have myelin. Their graded responses travel smoothly down their lengths. Because myelin is white in color, the tissue will appear white wherever there is a collection of axons in the nervous system. Wherever there is a collection of dendrites and cell bodies, the tissue will appear gray. For this reason, collections of axons are called *white matter,* and collections of dendrites and somas are called *gray matter.*

Summary

In order to summarize all this material, let's compare axons with dendrites and somas. Make sure you understand and can define all the italicized terms.

Axons	*Dendrites and Somas*
1. *Resting potential* of -90 mV.	1. *Resting potential* of -90 mV.
2. Produce an *action potential* (*spike, nerve impulse*) when sufficiently disturbed; increasingly intense disturbances produce more action potentials.	2. Produce a *graded potential;* increasingly intense disturbances produce larger graded potentials.
3. Obey the *All-or-None Principle;* they have *thresholds.*	3. Respond in a *graded* fashion; they do not have *thresholds.*
4. *Conduct nondecrementally.*	4. *Conduct decrementally.*
5. Require a *recovery period* after each action potential.	5. No recovery period is needed. They can perform *temporal* and *spatial summation.*
6. *Myelin* is present with its *nodes of Ranvier.*	6. *Myelin* is absent.

Axons	Dendrites and Somas
7. Have *saltatory conduction*.	7. Graded responses travel smoothly.
8. Conduct information away from the soma.	8. Conduct information toward the *axon hillock*.
9. *White matter*.	9. *Gray matter*.

Recommended Readings

Richard F. Thompson has written two exceptionally good texts that contain extensive material about neurons. I strongly suggest you get to know his books: *Introduction to Physiological Psychology* (Harper & Row, 1975), and his more advanced *Foundations of Physiological Psychology* (Harper & Row, 1967).

Scientific American carries high quality, well-written articles by experts in their fields. I will be recommending these articles often throughout the book. The articles can be found in the issues of *Scientific American* in which they originally appeared, or they can be individually ordered as Offprints from W. H. Freeman and Company. Whenever I recommend one of these articles, I'll indicate both the issue in which it first appeared and (in parentheses) the Offprint number.

For more information about the material in this chapter, try the following articles.

Katz, B. "The Nerve Impulse," *Sci. Amer.*, Nov. 1952 (Offprint #20).

Keynes, R. D. "The Nerve Impulse and the Squid," *Sci. Amer.*, Dec. 1958 (Offprint #58).

Solomon, A. K., "Pores in the Cell Membrane," *Sci. Amer.*, Dec. 1960 (Offprint #76).

2

The Synapse

Many neurons receive information from receptors or send information to effectors (muscles and glands). However, other neurons receive information from and send information to other neurons. On the basis of the source or destiny of the information, neurons are often divided into three functional groups:

afferent neurons, which receive information from receptors;

efferent neurons, which send information to muscles and glands; and

interneurons, which receive information from and send information to other neurons.

(It's sometimes hard to keep straight *afferent* and *efferent*. Try using a mnemonic device to help you. The one I use is *afferent* = *af*fection or feeling or the sensing side; *efferent* = *ef*fort or work or muscle action.)

The point of communication between neuron and receptor or effector or other neuron is called the *synapse*. Let's demonstrate with a neuron–neuron synapse.

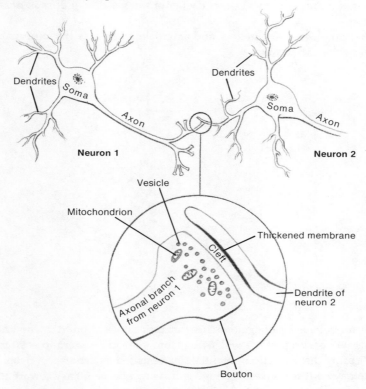

Each of the branches of the axon of neuron 1 has a swollen, knoblike ending called a *bouton*. Next to the bouton, there is a narrow space (called the *synaptic cleft*), and then there is a portion of a dendrite from neuron 2. These structures, taken together, form a synapse.

When you look at the diagram, can you figure out in which direction information will flow? Because you already know that axons carry information away from the soma and that dendrites carry information toward the soma, you should be able to tell that the information will flow from neuron 1 to neuron 2.

Think of the synaptic cleft as a marker that divides the synapse into halves: the information-inflow half and the information-outflow half. The inflow side (the bouton of neuron 1) is called the *presynaptic* side ("pre-" means "before," as in preschool); the outflow side (the dendrite of neuron 2) is called the *postsynaptic* side ("post-" means "after," as in postgraduate). In most synapses, certain structures are found in each half. Presynaptically, there are usually many mitochondria (energy suppliers) and small globular structures called *vesicles*. Postsynaptically, the membrane usually appears darker or thicker than it does in nearby regions.

Suppose we place meters and microelectrodes on the presynaptic and postsynaptic sides.

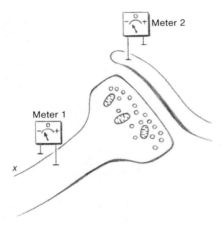

If we deliver a sufficiently strong electric shock at point x, you know what will occur: meter 1 will swing from -90 mV to zero to -90 mV, indicating that an action potential has occurred. After a short delay, as you may be able to guess, meter 2 will swing from -90 mV toward zero and then back to -90 mV, indicating that a graded potential has occurred.

When information flows across a synapse in this way, something takes place that is quite different from what we've previously discussed. Remember that, within a neuron, the information is self-propagating; as each segment of a neuron produces an action potential (in the case of axons) or a graded potential (in the case of dendrites and somas), it affects the neighboring segment by inducing ions to flow to or from the neighboring segment. Information flow across a synapse does not entail this kind of self-propagating activity. Instead, when an action potential reaches a bouton, some of the vesicles migrate to the surface of the bouton, toward the synaptic cleft. The vesicles briefly merge with the bouton's membrane and spill their contents out into the cleft. The contents of the vesicles are chemicals called *synaptic transmitters.* When the transmitters reach the postsynaptic side, they somehow disturb the thickened membrane there and a graded potential occurs. Notice that the original action potential does not directly produce the postsynaptic graded potential. The original action potential only produces the movement of the vesicles and the release of their contents. It is the synaptic transmitter that produces the postsynaptic graded response.

The synaptic transmitters are obviously important. A great many things are not known about them. What is known is the following.

1. In the nervous system, there are several different synaptic transmitters. However, it appears that each neuron produces only one transmitter for use at all its boutons.

2. The synaptic transmitters are manufactured in the soma and then sent down to the vesicles in the boutons via a network of extremely thin pipelines called *microtubules.*

3. Each time an action potential reaches a bouton, the same number of vesicles migrate to the surface where they release their contents. Each vesicle appears to contain the same amount of transmitter as every other vesicle.

4. Synaptic transmitters will continue to create a graded potential as long as they are in contact with the postsynaptic membrane.

The last point is important. Synaptic transmitters are not automatically "used up" in the process of creating a graded potential. If we want to make sure that the postsynaptic neuron stops reacting after a while, we need to find a way to remove the transmitters. (If the postsynaptic neuron keeps on reacting indefinitely, there will be serious problems. Imagine what it would be like if the neurons in the brain never stopped responding, or if they took a very long time to stop responding after receiving just one dose of synaptic transmitter.) The nervous system seems to have developed two main ways of dealing with the transmitters. At some synapses, the synaptic transmitter is reabsorbed by the bouton after it has remained in the cleft for awhile. The reabsorbed transmitter may then be recycled for later use. At other synapses, the postsynaptic membrane produces a neutralizing agent. The best-known example of such a synapse is the so-called *neuromuscular synapse.* If you take the word "neuromuscular" apart, you should be able to tell what kind of synapse it is: the information flows from a neuron ("neuro-") to a muscle ("-muscular"). Therefore, it's an efferent synapse.

At the neuromuscular synapse, the synaptic transmitter released by the neuron is *acetylcholine.* The postsynaptic side, in this case a muscle cell, produces a neutralizer called *acetylcholinesterase* (think of the "-esterase" suffix as meaning "destroyer of"). Chemicals that either block the production of acetylcholinesterase or "mimic" acetylcholine (that is, chemicals—such as nicotine—so similar to acetylcholine that they produce a postsynaptic graded potential) will seriously disrupt the normal workings of the synapse. Certain snake venoms operate in either or both of these ways, causing muscles to contract in a violent, prolonged manner. (Chemicals that block the manufacturing of other neutralizers or mimic other transmitters will affect other synapses.)

In afferent situations (a receptor sending information to a neuron), the receptor contains the mitochondria and vesicles. In efferent situations (a neuron sending information to a gland or muscle), the gland or muscle has the thickened postsynaptic membrane.

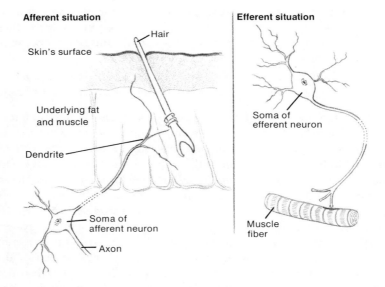

In interneuron situations, the presynaptic side is the bouton of an axon. The postsynaptic side is usually the dendrite or soma of another neuron. In a few cases, the postsynaptic side may be the axon of another neuron. Because synapses are named according to the direction of information flow, we have three possible interneuron situations:

1. *axodendritic synapse* (from the axon of one neuron to the dendrite of another);

2. *axosomatic synapse* (from the axon of one neuron to the soma of another);

3. *axoaxonic synapse* (from the axon of one neuron to the axon of another).

Postsynaptic Potentials

Let's go back to the situation in which we had an axodendritic synapse with meters and microelectrodes.

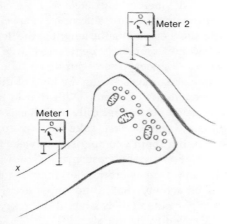

We said earlier that, if point x is stimulated strongly enough, an action potential will be produced; meter 1 will change from −90 mV to zero to −90 mV. After a delay, meter 2 will change from −90 mV toward zero and then back to −90 mV. Remember we said that, in the resting state, a neuron is *polarized* (that is, the interior and exterior are not equal). When the neuron is disturbed, it becomes depolarized. (Aha! Did you think of additional "de-" words back in the last chapter? If you did, you should be able to remember what "depolarized" means.) That is, the interior and exterior become more equal. In the case of axons, the interior and exterior do become equal. In the case of dendrites and somas, the interior and exterior never reach equality but, depending on the intensity of the disturbance, they become "more equal" (less different) than before.

With the meter placed on the postsynaptic side, we can record the depolarization that occurs after the synaptic transmitter is released. The more transmitter released, the larger the depolarization will be. Because the depolarization is occurring in the postsynaptic side of the synapse, it's called the *postsynaptic potential*. Don't be confused by this: we are still talking about a regular graded potential, just like any old graded potential that can be recorded from dendrites and somas. The term "postsynaptic potential" merely indicates that we are recording a graded potential at the postsynaptic side of a synapse, as opposed to recording one somewhere else along the length of the dendrite or soma.

Because axons become completely depolarized (the difference between interior and exterior goes to zero) during an action potential, we could talk about depolarizations as being the kind of thing involved in the activation or "excitation" of axons. With that in mind, a graded potential that is recorded postsynaptically and that is depolarizing is called an *excitatory postsynaptic potential*. Take the term apart: "potential" signifies that we're talking about a comparison between the interior and exterior of some part of a neuron; "postsynaptic" indicates the part of the neuron from which we are recording; "excitatory" means that we're studying the kind of activity that could end up exciting an axon. "Excitatory postsynaptic potential" is a mouthful to say and a handful to write; it's usually called by its initials, *EPSP*.

With all of this discussion of excitation and depolarization, you may have already guessed that there must be another kind of postsynaptic potential. There is. It is, in some ways, the opposite of the EPSP. It is *inhibitory* rather than excitatory, and it is a *hyperpolarization* rather than a depolarization.

Let's take this slowly.

If *de*polarization means a reduction in the difference between the interior and exterior, what must *hyper*polarization mean? (What does *hyper*active mean? *Hyper*sensitive?) Hyperpolarization means that the interior and exterior become even more different than they usually are.

Remember the resting potential? When a dendrite is undisturbed, its interior is some 90 mV less positive than its exterior. During the resting potential, all the positively charged sodium ions are on the exterior. Most of the positively charged potassium ions are on the interior. The negatively charged chloride ions are pretty well spread out. The result is that there are more positive ions on the outside than there are on the inside.

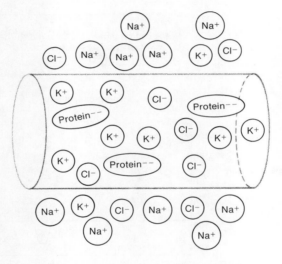

Now, how could you make the interior and exterior even less equal? How could you make the exterior even more positive and the interior even less positive? You could move any of those negative chloride ions found on the outside to the interior, and move the positive potassium ions to the exterior. That is precisely what happens during a hyperpolarization. The more negative ions we can move in and the more positive ions we can move out, the greater the hyperpolarization will be.

Depolarizations and hyperpolarizations are graded potentials. In other words, the greater the disturbance, the larger the response will be. Some disturbances cause depolarizations; others cause hyperpolarizations. It may be that different synaptic transmitters have a depolarizing or hyperpolarizing effect, depending on the particular nature of the postsynaptic membrane. But both kinds of response vary in size depending upon the intensity of the disturbance.

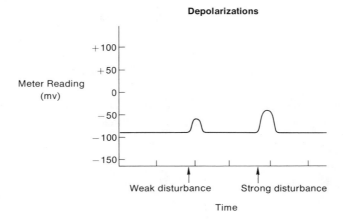

Depolarizations

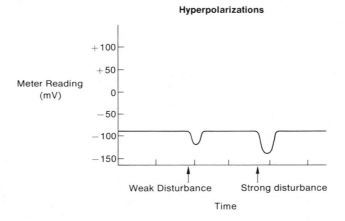

Hyperpolarizations

Hyperpolarizations are not the kinds of things that will activate or excite an axon to produce an action potential. In fact, hyperpolarizations do the reverse. They "inhibit" axons, making it less likely that an action potential will be produced. For that reason, a graded potential that is recorded postsynaptically and that is hyperpolarizing is called an *inhibitory postsynaptic potential,* or *IPSP.*

At many synapses, an IPSP can be recorded. The hyperpolarization moves along the length of the dendrite and the soma. The hyperpolarization gets smaller as it travels along (decremental conduction). If a dendrite is hyperpolarized twice in rapid succession, the hyperpolarizations are added up (temporal summation); if a dendrite is hyperpolarized at two different locations, the hyperpolarizations are added up (spatial summation).

Suppose we have three neurons.

If neuron A is disturbed enough, its axon will produce an action potential. Let's imagine that we can record an EPSP (a depolarization) at meter 1 each time neuron A is disturbed enough to produce an action potential. We know that, sometime later, we will be able to measure a smaller depolarization at meter 3. If that depolarization is large enough, neuron C will produce an action potential.

Now let's imagine that, when neuron B produces an action potential, we record an IPSP (a hyperpolarization) at meter 2. After a while, we will record a smaller hyperpolarization at meter 3, but neuron C will never produce an action potential as a result (remember that hyperpolarizations do not excite the axon).

Suppose now that we get neurons A and B each to produce an action potential. What will happen, a bit later, at meter 3? We will discover, at meter 3, the combined effect of the depolarization and the hyperpolarization.

Let's summarize these three situations.

When only neuron A produces an action potential, a bit later we will record the following at meter 3.

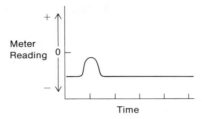

When only neuron B produces an action potential, a bit later we will record the following at meter 3.

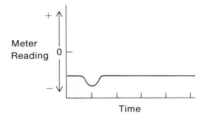

When both neuron A and neuron B produce action potentials, a bit later we will record the following at meter 3.

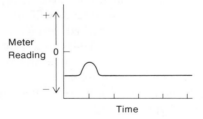

In the third case, the depolarization and the hyperpolarization are added up algebraically. Suppose that an action potential in neuron A is followed by a fairly large depolarization at meter 3, and an action potential in neuron B is followed by a fairly small hyperpolarization at meter 3. Then, if neurons A and B both produce action potentials at about the same time, we'll get a small depolarization at meter 3. (The small hyperpolarization partially, but not completely, counteracts the large depolarization.)

Now suppose that the depolarization recorded at meter 3 when only neuron A was active is just strong enough to produce an action potential in the axon of neuron C. Then, if both neurons A and B are active, the depolarization recorded at meter 3 probably will *not* be strong enough to create an action potential. Therefore, although an action potential in neuron A normally leads to an action potential in neuron C, the simultaneous arrival of an action potential in neuron B prevents (inhibits) the creation of the action potential in neuron C. In effect, neuron B acts as an inhibitor that can reduce the effectiveness of the signal normally passed along from neuron A to neuron C.

The Role of Inhibition

You might reasonably wonder why you would ever want to inhibit axons. Let me give you three situations to consider.

1. Suppose you're in a crowded room in which many different conversations are going on. You decide to "tune in" to one particular conversation. When you do, the other conversations seem to fade into the background.

    What we've described is what's often called the "Cocktail-Party Phenomenon." It's the ability to pay attention to some stimuli while ignoring others. Actually, we do this all the time. Just try to imagine what you would feel like if you were equally aware of all the sights, sounds, smells, touches, and so forth now impinging on you.

    What makes it possible for us to attend to certain stimuli and to shift our attention from stimulus to stimulus is a structure in the brain stem (the lower portion of the brain, where the brain and spinal cord meet) called the reticular formation. Evidently one of the properties of the reticular formation is that it can *inhibit* certain information (that is, the reticular formation can reduce the activity in some collections of axons) while enhancing other information.

2. We are built so that, each time one of our skeletal muscles is stretched, it automatically contracts. This automatic reflex contraction gives us what's usually called "muscle tone." When gravity pulls on the muscles of the arms, trunk, and legs, the muscles contract slightly in response. Without this device, we

would tend to be rather limp. Standing or sitting would require considerable concentration.

But now consider what happens if you bend your arm at the elbow. You contract your biceps muscle. That pulls the forearm up. But it also stretches the triceps muscle in the back of the upper arm. If muscles always contract whenever they're stretched, the triceps should contract. You shouldn't be able to keep your arm bent. In fact, your arm should continually unbend and bend, as first the triceps is stretched and it reflexly contracts, and then the biceps is stretched and it reflexly contracts, ad nauseum.

What happens instead is that, inside the spinal cord, there is an *inhibitory* interneuron. It synapses onto the efferent neuron that usually signals to the triceps that it should contract. This interneuron creates an IPSP in the efferent neuron and prevents it from producing an action potential. Because the efferent neuron doesn't produce an action potential, the triceps muscle doesn't reflexly contract.

3.   In the brain, there are neurons that produce regularly occurring action potentials. No one knows why or how these neurons keep producing action potentials but they do so at a steady rate. Usually we think of information in the nervous system as meaning the production of action potentials. However, if a neuron keeps producing action potentials at a steady rate, either an increase or a decrease in the number of action potentials could signal that "something happened." For this to work, the neurons that are producing the regularly occurring action potentials must be either excited (in the case of an increase in the number of spikes) or *inhibited* (a decrease in the number of action potentials). As we'll see later, this is precisely the method used in certain sensory systems, such as the visual system.

If you're having trouble with the concept that a decrease in activity can signal something, consider this analogy. If you have a heater or air-conditioner that produces a steady hum whenever it's on, you probably aren't even aware of the sound most of the time. You notice it most when the hum begins (an increase in activity) or when it ends (a decrease in activity). In essence, we notice change. In fact, our nervous system is designed to detect change. This is a point to which we will refer again and again. No matter which sensory system we discuss, there will be this important, underlying theme: we are built in such a way that changes in stimulation affect us more profoundly than steady-state situations do. We are attuned to beginnings and endings, to increases and decreases. We little notice constancy.

It turns out that inhibition is every bit as important as excitation in the nervous system. The interplay of the two allows us flexibility, subtlety, modifiability, and the ability to be especially aware of change.

Summary

Make sure you understand and can define all the italicized terms.

Synapses occur between receptors and *afferent neurons,* between *efferent neurons* and muscles or glands, and among neurons (*interneurons*). When the synapses are among neurons, they may be *axodendritic, axosomatic,* or *axoaxonic.*

Synapses usually contain a *presynaptic bouton,* a *synaptic cleft,* and a *postsynaptic membrane* that is thickened. The bouton contains *mitochondria* and *vesicles,* the storage sites for *synaptic transmitters.*

When released, synaptic transmitters may produce either an *EPSP* or an *IPSP.* The resulting *depolarizations* and *hyperpolarizations* are algebraically summed by the postsynaptic neuron. Depending upon their relative strengths, the axon of that neuron may be *excited* or *inhibited.*

Recommended Readings

There are two brief articles that will give you additional information about the synapse.

Eccles, J.   "The Synapse," *Sci. Amer.,* Jan. 1965 (Offprint #1001).

Gray, E. G.   "The Synapse," *Oxford Biology Reader #35.* Oxford University Press, 1973.

There is also an excellent, advanced book you may wish to scan.

McLennan, H.   *Synaptic Transmission,* 2nd ed. Saunders, 1970.

3

The Brain

Before we begin discussing the individual sensory systems, you'll need some information about the neuroanatomy (i.e., the geography) of the brain. This chapter is brief; it is intended to give you a basic vocabulary of neuroanatomical terms. The more specific neuroanatomy of the sensory systems will emerge later, in the course of the discussions of each system.

The brain is basically a large collection of neurons. Estimates of the numbers of neurons in a human brain range from the tens of billions to the hundreds of billions. Simply put, there are a lot of neurons. They tend to be grouped into functional units, and that makes the task of understanding the brain considerably less overwhelming. But the functional grouping is, in some ways, more apparent than real. For example, although most of the neurons involved in vision are clumped together in a few specific locations in the brain, visual information has a widespread impact on the entire brain. When you look at a word, recognize it, and understand it, far more than vision is involved. Also affected are the areas of the brain involved in speech and memory. (There really is no single location for memory in the brain. Memory is perhaps best regarded as something that occurs among neurons everywhere in the brain.) The areas of the brain involved in hearing, motor coordination, and so on are probably also involved. The same widespread impact occurs for any particular sensory system we consider. Thus, although we identify functional regions of the brain, try to keep in mind that the brain does not operate in small pieces—it works as a unit.

If the skull is removed, three very thin layers of tissue are found adhering to the bone and the brain. These tissues are collectively called the *meninges.* They line the entire brain and spinal cord, forming a kind of casing around the central nervous system. Deep within the brain, there are cavities called *ventricles.* They interconnect, and there is a continuation of them that runs down the length of the spinal cord as a thin canal. The ventricles produce a fluid that runs from them, down the spinal canal, and then up and around the outside of the spinal cord and brain. The meninges act as a container to hold in the fluid as it bathes the brain and spinal cord. If the brain and spinal cord were cut so that the ventricles and spinal canal were visible, they would appear as follows.

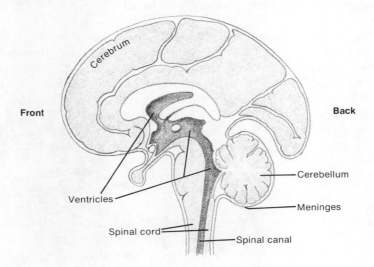

The fluid is constantly being manufactured by the ventricles. The old fluid is drawn off into the circulatory system to be carried to the kidneys and excreted. Reasonably enough, this fluid is called the *cerebrospinal fluid*. ("Cerebro-" refers to the brain; "-spinal" refers to the spinal cord. Thus, the name describes the fluid bathing the brain and spinal cord.)

The cerebrospinal fluid acts like a shock absorber, deadening any sudden impact and keeping the delicate brain and spinal cord from hitting their bony housings. In addition, the meninges and cerebrospinal fluid may serve as a filtering mechanism to keep some materials in the general circulatory system from reaching the central nervous system.

The brain and spinal cord do have rich blood supplies. Embedded in the meninges are numerous veins and arteries. Neurons (like other cells) require nutrients and produce waste products that must be carried off. In fact, neurons have a very high oxygen requirement. The large numbers of blood vessels that are found around and within the central nervous system reflect the need for a rich, constant supply of oxygen.

When the meninges are peeled away from the brain, there is no mistaking the deep and repeated folds in the brain's outermost layer. The whole surface of the brain appears to be made up of hills and valleys of gray matter. (Hmm, gray matter. That must mean lots of dendrites and somas but relatively few axons.)

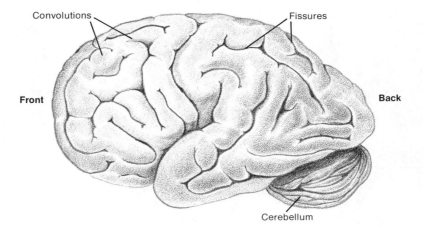

Convolutions   Fissures

Front   Back

Cerebellum

This deeply folded outer portion of the brain is called the *cortex*. The folds in the cortex are called *convolutions*, and the valleys between them are called *fissures*. It is not clear whether the convolutions and fissures come about because of an inherent property of the cortex or simply because, as the brain grows, it nearly fills the skull cavity. In the latter view, as more and more tissue is added during growth, the cortex begins to double up on itself, creating the folds.

Three of the fissures are particularly helpful in figuring out the brain's geography. The longest and deepest fissure runs down the middle of the brain, dividing it into left and right hemispheres. It could be called "the long fissure in the middle." In neuroanatomical terms, that gets translated into the *medial longitudinal fissure*. Extending out at right angles to the medial longitudinal fissure, there is another prominent fissure. This is the *central fissure,* so called because it is found about midway along (in the "center" of) the length of the medial longitudinal fissure. There is a central fissure on the left hemisphere and one on the right.

Finally, there is a fissure that comes up from the bottom of the brain and sweeps toward the back. Again, there is one on the left hemisphere and one on the right. It's called the *Sylvian fissure*.

In a simplified sketch of the left side of the brain, we can identify the central and Sylvian fissures.

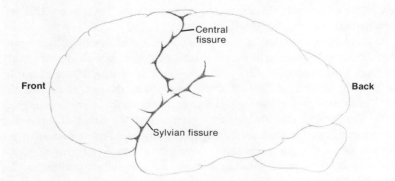

The medial longitudinal fissure can not be seen in this view; it runs along the top edge of the sketch.

These three fissures allow us (1) to divide the brain into left and right hemispheres, and (2) to divide each hemisphere into four regions or lobes.

The region of the brain in front of the central fissure is called the *frontal lobe*. There's a left frontal lobe and a right one. The region under the Sylvian fissure is called the *temporal lobe*. Again, there are two temporal lobes, a left one and a right one.

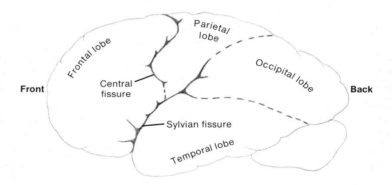

The area just behind the central fissure is the *parietal* (pronounced "par-ī'-et-al") *lobe,* and the remaining portion, at the rear, is the *occipital lobe*. These are also in duplicate; there's one of each on the left hemisphere and one on the right.

If an electric shock is applied to a collection of neurons, you know that action potentials will be produced when the shock is sufficiently intense. This procedure turns out to be very revealing. If, for example, an electric shock is delivered to the neurons in the occipital lobe, the individual will report seeing light, even if the room is kept competely dark. (Delivering electric shocks to regions of the brain of an awake person is a common practice during brain surgery. The responses of the person allow the neurosurgeon to be precise in determining which areas need to be removed. The person can remain awake during the surgery because the brain itself is insensitive to cutting. A local anesthetic is given to numb the scalp and skull.) Because we know the electric shock must have activated neurons in the occipital lobe, it would not be unreasonable to assume that the occipital lobe contains neurons that normally collect and interpret information coming from the eyes. This assumption receives added weight from the fact that, when the occipital lobe is intentionally removed from a laboratory animal, the animal has difficulty seeing. The animal is not blind, but it is obvious from the animal's behavior that vision has been seriously impaired.

If the temporal lobe is electrically stimulated, a person typically reports hearing music or other sounds. If one small region of the temporal lobe (typically somewhere on the left hemisphere in right-handed people) is stimulated, the person begins to make sounds that may or may not be intelligible speech. If the temporal lobes are damaged, hearing and speech are disrupted.

If the portion of the parietal lobe just behind the central fissure is stimulated, the person reportes feeling a tingling or touch sensation on the opposite side of the body. If this area is damaged, there is numbness on the opposite side of the body.

If the area just in front of the central fissure is stimulated, the person moves a portion of the opposite side of the body. Damage to the cortex just in front of the central fissure results in paralysis on the opposite side of the body.

Stimulating other portions of the cortex, such as the rest of the frontal lobes, does not produce any particular response. Damage to these areas results in subtle and complex changes in behavior that aren't easily categorized. Regions of the cortex that don't produce marked responses when stimulated or particular and specific deficits when damaged are usually called *association cortex*. The name suggests that these regions somehow link up or "associate" complicated material, thoughts, and relationships.

Let's go back to our simplified sketch of the left hemisphere and add functional names to the regions.

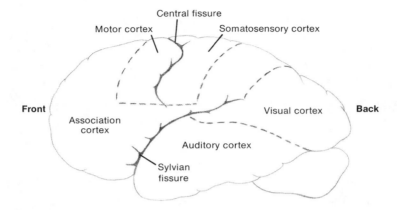

The areas we'll be most interested in are the following.

1. *Visual Cortex:* found in the occipital lobe. Seeing.

2. *Auditory Cortex:* found in the temporal lobe. Hearing.

3. *Somatosensory Cortex:* found in the parietal lobe. Bodily sensations ("somato-" refers to the body; "-sensory" refers to sensations).

For each of these areas, information does not flow directly from the appropriate receptors to the cortex. Instead, neurons collect the information, via their dendrites and somas, from the receptors. The axons of these neurons carry the information into the central nervous system. These axons synapse with a second set of neurons, which carry the information still further into the central nervous system. The process may be repeated several times before the information finally arrives at the cortex. The neurons that collect their information from the receptors are called the *first-order neurons.* The ones that collect information from the first-order neurons are called the *second-order neurons,* and so on.

At each of the synaptic areas along the way, information may be analyzed, modified, compared, sorted, dropped, etc. Because the synaptic areas contain lots of dendrites and somas, they appear as gray matter. The regions between synaptic areas are made up primarily of axons, and they appear as white matter. Let's sketch an imaginary chain from receptor to cortex.

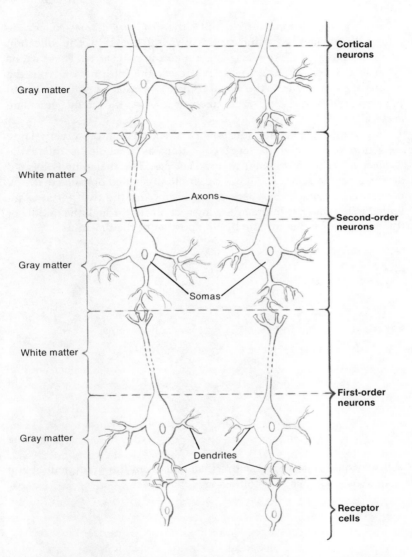

The synaptic areas (the gray matter) are often called *nuclei* (singular, *nucleus*). This is tricky because we're not talking about the nucleus of a cell. When the term "nucleus" is used in reference to a group of neurons, the word simply means an area in which there are many synapses, with lots of dendrites and somas. The axonal areas (the white matter) may be called *tracts* or *bundles* or *fibers* or *nerves*. Each of these terms means a collection of axons.

In the visual system, for example, the *first-order neurons* collect the information from the eye and carry it deep into the brain. The collection of all the axons of these neurons is called the optic *nerve*. These axons synapse onto *second-order neurons* that carry the information from the depths of the brain up to the visual cortex. The synaptic region between the first-order and second-order neurons is called the lateral geniculate *nucleus*.

The lateral geniculate nucleus is a subsection of a very large collection of nuclei. The large collection, as a whole, is called the *thalamic nuclei* or, more simply, the *thalamus*. The thalamus is located deep within the brain, and it has two football-shaped portions to it; one portion is in each hemisphere of the brain, and the two portions are linked in the middle. In the following section cut through the middle of the brain, we see the middle linking portion of the thalamus.

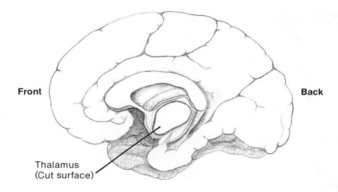

Front   Back

Thalamus
(Cut surface)

If we could remove the entire thalamus from the brain and view it from above, we'd see the following.

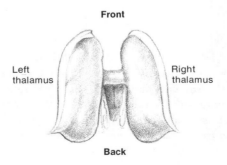

Front

Left   Right
thalamus   thalamus

Back

Keep in mind that the thalamus is deep within the brain. It is a collection of nuclei (therefore the thalamus is a large, funny-shaped piece of gray matter). What is most important for us is the fact that each sensory system, with the exception of olfaction (smell), has a subsection of the thalamus devoted to it. The subsections are each named and they come in "matched sets," with corresponding subsections in the left and right halves devoted to the same sensory system. As an example, you now know that the particular regions in the left and right halves of the thalamus devoted to vision are called the lateral geniculate nuclei.

At each synaptic region in the chain from receptor to cortex, information that started out on one side of the body is carried further into the central nervous system either on the same side or on the opposite side. Thus, we might have the following situations.

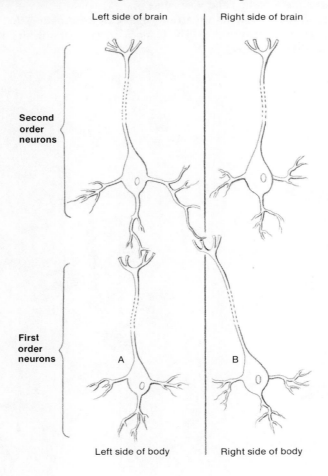

In this sketch, neuron A collects its information from the left side and feeds its information to a second-order neuron that stays on the left side. This kind of arrangement, in which the information remains on the same side, is called an *ipsilateral system* ("ipsi-" means same; "-lateral" means side). The kind of arrangement represented by neuron B, which collects information from one side but carries it to the opposite side, is called a *contralateral system* ("contra-" means opposite).

Remember the discussion of what occurs when the cortex is electrically stimulated. I said that, when the somatosensory cortex is stimulated, the person reports feeling something on the opposite side of the body. That's a perfect example of a contralateral system: the information coming from the left side of the body ends up in the right somatosensory cortex, and vice versa.

Some sensory systems are arranged so that information that begins on one side ends up being sent to both sides of the brain. We can diagram that as follows.

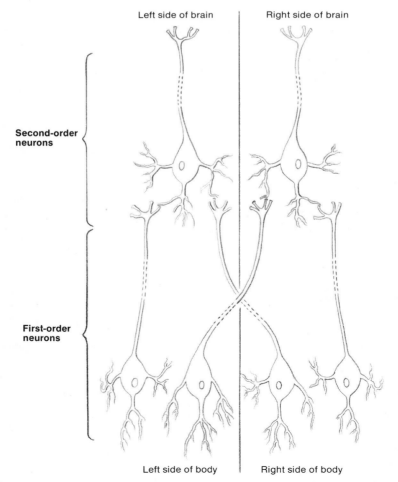

Left side of brain   Right side of brain

Second-order neurons

First-order neurons

Left side of body   Right side of body

Such a system is called a *bilateral system* ("bi-" means two, as in bicycle, "two wheels"). The visual system is a bilateral system. Each eye ends up sending information to both the left and right visual cortices. ("Cortices" is the plural form of "cortex.")

Summary

That's enough neuroanatomy for a while. The best way for you to summarize this chapter is to draw a sketch of the left side of the brain. Draw in the *central* and *Sylvian fissures*. (By the way, what's the name of the fissure that divides the brain into left and right hemispheres?) Find the *frontal, parietal, temporal,* and *occipital lobes*. Mark the *visual cortex, auditory cortex,* and *somatosensory cortex*. Think about what happens if each of these areas is electrically stimulated or is damaged.

Now think about how information gets from a receptor to the cortex. Make sure you understand and can define *first-order neuron, second-order neuron, nucleus* (as used in reference to a collection of neurons), and *nerve* or *tract* or *bundle* or *fiber*. Remind yourself that the *thalamus* is a large collection of nuclei intimately involved in almost all sensory systems.

Finally, figure out some mnemonic devices that will help you remember the meaning of *ipsilateral, contralateral,* and *bilateral systems*.

Recommended Readings

There is an outstanding book of illustrations of the nervous system. The illustrations are color-coded, informative, and clear. Please make sure you get to know this one.

Netter, F.   *The CIBA Collection of Medical Illustrations, Volume I: The Nervous System.* CIBA, 1962.

For a more thorough treatment of neuroanatomy, you can consult any introductory text. Two paperbacks you might consider are the following.

Matzke, H. A., and F. M. Foltz.   *Synopsis of Neuroanatomy,* 2nd ed. Oxford University Press, 1972.

Noback, C. R., and R. J. Demarest.   *The Nervous System: Introduction and Review.* McGraw-Hill, 1972.

For more information on the functioning of the nervous system, you can try the following paperbacks.

Butter, C. M.   *Neuropsychology: The Study of Brain and Behavior.* Brooks/Cole, 1968.

Wooldridge, D. E.   *The Machinery of the Brain.* McGraw-Hill, 1963.

There is an Offprint and a remarkable, poignant book that you may also want to read.

Luria, A. R.   "The Functional Organization of the Brain," *Sci. Amer.,* March 1970 (Offprint #526).

Luria, A. R.   *The Man With a Shattered World.* Basic Books, 1972. Paperback edition, Regnery, 1976. (This moving book is essentially the diary of a Soviet soldier, written after he received extensive brain damage in combat. It will provide you with considerable information about the functioning of the brain, as well as with much to ponder and, perhaps, regret.)

4

The Eye

The eye is a globe-shaped structure. The portion that you can see if you look at your own eyes in a mirror is the outside of the front of the globe. The white material called the *sclera* (pronounced "sklee'-ruh") covers the globe. It's a tough membrane that gives the eye support and shape. In the front of the eye, the sclera merges with a transparent membrane called the *cornea.* When you look at your own eye in the mirror, you can't see the cornea itself. Instead, you see what lies just beneath the cornea: the *iris* (the muscular ring of color) and the *pupil* (the black zone in the center of the iris). If you look at someone else's eye from the side while the person looks straight ahead, the cornea can be seen as a clear, curved surface.

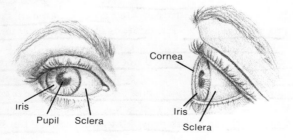

Light enters the eye through the transparent cornea and passes into the depths of the eye through the pupil. The pupil is actually a hole; it's just the opening in the middle of the iris.

The iris contains two kinds of muscles, plus the pigmentation that gives us "brown eyes," "green eyes," etc. One group of muscles runs around the circumference of the iris. These are the *circular muscles.* The other set runs like spokes, toward the pupil. These are the *radial muscles.* In a simplified sketch, they would appear as follows.

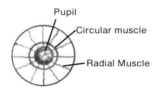

When the circular muscles contract, the pupil is made smaller. When the radial muscles contract, the pupil widens. If you stand in front of a mirror, with a light on nearby, your pupils will appear relatively small. Shade your eyes from the light for a few seconds. During this time, the pupils will widen. When you unshade your eyes and look into the mirror, you can see the pupils get smaller.

The principle behind the changes in pupil size is a simple one: the eyes require a minimum amount of light for comfortable vision. If the room is quite dim, the radial muscles contract, widening the pupil. This permits more of the available room light to enter the eye. When the eye is flooded by light, images become unclear because there is a great deal of scattered light in the eye. In a very bright room, the circular muscles contract, narrowing the pupil. This cuts down the amount of available room light that enters the eye. Thus, the size of the pupil is changed to permit the appropriate amount of light to enter the eye under varying conditions.

Although the principle is simple, the mechanism that implements it is not. Some of the axons in the optic nerve do not go to the thalamic nucleus involved in vision. Instead they go to an area of gray matter called the *pregeniculate nucleus.* The neurons of the pregeniculate nucleus, in turn, send their information to the muscles of the iris. The pregeniculate nucleus is influenced not only by visual information but also by emotional states; that is, portions of the nervous system involved in emotional responses send information to the pregeniculate nucleus. When a particularly interesting stimulus is presented, the pupils widen slightly. In a fear-provoking situation, the pupils narrow.

In fact, we tend to make unconscious note of the pupil size in other people and react accordingly. Women in ancient Egypt were aware of this; they applied a chemical (belladona) to their eyes in order to widen their pupils. The enlarged pupils presumably indicated that they were both interested and interesting. Contemporary eye make-up probably has much the same aim.

Notice that the two pupils are always approximately the same size. If you shade only one eye while looking in the mirror, you'll notice that the unshaded eye's pupil widens slightly. When you remove the shade, the pupils of both eyes narrow. Thus, when a change in the light level occurs in only one eye, the pupils of both eyes are affected. What this means is that we are dealing with a *bilateral system,* in which information from each eye ultimately affects both sides of the brain.

The eyes also tend to move together. Each eye has three pairs of *extraocular* ("extra-" meaning outside; "-ocular" meaning eye) *muscles* attached to the rear half of the globe. The pairs are formed by opposing muscles: one muscle pulls the eye in one direction, and the other member of the pair pulls the eye in the opposite direction. When you move your eyes to the right, the muscles of the right eye that move the eye toward the temple are contracted. The muscles of the left eye that move the eye toward the nose are simultaneously contracted. Once again, we're dealing with a *bilateral system.* However, in this case, the situation is a bit more complicated because the information is sent to different muscles of the two eyes.

Even when you do not shift your gaze, the eyes continue to move in a tremor-like fashion. These very tiny movements are not immediately apparent and can best be demonstrated with some fairly elaborate equipment. It has now been shown that the tremors are necessary for good vision. When the tremors are artificially stopped, images tend to fade from view within a short time. Apparently the tiny movements keep the image moving so that different receptor cells in the eye are affected with each movement. In a sense, we see best when the image changes position very slightly. Recall that in Chapter 2 we noted that the nervous system seems to respond best to change; here is just one example of that theme.

Internal Structure of the Eye

Just underneath the sclera, there is a rich blood-supply layer. It contains large numbers of small veins and arteries, as well as a dark brown pigment. The layer, with all its components, is called the _choroid_ (pronounced "core'-oid"). It provides nutrients for the neural cells in the eye, and its pigment helps to absorb scattered light within the eye.

If the choroid is peeled away, we finally come to the neural layers of the eye, collectively known as the _retina_. It is within the retina that light is absorbed and translated into neural information.

A view of an eye sectioned down the middle (looked at from the cut side) would reveal the following.

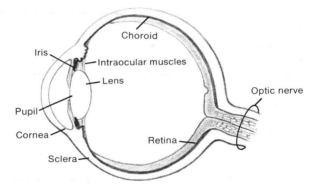

Before we describe the retina in detail in the next chapter, let's identify some of the other internal structures.

Just behind the iris is a _lens_, which is held in place by fine muscles called the _intraocular muscles_ ("intra-" meaning within; "-ocular" meaning eye). The area in front of the iris and lens (that is, between them and the cornea) is called the _anterior_ ("front") _chamber_. It is filled with a clear, watery substance called the _aqueous humor_ ("aqueous" meaning watery; "humor" meaning material). The area in back of the iris and lens is called the _posterior_ ("back") _chamber_. It is filled with a relatively thick, semisolid substance called the _vitreous humor_ ("vitreous" meaning thick or viscous). Light enters the eye through the cornea. It passes through the aqueous humor. Depending upon the size of the pupil, a certain amount of light reaches the lens. Light then travels through the lens and the vitreous humor. Some of the light is absorbed by the retina. The stray light is absorbed by the pigment in the choroid.

Bending Light

The <u>cornea is denser than air, and it is curved</u>. These two properties result in a <u>bending of light by the cornea</u>. In order to understand what's going on, let's use an analogy. Imagine that you have five marbles. If you line them up on a table and push them all with the same force at the same time, they will all move at approximately the same rate. If you place sand in the path of some of the marbles, their speed will be slowed by the sand.

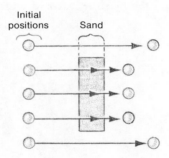

When they emerge from the sand, they will be moving more slowly than the other marbles.

Imagine now that you place an arc of sand in the path of the marbles.

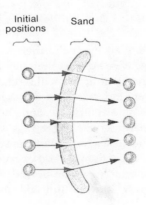

The three marbles in the middle will run into the sand sooner than the ones on the top and bottom. The ones in the middle will be slowed first. As the marbles keep moving forward, the outer ones will reach the sand and also be slowed.

The middle marble goes through the sand head-on. When it emerges on the other side, its speed is slower but its direction of movement is unchanged. The other marbles hit the sand at odd angles. When they emerge, both their speed and direction are changed. In order to understand why the direction changes, consider the marble on top in the sketch. Before it hits the sand, it is spinning over itself again and again. If we looked down on the marble, it would appear to be spinning as follows.

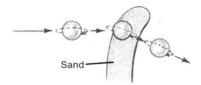

Sand

As it hits the sand at an angle, the half of the marble on the bottom in the sketch will be slowed first, because it reaches the sand first. The top half keeps moving at its original speed. Finally, the top half also enters the sand. Its movement is slowed. But by the time this occurs, the top half is ahead of the bottom half and the marble has turned slightly. When it emerges from the sand, the marble's speed is slower and its direction has changed.

The more sharply curved we make the arc of sand, the more the direction will be changed. The denser the sand, the more the speed will be slowed and the more the direction will be changed. The latter is true because, the denser the sand, the more one side of the marble will be slowed before its other side enters the sand.

Now replace the marbles with light rays and the sand with the cornea. The light rays move at a fairly uniform speed toward the cornea. Because the cornea is denser than air and because it is curved, the light rays going through the middle will be slowed, and the light rays going through the edges will be slowed and will also have their direction altered. Rays that strike the cornea further out toward the edges will be bent more because they will strike the cornea at greater angles.

The direction of the light rays is changed in such a way that they will all eventually meet. The meeting point is called the *focal point*.

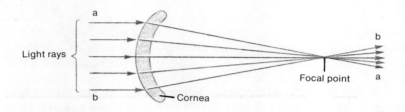

Past the point where they all meet or *converge*, the rays will spread out again as they continue on in their paths.

The denser the cornea or the more sharply angled it is, the sooner the rays will converge.

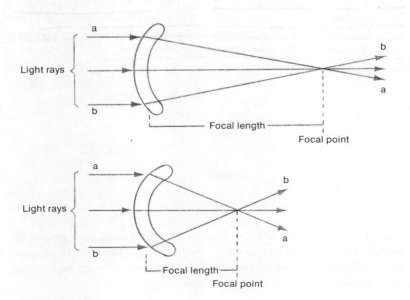

The distance between the cornea and the focal point is called the *focal length*. A denser or more sharply angled cornea will have a shorter focal length. The size of the focal length tells us how much bending power the cornea has. The average cornea has a focal length of approximately 0.022 meter (2.2 centimeters).

Any substance that is relatively transparent, that is different in density from the material through which the light had been traveling, and that is curved will bend light rays; all such substances are called *lenses*. Thus, the cornea is a kind of lens. The structure in the eye called a lens also fulfills all of these qualifications, and it too bends light. The eye's lens is located close enough to the cornea so that light rays pass through it before they have completely converged.

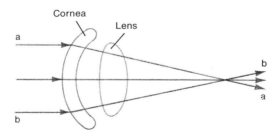

If we want to know the bending power of the lens, we remove the cornea and allow the lens to do all the bending. Then we can measure its focal length. The focal length of the lens turns out to be approximately 0.0833 meter (8.33 centimeters).

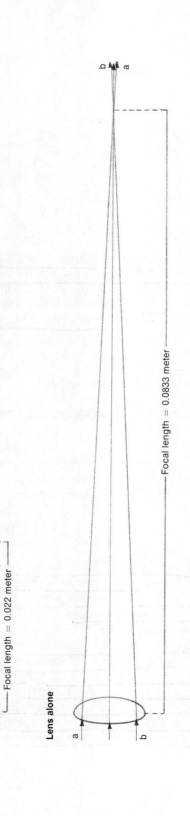

Cornea alone

Focal length = 0.022 meter

Lens alone

Focal length = 0.0833 meter

The cornea has a shorter focal length; it bends the light rays more sharply than the lens; it has greater bending power. The easiest way to summarize this is to figure out a way to describe bending power. A unit, called the *diopter,* is designed to do just this. The number of diopters for a lens is found by dividing the focal length (in meters) of the lens into one:

$$\frac{1}{\text{focal length (m)}} = \text{number of diopters.}$$

Thus, we can readily compute the bending power of the cornea,

$$\frac{1}{0.022 \text{ m}} = 45 \text{ diopters,}$$

and of the lens,

$$\frac{1}{0.0833 \text{ m}} = 12 \text{ diopters.}$$

The greater the number of diopters, the more the light is bent. Thus, in our eye, the cornea (with its bending power of 45 diopters) does most of the light bending. The lens (with its bending power of 12 diopters) adds a small amount of bending.

What is important about the lens is its ability to change shape. When the muscles that hold it in place (the intraocular muscles) contract and relax, the lens becomes thicker and thinner. The thicker it becomes, the more sharply it will bend light. At its thickest, the lens has a bending power of approximately 15 diopters. It is when the lens is at its thinnest that it has a bending power of about 12 diopters.

Light rays that come to the eye from a distant source tend to be parallel to each other when they reach the cornea. But light rays that

come to the eye from a nearby source tend to be diverging from each
other when they reach the cornea.

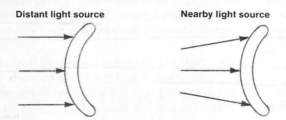

If we want both sets of rays to converge at the same point, we'll have
to add more bending power to the situation on the right. The lens does
just that.

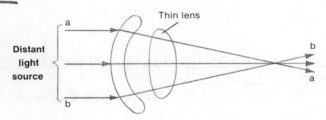

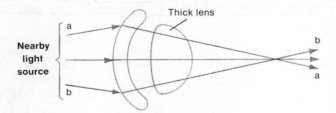

When we focus on nearby objects, the lens becomes thick. It gives
the additional bending power that's needed. The more distant the
object we focus on, the thinner the lens becomes (within limits, of
course). The process of changing the shape of the lens in order to keep
the focal length the same is called *accommodation*. During the "eyestrain"
that comes after a great deal of close work (such as reading, sewing,
etc.), it's really the intraocular muscles, which hold the lens in place and

change its shape, that become "strained." Like all other muscles, they fatigue after prolonged use.

Despite the accommodation performed by the lens, the focal points of very distant and very close objects will not be precisely the same. The lens' ability to change shape, remarkable as it is, is simply not sufficient to bring both parallel light rays and very divergent light rays to convergence at exactly the same point. The focal point of very distant objects is always slightly closer to the lens than the focal point of very close objects.

If the cornea or the lens is not smoothly curved, all the light rays will not converge at the same point. The rays going through the uneven areas will not meet at the same place as the rays that have gone through the rest of the structure. The result is the condition called *astigmatism*, in which portions of images are blurred. Corrective glasses supply the appropriate bending power that's needed to get all the rays to converge at one point.

Focus

The purpose of all this bending of light is to have an image that is in focus when it reaches the retina. The simplest way to think of focus is to consider that an image is in focus when its lines or edges are distinct and clear.

Suppose you are looking at a spot of light. The image of the spot will be in focus when all the light rays coming from it converge on your retina; that is, the image will be in focus when the focal point falls on your retina.

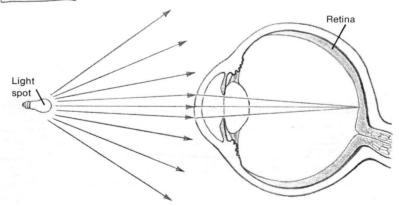

If the retina is located in front of the focal point, the light rays from the spot will strike the retina before they completely converge. If the retina is behind the focal point, the light rays from the spot will strike the retina after they have converged. These rays will therefore be spread out by the time they reach the retina.

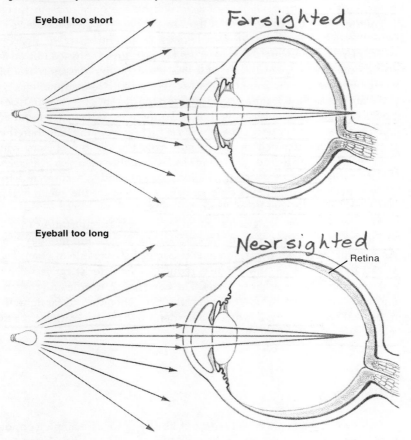

Eyeball too short

Farsighted

Eyeball too long

Nearsighted

Retina

In either case, the image of the light spot will be a blurred area on the retina rather than a sharp spot. However, if the retina is located exactly at the focal point, the rays from the light spot will form one distinct point of light on the retina. Then the spot will be seen distinctly; the image will be in focus. Thus we see that, even if an individual's cornea and lens are smoothly and correctly curved, images will still be blurry if the eyeball is too short or too long.

When the eye is too short, the focal point for nearby objects is located in back of the retina. Distant objects will be the only ones in focus (remember that the focal point of light rays from very distant objects is closer to the lens than the focal points of intermediate or nearby objects); nearby objects will always tend to be blurred. This condition is commonly called *farsightedness,* and it is corrected by glasses that add more bending power, making light rays converge closer to the lens.

When the eye is too long, the focal point for distant objects is in front of the retina. Nearby objects will be the only ones in focus (remember that the focal point of very close objects is further from the lens than the focal point of intermediate or distant objects); distant objects will always tend to be blurred. This condition is usually called *nearsightedness* (in its more extreme form it's called *myopia*), and it's corrected by glasses that make light rays diverge before they enter the eye, moving the focal point further away from the lens.

The lens keeps growing continually. New layers are constantly added to the outside, and the interior layers become denser and less flexible. As a result, as we get older, the lens becomes less capable of changing shape. Its ability to accommodate is reduced. Characteristically, nearby objects cannot be brought to focus. The newspaper, needle and thread, and watch dial are held further from the eye. This kind of farsighted-ness is called *presbyopia;* it is due to a hardening of the lens rather than to a change in the shape of the eye.

Visual Acuity

Usually we are *not* concerned with our ability to focus a single spot of light. Instead we care about our ability to see clearly objects of particular shapes, textures, sizes, and so on. The principles involved in bringing an object to focus are the same as those involved in bringing a spot of light to focus. To understand this, you need to consider that an object can be regarded as an array of individual spots. For example, imagine that you are looking at a neon sign in the shape of an arrow.

Each portion of the arrow can be thought of as a spot of light. Let's consider just two such spots.

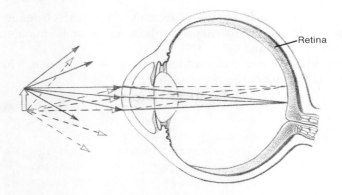

Each spot will be brought to focus. Had we drawn in all the spots, they would appear as an array with an overall shape of the arrow. If all the spots are not brought to focus on the retina, some of the edges or details of the arrow will appear blurry. Now we can say that the object will appear in focus when each of the individual spots making up the object is brought to focus on the retina. If the eyeball is too short or too long, no individual spot will be brought to focus on the retina. If there are irregularities in the cornea or lens, *some* of the spots will not be brought to focus on the retina.

Let's simplify our sketch by allowing one ray of light to stand for the entire collection of rays coming from each spot.

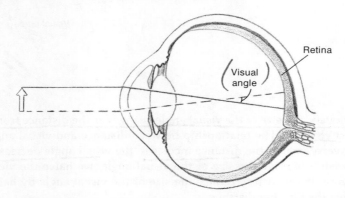

The angle formed by these two rays as they cross each other is called the *visual angle*. It is measured in the same terms as other angles:

degrees, minutes, and seconds (60 seconds = 1 minute; 60 minutes = 1 degree; or to use the common symbols for seconds, minutes, and degrees, 60″ = 1′ and 60′ = 1°).

If the arrow is moved closer to the eye or further from it, what will happen to the size of the visual angle?

It gets bigger.

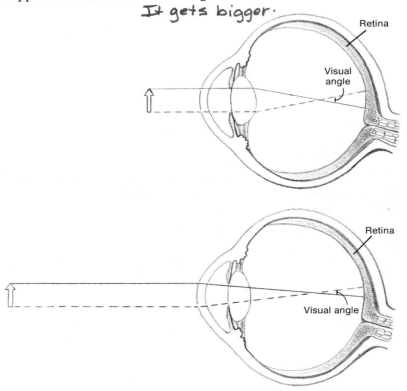

Obviously, the size of the visual angle changes as the distance from the object changes. The relationship between distance and visual angle is an inverse one: as the distance increases, the visual angle decreases. If we wish to double the size of the visual angle, we halve the viewing distance. If we wish to reduce the size of the visual angle by half, we double the viewing distance.

There is another factor that determines the size of the visual angle: namely, the size of the object. If we look at large and small arrows from the same viewing distance, the visual angles they form will not be the same size.

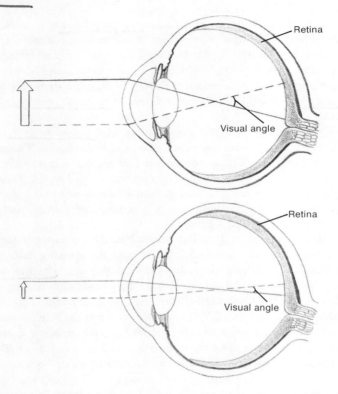

Obviously, larger objects form larger visual angles than smaller objects viewed from the same distance. If we wish to double the size of a visual angle, we double the size of the object. If we wish to reduce the size of a visual angle by half, we halve the size of the object.

Notice that the viewing distance and size of the visual angle are inversely related, while the object size and size of the visual angle are directly related. This means that a small, nearby object can form a visual angle that is exactly the same size as a larger, more distant object.

Almost all of us can clearly see objects that *subtend* (form an angle of) less than one degree. In fact, most of us can see objects that subtend even less than one minute. The smallest visual angle that can be clearly seen is a measure of what's called *visual acuity*. If you require rather large visual angles (that is, you are nearsighted), your visual acuity is poor. If you can clearly see objects that subtend very small visual angles (that is, you are farsighted), your visual acuity is good. You have probably had your visual acuity checked with an eye chart made up of rows of letters that get smaller and smaller.

The original eye chart, developed by Hermann Snellen, consisted of the capital letter E printed many times in various sizes. Viewed from a fixed distance, the different-sized letters form different-sized images on the retina. Snellen tested individuals by having them stand 20 feet from the chart and indicate the smallest E they could see clearly. He found that most people could clearly see an E that subtended a visual angle of 5 minutes.

Snellen therefore used the visual angle of 5 minutes as a norm, against which to compare the visual acuity of individuals. If someone could clearly see an E that subtended less than 5 minutes, Snellen described that person as farsighted. If a person needed an E subtending more than 5 minutes for clear vision, Snellen described that individual as nearsighted. He also worked out a method of stating just how farsighted or nearsighted a person is.

The easiest way to understand this method is to suppose that we label each letter E on the Snellen chart with the viewing distance at which that E will subtend 5 minutes. Let's call this the "distance norm" for the E. For the very large letters, the "distance norm" will be more than 20 feet. For the very small letters, the "distance norm" will be less than 20 feet. If a person with "normal" visual acuity (as Snellen defined it) views the chart from a distance of 20 feet, the smallest E clearly visible to that person will be the one with a "distance norm" of 20 feet. If the smallest E clearly seen is one with a "distance norm" of more than 20 feet, the person is nearsighted. If the smallest E clearly seen is one with a "distance norm" of less than 20 feet, the person is farsighted.

To calculate the visual acuity of the individual, Snellen used a ratio:

$$\frac{\text{Actual viewing distance}}{\text{"Distance norm" of smallest E clearly seen}}$$

For example, consider the person with "normal" visual acuity. Standing 20 feet from the Snellen chart, this person will find that the smallest E clearly seen is the one with a "distance norm" of 20 feet—that is, the E that subtends a visual angle of 5 minutes at a distance of 20 feet. Therefore, using Snellen's system, we say that this person has a visual acuity of

$$\frac{\text{Actual viewing distance}}{\text{"Distance norm" of smallest E clearly seen}} = 20/20.$$

Now consider a nearsighted person. The smallest E clearly seen by this person (at a viewing distance of 20 feet) will be a relatively large one, perhaps one with a "distance norm" of 40 feet. (In other words, at a viewing distance of 40 feet, this E would subtend 5 minutes. Remember that viewing distance and visual angle are inversely related; thus, halving the viewing distance doubles the visual angle. Therefore this E, when seen from the actual viewing distance of 20 feet, subtends 10 minutes.) We can describe the visual acuity of this nearsighted person by the ratio

$$\frac{\text{Actual viewing distance}}{\text{"Distance norm" of smallest E clearly seen}} = 20/40.$$

What about a farsighted person? The smallest E clearly seen by this person (from 20 feet) will be a relatively small one, perhaps one with a "distance norm" of 10 feet. (You should be able to satisfy yourself that this E actually subtends $2\frac{1}{2}$ minutes when seen from the actual viewing distance of 20 feet.) The visual acuity of this farsighted person is described by the ratio 20/10. (Be sure you understand just how this ratio is determined.)

It is important to realize that Snellen's system is not suitable for describing the vision of people who have problems such as astigmatism (where part of the image is clear and part is blurred). It merely suggests the extent to which the image is focused in front of or behind the retina at a standard viewing distance (usually 20 feet).

Let's review the meaning of the Snellen ratio. A person with visual acuity of 20/10 is farsighted. This person can see clearly from 20 feet an E that is clearly visible to a "normal" person only up to a distance of 10 feet. In other words, this person with 20/10 vision can see clearly a letter E that subtends only $2\frac{1}{2}$ minutes.

A person with visual acuity of 20/20 has "normal" vision (by Snellen's definition). This person can see clearly an E that subtends 5 minutes.

A person with visual acuity of 20/40 is nearsighted. The smallest E clearly visible to this person (at 20 feet) is one that a "normal" person could see clearly from 40 feet away. In other words, this person with 20/40 vision cannot see clearly a letter E that subtends less than 10 minutes.

Test your understanding by trying the following exercises.

1. Viewing the chart from a distance of 20 feet, an individual finds that the smallest E clearly seen is one that subtends 20 minutes. What is this person's Snellen ratio?

2. The visual acuity of an individual is described as 20/5. How many minutes are subtended by the smallest E this person can see clearly?

Contemporary eye charts use the same principles as the Snellen chart. However, a variety of symbols (not just E) are usually used to be sure that the person accurately reports what is seen.

You should realize that 20/20 is not necessarily the "best" vision. If you have 20/20 vision, you can comfortably read most printed material without moving the paper unusually close or far away. However, if you work a lot with small objects at close range, you may find it an advantage to be slightly farsighted. (Because you will be able to see clearly images that subtend very small angles, you will do better than if you had 20/20 vision.) On the other hand, because we all become farsighted as we grow older (*presbyopia*), a young person who is slightly nearsighted will not need glasses as soon as a young person whose vision is rated as 20/20.

To give you an idea of the size of an image produced by a known object, the full moon subtends a visual angle of approximately $\frac{1}{2}$ degree (or 30 minutes).

That sounds simple enough. There is one problem: which full moon? Is it the one at the horizon that appears so enormous, or is it the overhead full moon which appears rather small? The answer is "both." Whether the full moon is at the horizon or directly overhead, its image subtends about $\frac{1}{2}°$.

There are only three ways in which the visual angle could actually change size when the moon is seen at the horizon or overhead. (a) If the moon literally shrunk when overhead and expanded when at the horizon, the image size would certainly change. But the moon does not shrink and expand. (b) If the moon stayed the same size but got closer to us at the horizon and further away from us when overhead, the image size would change. But we are at essentially the same distance from the moon whether it's at the horizon or overhead. (c) If the atmosphere at the horizon somehow made the rays of light coming from the moon diverge, while the rays of light coming from the overhead moon did not diverge as much, the image would change size. In fact, there is a very slight effect of the atmosphere along these lines. But it is only a very slight effect, and it doesn't come close to accounting for the very large changes we see.

The answer to the puzzle has to do with the way in which we perceive things. When we know that an object is far away, we tend to perceive it as being larger than its physical image indicates. When we look at the moon on the horizon, we simultaneously see lots of other objects: trees, buildings, the ground, etc. The scenery is rich in all kinds of signals that tell us that the moon is very far away. When the moon is viewed overhead, there is little in the way of information about the moon's relative distance from us. When the moon is at the horizon, we overestimate its size because we know it is very distant. When the moon is overhead, we tend to calculate its size simply on the basis of the actual size of its image.

There is a simple, convincing way to demonstrate what's happening. The next time you see a full moon at the horizon, use your hands to block out as much of the rest of the scenery as possible. The easiest way is to cup your hands as if you held an imaginary telescope and then look through with one eye. When your hands block out the scenery with all its information about the moon's distance, the moon appears to be the same size as it appears when it's overhead. When you remove your hands, the moon appears large once again.

The puzzle of the large rising or setting moon has intrigued people for centuries. It's referred to as the _moon illusion_. It's startling to have the moon "shrink" when the scenery is blotted out. Most importantly, it's a good example of something we discussed in the Introduction: our sensory systems interpret and modify the information received by receptors. You should realize that we overestimate the size of all objects that appear to be far away. It's just that the moon illusion is a dramatic example of this overestimation.

Summary

Make sure you can understand and define the italicized terms.

The exterior of the eye is formed by the _sclera_ and _cornea_. Attached to the sclera are three pairs of _extraocular muscles_. These muscles allow the gaze to be shifted, and they produce tiny, tremor-like movements necessary for clear vision.

When light enters the eye, it is bent by the cornea. The cornea has a bending power of some 45 _diopters_. The light then passes through the _aqueous humor_, the _pupil_, and the _lens_. The pupil can vary in size, depending upon the contraction of the *circular* and *radial muscles* of the *iris*. At the lens, the light is bent again. The lens, held in place by the *intraocular muscles*, bends light to a varying degree in order to *accommodate* to objects at different distances. Once past the lens, the light passes through the *vitreous humor*. In the *posterior chamber*, light comes to a *focal point* as it reaches the *retina*. Some of the light is absorbed by the retina and translated into neural information. Stray light is absorbed by the pigment in the *choroid*.

Images may not be brought into *focus* on the retina for several different reasons, such as *astigmatism, nearsightedness, farsightedness,* and *presbyopia*. The degree of nearsightedness or farsightedness can be measured in tests of *visual acuity* such as the Snellen eye chart. Calculations of rated vision depend upon determining whether an object that *subtends* a particular *visual angle* can be clearly seen.

Recommended Readings

There are two books dealing with vision that are well worth knowing. One is a brief paperback.

Gregg, J. R., and G. G. Heath.   *The Eye and Sight.* Heath, 1964.

The other is a book containing extensive and excellent illustrations as well as a very readable text.

Mueller, C. G., and M. Rudolph.   *Light and Vision.* Time, 1966.

If you would like to read a fuller account of the way in which lenses work, there is a fine and mostly nonmathematical discussion in the following paperback.

Asimov, I., *Understanding Physics, Volume II: Light, Magnetism and Electricity.* Signet, 1969.

You might also want to read the following articles.

Fender, D. H.   "Control Mechanisms of the Eye," *Sci. Amer.,* July 1964 (not available as an Offprint).

Kaufman, L., and I. Rock.   "The Moon Illusion," *Sci. Amer.,* July 1962 (Offprint #462).

Pritchard, R. M.   "Stabilized Images on the Retina," *Sci. Amer.,* June 1961 (Offprint #466).

5

The Retina and Light

The retina lines the interior of the posterior chamber of the eye. It's composed of three layers of cells.

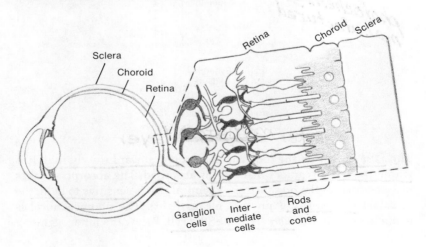

The layer closest to the choroid coat contains the *rods* and *cones.* These receptor cells absorb light and convert it into neural information. The rods and cones synapse onto cells in the *intermediate layer.* In turn, the cells of the intermediate layer synapse onto the *ganglion cells* in the innermost layer. The ganglion cells throughout the eye have axons that run along the inner surface of the ganglion cell layer and that leave the eye, as a group, to form the *optic nerve.*

Rods and Cones

Because the rods and cones provide the neural information, they are of interest and they deserve special attention. Under the light microscope, rods and cones appear to be made up of four parts.

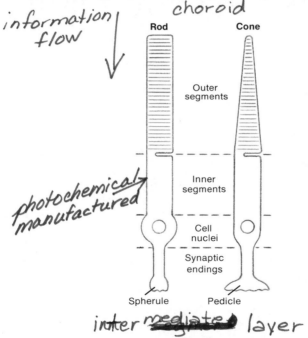

The *outer segments* of the rods and cones point toward the choroid. It is within the outer segment that light is absorbed. The absorption takes place because of the presence of a chemical that is sensitive to light, the so-called *photochemical* ("photo-" means light). The photochemical is manufactured in the *inner segment* of the cell. Below the inner segment, the cell *nucleus* is found (like most cells, rods and cones require a nucleus to produce nutrients and direct the cell's activities). Pointing toward the intermediate layer, the *synaptic endings* of the rods and cones are found.

Rods and cones certainly do not look like typical neurons. They are not true neurons, but they have some important neuron-like properties. First, they react to disturbances (especially the absorption of light) by producing a graded potential that moves down the length of the cell toward the synaptic ending. Second, at their synaptic endings, they have synaptic vesicles, and they are able to activate postsynaptic cells by having the contents of the vesicles spill out into the synaptic cleft.

Rods and cones do not have true dendrites and axons. However, information does tend to flow in one direction: from outer segment to inner segment to nucleus to synaptic ending. The information they carry is always in the form of a graded potential; they do not produce action potentials. The information, like all graded potentials, is decrementally conducted. The rods and cones are capable of spatial and temporal summation, and the size of the graded potential reflects the intensity of the disturbance (the amount of light absorbed).

Notice that there are clear structural differences between rods and cones. The outer segments of rods are club-shaped, while the outer segments of cones are more pointed, almost suggesting the shape of an inverted ice-cream cone. And the synaptic ending of the rods is a small, knobbed structure. It's called a *spherule* (pronounced "sphere'-ule"). The synaptic ending of cones is a broader structure called the *pedicle* (pronouned "ped'-i-kul").

There are two extremely important differences between rods and cones. First, they are activated under different conditions. Rods react during *dim* light conditions. They are extremely sensitive to light, and very little light is required to disturb them (another way to say this is to state that rods have *low thresholds*). Because they are so sensitive, they soon reach their maximum level of responding as the intensity of light is increased. They work best under dim light conditions, and they are the cells that allow us to see in nighttime situations. Cones, on the other hand, are less sensitive (they have *higher thresholds*). They require a greater intensity of light before they become disturbed. Thus, cones operate best under *bright* light conditions.

The second difference is that rods and cones are not equally distributed throughout the retina. The greatest concentration of rods is found away from the center of the retina; the greatest concentration of cones is found in the center of the retina. Imagine that we could remove a retina and place it flat on a piece of paper. The retina would be roughly circular in shape and we could count the number of rods and cones in a strip at the equator.

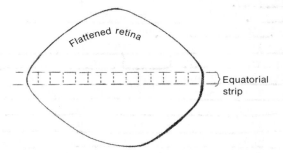

We could divide the strip into a series of sections of some arbitrary size and, starting with the first section on the left, we could count the numbers of rods and cones. Moving on to the next section, we could make the same counts. As we continued the process, we would find that the sections in the middle contain mostly cones. The sections toward the left and right contain more rods than cones. We can represent the results in a graph.

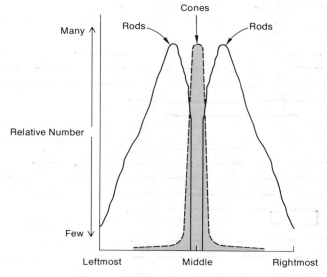

In one section near the middle, no rods at all are found, but there is an enormous number of cones. This area, called the *fovea*, is the region of best visual acuity. When you read or do other detailed work in good light, your eyes gaze at the material in such a way that the image falls on the fovea.

Because there are no rods in the fovea, this area of the retina is not very helpful for seeing under dim light conditions. Under dim conditions, the rod-rich areas located above, below, and to the sides of the fovea are best for seeing. You can demonstrate this for yourself. In the evening, find a location away from bright lights. When you look up at the sky, notice that you can often see dim stars off to the left or right of your direct gaze. If you shift your eyes to look directly at one of the dim stars, it seems to disappear. As you shift your eyes slightly to one side, it reappears. What is happening is that, when you look directly at the star, its image falls on the fovea. Because the fovea contains only cones and because cones require bright light conditions to operate, the star is not visible. When you shift your gaze to one side, the image of the star falls on a rod-rich area of the retina. Because rods are very sensitive, the star becomes visible.

When you look directly at something so that its image falls on the fovea, you are said to be using *central* vision. When you look off to one side so that the image falls on the rod-rich areas, you are said to be using *peripheral* vision.

There is one spot on the retina where no rods and no cones are found. The spot is located below the fovea and toward the nose. It is the spot where all the axons of all the ganglion cells in the retina gather and leave the eye to form the optic nerve. Because there are no rods or cones, but only ganglion cell axons, the spot should be insensitive to light. And it is. For that reason, the spot is often called the *blind spot*. An alternative and frequently used name for it is the *optic disc*. Normally, you are not aware that there is a tiny blind spot in each eye. Certainly when you look at the world around you, you don't see two small black holes. You can see the blind spot if you close your right eye and, with your left eye, focus on the X below. As you move the page toward you, at some point the O will seem to disappear.

———O———————X———

You can see the blind spot of the right eye by closing the left and staring at the O with the right.

Notice that, when you have the page at the correct distance, not only does the O or X seem to disappear, but also the line appears to run continuously through the area where the O or X should be. That is, we seem to automatically "fill in" the missing information, and we fill it in with material that is similar to the nearby, visible material. This is part of the reason why you're not normally aware of the blind spot: you automatically supply the missing information. Imagine that you're looking at a regular, repeating pattern such as wallpaper or a brick wall. The portion of the image that falls on the blind spot will be "filled in" with the same pattern you can see.

There is a second reason why the blind spot is not usually apparent. Notice that you cannot locate the blind spot if you keep both eyes open, look at the X or O, and move the page. The reason for this is that the two eyes each receive slightly different views. The portion of the view that falls on the blind spot of the left eye will not fall on the blind spot of the right eye, and vice versa. The brain collects and interprets the information supplied by both eyes; details that are missing in the information from one eye will be supplied by information from the other eye.

The Retinas of Other Animals

Not all animals have both rods and cones. Some animals have pure rod eyes; others have pure cone eyes. Because rods work extremely well under dim conditions, nocturnal animals tend to have pure rod eyes or eyes that are dominated by rods. Many species of cats, for example, have pure rod eyes.

Nocturnal animals need to take advantage of all the available light. To do this, they not only invest in rods; they also have a reflecting layer located between the rod outer segments and the choroid.

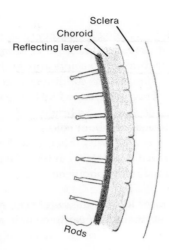

When light comes into the eye, some of it is absorbed by the rod outer segments. Any light that is not absorbed hits the shiny reflecting layer and bounces back toward the outer segments. As it passes the outer segments for a second time, some of it will be absorbed. It's as if the outer segments get two chances to collect the light. Some of the reflected light does not get absorbed during the second chance, and it actually escapes from the eye through the pupil. This is the "eye shine" you see when your headlights shine into the eyes of some animals. By the way, the name of the reflecting layer is the *tapetum lucidum*. Freely translated, it means a "carpet of light."

Animals that spend most of their waking hours in daylight—and that require a very high level of visual acuity—tend to have pure cone or predominantly cone eyes. Many birds of prey, for example, have pure cone eyes.

Humans have both rods and cones: in each eye we have about 6 million cones and about 120 million rods. That means that we have good daylight vision and good acuity (although not as extraordinary as the acuity of some animals), and that we have adequate night vision (although not nearly as keen as some animals). It also means that there might be a light level too dim for the cones but a bit too bright for the rods. At that light level, we should have more difficulty seeing than if the light were just slightly brighter or dimmer. Indeed there is such a light level. It occurs near dawn and at dusk and, as you might expect, automobile accident rates tend to be higher during these periods than at any other time.

Photochemicals

Under dim conditions, everything looks gray to us. At night (away from bright lights), the grass, trees, buildings, everything appears in shades of gray. Under brighter conditions, colors appear. Because you already know that rods operate under dim conditions and cones under bright conditions, it should not surprise you to find out that cones permit us to see in color. Rods can only signal how bright or dim something is. They cannot supply any information about color.

It will take a while to explain why this is true. Some of the explanation will have to be delayed until later chapters, but the beginning of the explanation is to be found in the photochemicals of the outer segments of rods and cones.

Let's take a much closer look at the outer segments. In the electron microscope, the outer segments appear to contain a stack of disks.

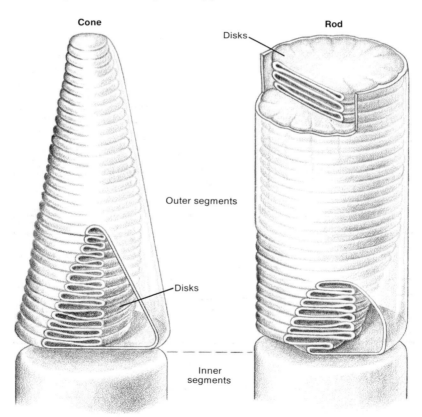

The disks contain the photochemical. The photochemical is manufactured in the inner segment and is sent through a narrow stalk to the outer segment. In the case of rods, the lower part of the outer segment keeps producing new disks. The new disks are filled with photochemical and take their places at the bottom of the stack. Because this process is repeated continuously, the disks are pushed steadily up the stack. When the disks reach the tip of the outer segment, they break off and are engulfed and destroyed within the choroid.

In the case of cones, new disks are not continuously made. Once the cone has developed its complete set of disks during the cone's growth, photochemical is supplied to the same set of disks on a continuing basis.

A great deal is known about the photochemical found in rods. There is less information about the cone photochemicals, but there is enough to allow us to begin understanding the nature of photoreception. For now, let's concentrate on the photochemical found in rods and what happens to it when light strikes it.

The photochemical in all our rods is called *rhodopsin*. It is made of a vitamin A derivative and a protein, called an *opsin*. When a molecule of rhodopsin absorbs light, the molecule changes shape. This process of changing shape is called *isomerization*. The isomerized rhodopsin molecule behaves differently from the original rhodopsin molecule; the isomerized molecule is called *prelumirhodopsin*. That is all that light does to rhodopsin: it isomerizes (changes the shape of) the molecule. It turns out that prelumirhodopsin is not very stable. It rapidly decays into a substance called *lumirhodopsin*. (If you can remember the term "lumirhodopsin," the word "prelumirhodopsin" should be easy to remember. "Pre-" means "before," and prelumirhodopsin is the stuff you get before lumirhodopsin.) Lumirhodopsin is also unstable, and it soon becomes *metarhodopsin I*, which is unstable and soon becomes *metarhodopsin II*, which—you guessed it—is also unstable. Molecules of metarhodopsin II soon split apart into the original constituents, a vitamin A derivative and the opsin.

All of the changes from prelumirhodopsin to the splitting of the molecule occur because the intermediate stages are unstable. Light does not cause these changes. Light only changes rhodopsin to prelumirhodopsin. In fact, if light strikes any of the intermediate stages, the substance is turned back into rhodopsin. So light supplies the energy needed to isomerize rhodopsin, but it can also supply the energy needed to re-isomerize rhodopsin from the intermediate stages. Once the final stage is reached, light alone is not enough to get the split molecule back together; enzymes are required.

A summary of the chain of events might appear as follows.

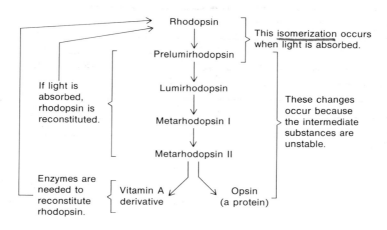

Notice that vitamin A is needed in order to manufacture rhodopsin initially. Because our bodies don't create vitamin A, a new supply of it is needed regularly. Without vitamin A, rhodopsin cannot be made and rods cannot function. The result is a condition called *night blindness*. It should be clear to you that an individual with night blindness cannot see under dim conditions. If the vitamin A deficiency is not rapidly corrected, the outer segments of the rods disintegrate. Once damaged, the rods do not recover and the individual has permanently impaired vision. Because carrots are a good source of Vitamin A (so are liver and spinach), your mother was right when she kept telling you to eat carrots if you wanted to be "bright-eyed."

When rhodopsin is isomerized, it changes color. Initially, rhodopsin is deep purple. As we get prelumirhodopsin, then lumirhodopsin, and so on, the material becomes lighter in color. Therefore, rhodopsin is often said to be *bleached* by light.

The initial step—the change from rhodopsin to prelumirhodopsin—somehow triggers a graded potential in the rod. No one understands precisely how this critically important even occurs. Some theories suggest that the isomerization punches a hole in the rod's membrane, permitting some ions to enter or leave the cell. Others suggest that the isomerization produces tiny vibrations of the outer segment's disks. We know what happens when light strikes rhodopsin, and we know what happens once a graded potential occurs in the rod; but, in the world between the physical energy of light and the neural response of the cell, we are lost. The mystery is fascinating. Without the mechanism for converting an isomerization into a graded potential, all the corneas, lenses, rods, intermediate cells, ganglion cells, lateral geniculate nuclei, and visual cortices would be for nought. It's a mystery worth pondering and unraveling.

The Graded Potentials of Rods and Cones

In order to record the responses of a rod or cone to light, the tip of a microelectrode must be placed inside the receptor cell. Usually when recordings are made from tissue, the microelectrode is mechanically lowered into place. However, microelectrodes thin enough to penetrate the extremely small receptor cells are themselves very fragile and pliable. When a very skinny microelectrode is lowered against a receptor cell, it tends to slip around the cell. In order to make the microelectrode more rigid, its size must be increased; it then becomes too large to enter the receptor cell without killing it in the process. Obviously, recording the responses of rods and cones is a tricky business. It has been accomplished, thanks primarily to the efforts of an ingenious researcher named Tsuneo Tomita.

Tomita reasoned that—if the thin, pliable microelectrode could not simply be lowered into the receptor cell—perhaps the microelectrode could be lowered while the receptor cells were suddenly hurled against it. He placed a piece of a retina on a modified loudspeaker. When the speaker was abruptly and briefly turned on, it bounced and threw the lightweight retina into the air. He mounted a microelectrode above the speaker and found that, on occasion, the tossed retina would impale itself on the microelectrode. In some of these cases, Tomita's microelectrode ended up inside a rod or cone. When it did so, he quickly shone various lights on the rod or cone and measured the cell's responses. Tomita's patience is matched only by his enormous technical skill. Using this method, he was able to record the graded potentials of rods and cones. His findings have now been verified by others.

All the recordings have indicated something that is rather surprising: in response to light, rods and cones produce graded potentials that are *always hyperpolarizations*. These hyperpolarizations sweep down the receptor cells and, unlike hyperpolarizations elsewhere in the nervous system, they cause the synaptic vesicles in the spherule or pedicle to spill their contents out into the synaptic cleft.

It is not at all clear why rods and cones hyperpolarize in response to light, or why these hyperpolarizations cause the release of synaptic transmitters. What is clear is that rods and cones operate in very similar ways.

Cones also contain photochemicals made up of a vitamin A derivative and an opsin. (Vitamin A deficiency will result in the malfunctioning and eventual disintegration of cones as well as rods. "Night blindness" is so called because the individual is usually first aware of a loss of vision under dim conditions.) Light isomerizes the photochemical, and that isomerization is the event that triggers the hyperpolarization.

Cones, however, do not all contain the same photochemical. Each cone contains only one photochemical but, taken together, there are three different cone photochemicals in our retina. The photochemicals differ from each other and from rhodopsin in the nature of the opsin they have. The different opsins determine the sensitivity of the photochemical to different colors of light. Before we can describe these differing sensitivities of the cone photochemicals, we'll need to examine the nature of light.

The Nature of Light

Light is energy; it can be used to perform work. The energy we call light is packaged in an odd way. In some situations, light behaves as if it were made up of individual packets called *quanta* (singular, *quantum*). In other situations, light behaves as if it were made up of waves. The truth is that we don't have a single, all-encompassing description of the behavior of light. All we can do is describe the way it behaves in various circumstances.

Let's consider a situation in which light behaves as if it were made up of waves, similar in many ways to waves on water. Suppose we have a shallow tank of water. When the water is undisturbed, the surface is smooth. If you slap the water at both ends at about the same time, the waves from each end travel toward the middle. Where the waves meet each other, a complicated pattern of waves appears. Depending on the timing, intensity, and frequency of the slaps at each end, the water waves might pile up on each other, forming a very large wave, or cancel each other out in the middle of the tank. In an analogous situation, light behaves the same way. Under the right conditions, lights can either reinforce or cancel out each other when they cross. Instead of seeing the peaks and valleys of water waves, we'd see a *regular* pattern of bright areas (where the lights reinforce each other) and dark areas (where they cancel out each other).

Light waves can differ from each other in two ways. First, the waves may have different frequencies. That is, some waves may have more "peaks" in them than others. In a side view of some waves, we could have the following situation.

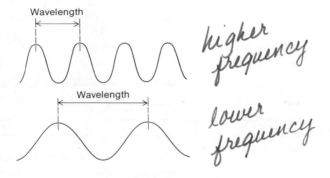

The first wave has a higher frequency than the second. Another way to say this is to note the fact that the distance between successive peaks in the first wave is shorter than that in the second wave. The distance from peak to peak is called the *wavelength*, and it is measured in very small distance units called *nanometers* (abbreviated *nm*). One nanometer is equal to one ten-millionth of a centimeter (again, let me invite you to look at the Measurement Units information at the back of the book).

If our eyes receive light of short wavelengths (about 400 nm), we see blue light. Medium wavelengths (about 525 nm) are perceived as yellow or yellowish-green. Long wavelengths (about 650 nm) are seen as red.

Two waves may have the same wavelength, but the height of their peaks may differ. Thus, the second way in which waves differ is in their height, or *amplitude*.

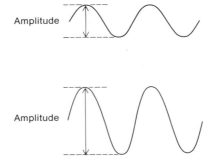

When light waves of greater amplitude reach our eyes, the light appears brighter to us. If we receive a mixture of all wavelengths in which the amplitudes of the various wavelengths are about equal, we see white light. If all the amplitudes are equally increased, the light will appear brighter.

All this seems fine and sensible: when lights interact with each other, they behave as if they were made up of waves. However, there are other situations in which lights do not behave as if they were made up of waves. Let's consider two of these situations.

The first is rather straightforward. It involves the fact that, whenever we are dealing with waves, we must have a medium that does the "waving." For example, we can't have water waves without water. Similarly, we can't have sound waves without air or some other substance through which the sound can travel. Thus, if a ringing alarm clock is suspended in a container and all the air is evacuated from the container, we can no longer hear the ringing. But here's the problem: light can travel through a vacuum. Light does not require any medium through which it must travel, and this does not make any sense if light is truly made up of waves.

The second situation is a bit more complicated. It involves what's called the *photoelectric effect.* To begin, imagine we've arranged two shiny metal plates, a battery, a meter, and some wires as follows.

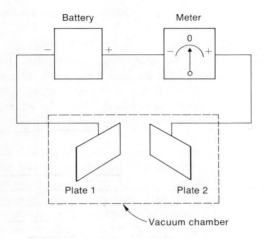

As things stand in the sketch, no current will flow through this circuit because nothing links the two metal plates. The meter reading will be zero. If, however, we shine an appropriate light onto plate 1, current will flow through the circuit; the meter will no longer read zero.

What's happening? Well, electrons travel from the negative side of the battery, through the wire, to plate 1. When a light shines on plate 1, the plate absorbs the light's energy. This energy releases some of the electrons from the plate's surface. Because they are negatively charged, the electrons will be attracted to any surface that is less negative (more positive) than they. Plate 2 does not have a build-up of electrons, and it is therefore not negatively charged. Some of the freed electrons will be attracted to it. As a result, there will be excess electrons that can travel from plate 2, through the wire and meter, to the battery. As long as we continue to shine a light on plate 1, electrons will move through the circuit, and the meter will register the fact that a current is flowing.

What is interesting about this photoelectric effect is the fact that only particular lights will produce a flow of current. The particular lights that work depend on the metal we've used for our plates. For example, if the plates are made of copper, only ultraviolet light will work.

In the wave view of light, ultraviolet light is described as being of a very short wavelength (less than 400 nm). Therefore, when we shine an ultraviolet light on the copper plate, waves arrive in rapid succession.

When they have provided enough energy, electrons are freed from the plate.

But why shouldn't lights of other wavelengths also work? For example, suppose we use red light (long wavelength). The waves will arrive less frequently, but if we make the individual waves large enough (a very intense red light), we ought to be able to deliver whatever amount of energy is required to free the electrons. But we can't. A red light, no matter how intense, will never produce current in the circuit.

These kinds of phenomena led physicists to consider a very different view of light. They proposed that light is composed of individual packets of energy. These packets, or quanta, differ from each other in the energy they contain. "Small" packets are low in energy; "large" packets are high in energy. Furthermore, the quanta are only of particular sizes. There are no half or three-quarter or one-and-an-eighth sized packets; that is, quanta come in whole sizes only.

The energy levels of quanta have a particular significance for us. If a whole group of higher energy quanta is delivered to our eyes, we see a blue light. If lower energy quanta arrive, we see yellow light. Still lower energy quanta are perceived as red light. The greater the number of quanta we receive, the brighter the light will appear. If we receive a mixed group containing about equal numbers of high, medium, and low energy quanta, we perceive white light. The more quanta there are, the brighter the white light will appear.

If we think of light as being composed of quanta, we no longer have any difficulty with the fact that light can travel through a vacuum. Quanta don't require any medium in which to travel; just as we could throw pebbles through a vacuum, so we can send quanta through a vacuum.

According to the quantum view, light is emitted and absorbed as individual packets of energy. In the photoelectric effect, the copper plate absorbs quanta. If a quantum contains sufficient energy, it can free an electron from the plate. If the quantum does not contain sufficient energy, no electron will be freed. An electron can't hold on to the energy supplied by one quantum, wait for a second quantum to come along, add the energy of the second quantum, and then escape from the plate. The energy supplied by each quantum is either immediately used to free an electron, or it is dissipated.

Now it should begin to become clear why only ultraviolet light frees electrons from the copper plate. Each quantum of ultraviolet light contains sufficient energy to free an electron. Quanta of lower energy levels (such as those making up red light) do not contain sufficient energy to free electrons. No matter how many lower energy quanta we provide, no electron will receive enough energy; thus, even a very intense red light will not free electrons.

Notice that, if light were truly energy in the form of quanta, we shouldn't be able to make lights reinforce or cancel out each other when they cross. Most of the quanta, because they're extremely small, should miss each other and have no effect on each other. Once in a while, quanta might collide, but collisions should only occur here and there, at random, in the area where the lights cross. When collisions occur, the quanta certainly wouldn't reinforce or cancel out each other; they would just change their directions and their speeds. As an analogy, think about what would happen if you rolled two handfuls of marbles at each other. Most of the marbles would not be struck, and those that collided would be found at odd locations, here and there. Where marbles did collide, we wouldn't find one double-size marble (they wouldn't reinforce each other) or the annihilation of both marbles (they wouldn't cancel out each other). Yet as you already know, when lights cross each other under the right conditions, a *regular* pattern of bright and dark areas is found.

We are forced to conclude that some situations are best understood if we view light as quanta, while other situations are best understood if we view light as waves. The fact that light sometimes behaves like quanta and sometimes like waves shouldn't bother you. Keep in mind that we are describing light's behavior and not the essence of, the true meaning of, the basic nature of light. Its essence, true meaning, and basic nature are "energy." A physicist friend of mine often uses an analogy. He says that a child may behave in a sweet, pleasant, endearing way in some situations. Then we say the child is behaving like an angel. In other situations, the same child may be quarrelsome, nasty, and cruel. In that case, we say the child is behaving like a devil. The child is neither angel nor devil. Its behavior may be angelish or devilish, depending on the situation. Similarly, light may be "quanta-ish" or "wave-ish," depending on the situation.

Whether we choose to talk about light as quanta or as waves, two properties are important because they give rise to our perceptions of color and of brightness.

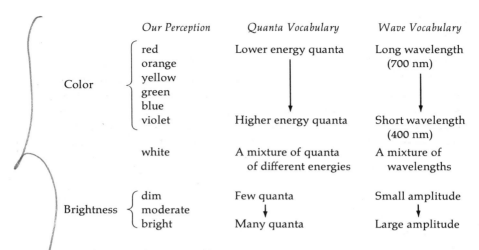

	Our Perception	Quanta Vocabulary	Wave Vocabulary
Color	red orange yellow green blue violet	Lower energy quanta ↓ Higher energy quanta	Long wavelength (700 nm) ↓ Short wavelength (400 nm)
	white	A mixture of quanta of different energies	A mixture of wavelengths
Brightness	dim moderate bright	Few quanta ↓ Many quanta	Small amplitude ↓ Large amplitude

Let's return now to the topic of the graded potentials of rods and cones. For the moment, let's use the wave vocabulary. When any wavelengths of light fall on rods or cones, the cells hyperpolarize. However, some wavelengths produce larger hyperpolarizations than others.

With a microelectrode placed in a rod, we can examine what happens when lights of different wavelengths are shone on the cell. We'll use wavelengths that all have the same amplitude. (In other words, we're going to turn on lights of different colors that are equally intense). The rod hyperpolarizes in response to all of the lights, but it produces larger hyperpolarizations to lights in the region of 480 nm (the green-blues) than to any other light. All rods react in the same way.

With a microelectrode placed in a cone, we can also record hyperpolarizations in response to equal amplitude lights of different wavelengths. However, unlike rods, cones do not all react in the same way. Some cones produce their greatest hyperpolarization in response to 570 nm (orange-red); others react most to 550 nm (green); still others react most to 440 nm (blue-violet).

During the day, when light conditions are bright, we have three different kinds of cones that can react well to lights of varying wavelengths throughout the *visible spectrum* (all the colors we can see). At night, under dim conditions, only the rods work. They respond to wavelengths throughout the spectrum, but they react best to lights in the blue-green region. For this reason, objects that are blue-green in color will appear brighter at night than objects of other colors. Everything will be in shades of gray, but the blue-green objects will appear brighter. The increased brightness of blue-green objects at night was noted hundred of years ago; it's called the *Purkinje effect* (pronounced "purr-kin'-gee"). Recently, fire trucks and ambulances in some cities have been painted a bright, sickly looking green instead of the traditional red. The change has occurred because of a long overdue recognition that Purkinje was right: under dim conditions, it's easier to see something in the green-blue portion of the spectrum than to see something red. In daylight conditions, either can be seen well. (By the way, automobile accident rates are lower for light blue or green cars than for cars of other colors, probably because of their increased visibility.)

The Intermediate Cells of the Retina

The rods and cones synapse onto the cells of the intermediate layer of the retina. The intermediate layer contains three kinds of cells: the *bipolar cells* carry information primarily from the rods and cones to the ganglion cells; the *horizontal cells* carry information horizontally through the intermediate layer; the *amacrine cells* are large cells that may collect information from rods, cones, bipolar cells, or horizontal cells and may send information to bipolar cells, horizontal cells, or ganglion cells. A schematic drawing of these cells might appear as follows.

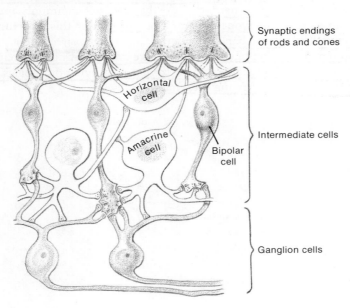

Synaptic endings of rods and cones

Horizontal cell

Amacrine cell

Bipolar cell

Intermediate cells

Ganglion cells

Close examination of the synaptic endings of the rods and cones reveals that often bipolar cells, amacrine cells, and horizontal cells all receive information from the receptor cells. In the electron microscope, both the spherules of rods and the pedicles of cones appear to have a series of indentations facing the synaptic cleft.

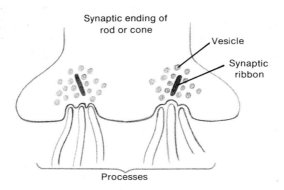

In most of the indentations, from 2 to 4 processes are found per indentation. When the processes are traced to their cell bodies, it becomes clear that some belong to bipolar cells, some to amacrine cells, and some to horizontal cells.

On the presynaptic side, numerous synaptic vesicles are found. In addition, there is a prominent structure that does not commonly appear at synapses in the nervous system. The function of this structure is unknown; it is a dense band of material called the *synaptic ribbon*.

Throughout the intermediate layer, there are a great many synapses among the bipolar, amacrine, and horizontal cells. Synaptic vesicles and synaptic ribbons identify the presynaptic sides.

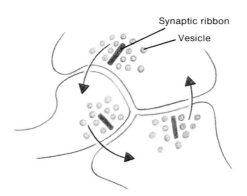

In this sketch (a representation of what can be seen in an electron microscope), there are three synapses among three cell processes. The direction of information flow is indicated by arrows. Notice that the three processes all influence each other and that, once a disturbance has begun in any of the processes, the other two will eventually be disturbed. Furthermore, these processes will send information back to the first process. And so it will go. Because each cell in the intermediate layer produces only *graded potentials,* the disturbance will gradually die out as a result of decremental conduction. This kind of arrangement, often called a *feedback loop,* allows a single disturbance to have a relatively sustained effect.

The synapses between the cells of the intermediate layer and the ganglion cells also contain synaptic vesicles and synaptic ribbons, and they too may form feedback loops.

The intermediate layer certainly appears to be a place where information is collected, compared, modified, sustained, etc. Two prominent features of this complicated set of cells and synapses bear mentioning: in the intermediate layer, information *converges* and information *diverges. Convergent arrangements* mean that information from several cells feeds into one cell. As an example, several receptor cells may send information to one bipolar cell, or several bipolar and horizontal cells may send information to one amacrine cell. Convergence must occur because there are about 126 million receptor cells but only 1 million ganglion cells in each retina. The information from all the receptor cells must eventually be collected by the comparatively few ganglion cells, and the convergence of the information occurs in the intermediate layer.

At the same time that convergence is taking place, divergence occurs. *Divergent arrangements* mean that information from one cell feeds into several cells. As an example, one receptor cell may send information to many different intermediate cells, or one horizontal cell may send information to several amacrine and bipolar cells.

Convergent and divergent arrangements are found throughout the nervous system. These arrangements turn out to be extremely important because they permit information to be shared among cells. As we discuss the various sensory systems, you may want to be on the lookout for other examples of these arrangements. To help you keep them in mind, we can sketch general plans for convergence and divergence.

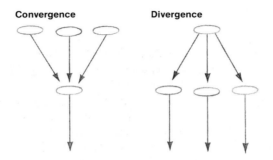

In both cases, information can be compared, analyzed, and modified.

The Graded Potentials of the Intermediate Cells

When a microelectrode is placed in the intermediate layer and lights are shone on the rods and cones, graded potentials can be recorded from the intermediate cells. It is not clear which of the three kinds of intermediate cell produces the graded potentials, although it may be reasonable to guess that most recordings are actually taken from the amacrine cells because they are, relatively speaking, so large.

The graded potentials may be either hyperpolarizations or depolarizations. Because the rods and cones always hyperpolarize in response to light, an important event has occurred: what began as only hyperpolarizations has been transformed into some hyperpolarizations and some depolarizations. The change occurs in the course of the multitude of synapses between and among the receptor cells and the cells of the intermediate layer.

All the graded potentials that can be recorded from the intermediate layer, whether they are hyperpolarizations or depolarizations, are called *S-potentials*. Some cells in the intermediate layer only produce hyperpolarizing S-potentials; others produce only depolarizing S-potentials; still others produce hyperpolarizing S-potentials in response to some wavelengths of light, while producing depolarizing S-potentials in response to other wavelengths. Let's see if we can figure out what's going on.

If an intermediate cell always produces a hyperpolarizing S-potential or always produces a depolarizing S-potential, regardless of the wavelength of light shone on the receptor cells, that intermediate cell is not signaling any color information. Because rods do not signal color, it is reasonable to suppose that the intermediate cell is collecting information from rods. Rods do signal the intensity of light: hyperpolarizations of the rods are larger when the light is made more intense. Similarly, these intermediate cells also signal light intensity: the size of the hyperpolarization or depolarization is determined by the intensity of the light falling on the receptors. Because these cells supply information about the intensity or luminosity of light, they are called *Luminosity-units*, or (shortened) *L-units*.

If an intermediate cell sometimes hyperpolarizes and sometimes depolarizes, depending upon the wavelength of light falling on the receptors, it is supplying color information. Because cones signal color, it is reasonable to suppose that such an intermediate cell is collecting information from cones. Cones also signal light intensity. Don't be misled here: cones signal color by responding maximally to certain wavelengths, but they also hyperpolarize more when the light is made more intense. As an example, let's consider the cones whose photochemical reacts most readily to 440 nm (blue). If lights of different wavelengths that are all of the same intensity fall on these cones, these cones hyperpolarize most to a wavelength of 440 nm. But if the amplitudes of all wavelengths are increased, the cones hyperpolarize more in response to all the lights, although they continue to respond most to 440 nm.

The same is true of some of the cells in the intermediate layer. A particular cell may always depolarize when short-wavelength lights fall on the receptors, and always hyperpolarize in response to long wavelengths. In that sense, the cell is signaling something about color. If the intensities of the lights are increased, the cell will continue to respond in the same fashion, but both the depolarizations and the hyperpolarizations will be larger. The cell is signaling both color and intensity information.

Because the feature that distinguishes these cells from the others in the intermediate layer is their ability to react differently to different wavelengths, they are called *Chromaticity-units* (that is, "color-units"), or *C-units* for short.

Let's summarize this section with the use of a few graphs. Each graph shows what can be recorded if a microelectrode is placed in the intermediate layer and then lights of different wavelengths are, briefly and individually, shone on the receptors.

The S-Potentials of L-Units

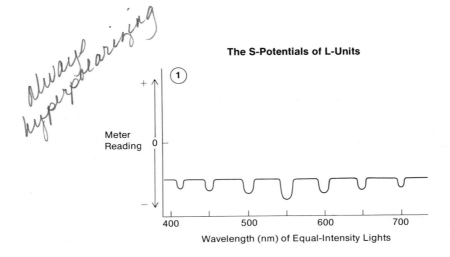

①

Meter Reading

400   500   600   700

Wavelength (nm) of Equal-Intensity Lights

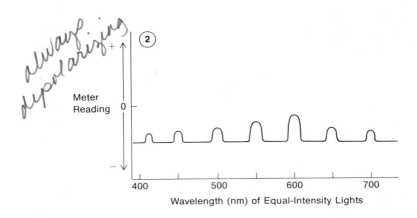

②

Meter Reading

400   500   600   700

Wavelength (nm) of Equal-Intensity Lights

The S-Potentials of a C-Unit

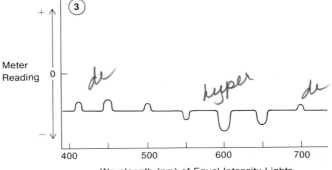

③

Meter Reading

de   *hyper*   *de*

400   500   600   700

Wavelength (nm) of Equal-Intensity Lights

The responses of two different L-units are shown in graphs 1 and 2. Graph 1 shows the responses of a cell that always hyperpolarizes; graph 2 shows the responses of a cell that always depolarizes. Notice that, even though the lights are equally intense, graphs 1 and 2 indicate that the cells produce a larger response when some wavelengths are used. In other words, each cell is more sensitive to some wavelengths than to others. If all the lights were made more intense, all the responses would increase proportionately. But no matter how intense the light or what particular wavelength is used, each L-unit either always hyperpolarizes or always depolarizes.

Graph 3 shows the responses of a C-unit. It depolarizes in response to either short or long wavelengths, but it hyperpolarizes in response to wavelengths in the middle of the spectrum. Again notice that some of the hyperpolarizations are larger than others, and some of the depolarizations are larger than others, despite the fact that the lights are of equal intensity. If all the lights are made more intense, all the responses will be larger. But, no matter how intense the lights are, the cell will react to some wavelengths by depolarizing and to others by hyperpolarizing.

The Ganglion Cells

Ganglion cells collect their information from the intermediate cells. Each ganglion cell has a long axon that runs along the inner surface of the retina to the *blind spot (optic disc)*. Where all the axons from all the ganglion cells leave the eye, they form a bundle called the *optic nerve*. Just where the axons leave the eye, they acquire a *myelin* coating. Thus, the ganglion cells are like the typical neuron described in Chapter 1: each ganglion cell has dendrites and a soma that collect information, via synapses, from the intermediate cells, and each ganglion cell has an axon whose length outside the eye is myelinated. The axon sends information to the portion of the thalamus devoted to vision (the lateral geniculate nuclei).

The rods and cones are receptor cells. They have some properties in common with neurons, but they are not "true" neurons. The intermediate cells are not "true" neurons either: they produce only graded responses, and all their processes behave most like dendrites. The ganglion cells, on the other hand, have all the characteristics of "true" neurons, and they deserve to be designated the *first-order neurons* of the visual system.

We'll discuss the activities of the ganglion cells in the next chapter.

A Final Word About the Retina

As I hope you'll recall, the retina is arranged so that the rods and cones point toward the choroid. The intermediate cells lie in front of them (toward the lens), and the ganglion cells are in front of the intermediate cells. When light enters the eye, it must pass through the ganglion cells, intermediate cells, and the cell nuclei and inner segments of the rods and cones before reaching the all important outer segments. At first glance, this seems to be a strange arrangement: there is a substantial amount of material through which light must pass before reaching the photochemicals. The fact that the material is virtually transparent means that most of the light will, indeed, reach the outer segments. But that doesn't explain why the outer segments should be in the back of the retina, pointing toward the choroid. Why not place the rods and cones at the innermost surface of the retina with their outer segments pointing toward the entering light?

The answer has to do with the fact that rods and cones have extremely high oxygen requirements. And the outer segments, housing the critical photochemicals in their disks, have the highest oxygen requirements of all. In order to provide enough oxygen, a rich blood supply must be located near the outer segments. Indeed, the choroid has just such a blood supply.

If the retina were turned around so that the rods and cones were on the inner surface of the retina, facing toward the entering light, the blood supply would also have to be moved to the interior of the eye. But blood vessels are not transparent. They absorb and scatter light.

Having the receptors located at the back of the retina, near the choroid, allows the rods and cones to receive their oxygen without placing blood vessels in the path of the incoming light.

Summary

This has been a long and complicated chapter. By way of summary, you should think carefully about the structure of the retina. Picture the three layers of the retina: the *rod-and-cone layer,* the *intermediate layer,* and the *ganglion-cell layer.* Think about light reaching the rods and cones, and then—step by step—trace the sequence of events that will occur.

1. Light absorbed by *rhodopsin.*

2. *Isomerization* to *prelumirhodopsin.*

3. *Hyperpolarization* of the rod or cone.

4. Release of synaptic vesicles at the *spherule* or *pedicle.*

5. Graded potentials in the *amacrine, bipolar,* and *horizontal cells.* The graded potentials are called *S-potentials,* and they occur in *L-units* and *C-units.*

6. Combining, collecting, analyzing, and modifying (created in large part by *convergence* and *divergence*) of information in the intermediate layer.

7. Synapses between the intermediate cells and the ganglion cells.

8. Graded potentials in the dendrites and somas of the ganglion cells; action potentials in their axons that collectively leave the eye to form the *optic nerve.*

As you think about this sequence, ask yourself questions about each step. For example, when you consider step 1, ask yourself about the nature of light and ask yourself about rhodopsin. (Where is it found? How is it made?) For step 2, ask yourself what happens after rhodopsin becomes prelumirhodopsin. For step 3, what are the differences between rods and cones? Etc.

Each time you think about this sequence, ask yourself tougher and more detailed questions.

Recommended Readings

There is an interesting little paperback that describes the eyes of various animals.

Tansley, K. *Vision in Vertebrates.* Science Paperback (Chapman and Hall Ltd.), 1965.

There is also an excellent, large volume that contains a fantastic amount of information on the eyes of many animals.

Walls, G. L. *The Vertebrate Eye.* Hafner, 1942.

For more information on the photochemicals and the receptors, see the following articles.

Dowling, J. E.   "Night Blindness," *Sci. Amer.,* Oct. 1966 (Offprint #1053).

Hubbard, R., and A. Kropf.   "Molecular Isomers in Vision," *Sci. Amer.,* June 1967 (Offprint #1075).

MacNichol, E. F.   "Three-Pigment Color Vision," *Sci. Amer.,* Dec. 1964 (Offprint #197).

Rushton, W. A. H.   "Visual Pigments in Man," *Sci. Amer.,* Nov. 1962 (Offprint #139).

Young, R. W.   "Visual Cells," *Sci. Amer.,* Oct. 1970 (not available as an Offprint).

For more information on light, again I'd suggest the Isaac Asimov book recommended in Chapter 4, or this excellent, enjoyable, and very readable paperback.

Baker, A.   *Modern Physics and Antiphysics.* Addison-Wesley, 1972.

6

The Visual System

Where the axons of the ganglion cells leave the eyes, they form two large bundles, the *optic nerves*. The axons of the optic nerves travel into the brain until they reach the thalamus. There these axons, which originated in the retina, synapse onto second-order neurons that carry the information to the visual cortex.

Let's take a close look at these components of the visual system.

Optic Nerves

Each eye gives rise to an optic nerve that contains about 1 million axons. Each optic nerve runs along the underside of the front of the brain. At a location several inches above the roof of the mouth, the two optic nerves cross. The crossing point is called the *optic chiasma*. (In the Greek alphabet, an X is pronounced "chi," and the two optic nerves form an X where they cross.) At the optic chiasma, some of the axons that originate in the left eye cross over to the right side, and vice versa. In particular, the axons that begin in the right half of the left eye cross over, and the axons that begin in the left half of the right eye cross over. The easiest way to keep this straight is to say that the axons from the left halves of both eyes end up on the left side of the brain after the optic chiasma; the axons from the right halves of both eyes end up on the right side.

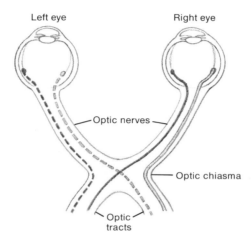

In this simplified sketch, only a few axons have been drawn in. Notice that, after the optic chiasma, the two bundles of axons are called the *optic tracts*. These are the same axons as the ones in the optic nerve; the term "optic tract" signifies that we are past the chiasma and that each bundle now contains axons from both eyes.

To be sure that you understand what's going on, let's go through a series of questions.

1.   What would happen if the left *optic nerve* were cut?
     Because the left optic nerve carries all the information from the left eye into the brain, cutting the left optic nerve would result in complete blindness in the left eye.

2.   What would happen if the left *optic tract* were cut?
     Because the left optic tract carries information from the left halves of both eyes into the brain, the left halves of both eyes would be blind.
     Do you recall, in Chapter 4, the discussion of how the cornea and lens bend light? You may have noticed that light rays that come into the eye through the top part of the cornea end up on the lower part of the retina, and vice versa. Thus, the image that is formed on the retina is upside down as compared to the

original object. The left and right sides of the image are also reversed. When you look at the world, the images formed on the retina are upside down and backwards; the image of the ceiling is on the lower parts of your retinas, and the image of the floor is on the upper parts. The images of objects on your left fall on the right halves of your retinas; the images of objects on your right fall on the left halves of your retinas. This inversion of the image occurs in any optical system that uses a lens similar in shape to our own. If you use a slide projector, you know that you must load the slides upside down and backwards if you want to see the pictures correctly. The lens in the slide projector inverts the image it is given, just as our lens does.

All this is important because, if the left optic tract is cut, the left halves of both eyes will be blind but, because the images are reversed on the retina, the individual will be blind to objects on the right. (Remember that the images of objects located on the right fall on the left side of the retina.)

3. What would happen if the *optic chiasma* were cut right down the middle?

Because axons from the inner halves of both eyes cross at the optic chiasma, the information coming from the inner halves would not be carried into the brain. The inner halves of both eyes would be blind. The information coming from the outer halves of both eyes would continue into the brain.

Keeping in mind the fact that the image on the retina is upside down and backwards, how would the world look to a person whose optic chiasma had been cut down the middle?

Because the images are reversed, objects off to the left of the left eye and to the right of the right eye will have their images fall on the inner halves of the two retinas. The person will be blind to objects located out at the sides.

The fact that the image is reversed sometimes confuses people. They want to know where the image is turned rightside up again. The answer is, it isn't. The light reaching the rods and cones is converted into neural information. The image itself is not passed on to the brain; only the neural information is. The brain does not "reconstruct" the image. It simply interprets and analyzes the neural information. The interpretation and analysis depend, in large part, on experience. Somehow we learn to call the ceiling "up" and the floor "down." We learn the direction of objects with reference to gravity and to our bodies. The process by which we learn to make these interpretations of neural information is poorly understood, at best.

The fact that we learn to interpret visual information has been vividly demonstrated in studies in which people wear prism-glasses. These glasses reverse the visual world: the floor appears "up" and the ceiling appears "down," left appears "right" and right appears "left." Initially, the individuals wearing the glasses become dizzy and confused, and they are extremely awkward. After a few days of continuous use, however, the individuals find that the world begins to look normal again. The floor is "down," the ceiling is "up," left is "left," and right is "right." The glasses don't change during their use; the interpretation of visual information by the brain changes. When the individuals remove the glasses, they are again dizzy, confused, and awkward. The world appears upside down and backwards again, and the individuals often become extremely depressed. (The reason for the depression is not clear; perhaps the amount of effort involved is just a bit overwhelming. Although the reason isn't clear, the depression is typically severe enough to indicate that people should not try this procedure on their own.) After several days, the world again appears rightside up. The brain has relearned the original set of rules for interpreting visual information.

If you are one of those who thought the image has to be turned "rightside up" again by our eyes, take heart. Leonardo da Vinci thought so too, and he drew many sketches of the eye—trying to figure out a way to get the image reinverted before it reached the retina.

Lateral Geniculate Nuclei

The axons of the optic tract terminate in the portion of the thalamus devoted to vision: the *lateral geniculate nuclei* (one nucleus on the left side of the brain; one on the right). Each lateral geniculate nucleus is composed of the dendrites and somas of the second-order neurons. Their axons carry information on to the visual cortex.

The dendrites and cell bodies are arranged in six layers. The first, fourth, and sixth layers receive information from axons that originate in the eye on the opposite side. (That is, layers 1, 4, and 6 of the left lateral geniculate nucleus receive information from the right eye.) The second, third, and fifth layers form synapses with the axons that originate in the eye on the same side. None of the second-order neurons receives information from both eyes.

The lateral geniculate nuclei analyze information about color. We'll discuss their functioning in detail in the next chapter. For now, it will be enough to recognize that, in the lateral geniculate nuclei, the information coming from the two eyes is kept separate.

The axons leaving the lateral geniculate nucleus travel in groups (called the *optic radiations*) through the depths of the brain. They synapse onto neurons on the surface of the brain in the visual cortex.

Before going on to describe the visual cortex, let me remind you that some axons of the optic nerve do not go to the lateral geniculate nuclei. Some of the axons go to the *pregeniculate nuclei*—which, in turn, control the muscles of the iris (remember we talked about that in Chapter 4). In addition, some of the axons go to other areas of gray matter, the *superior colliculi* (singular, colliculus). The superior colliculi control the extra-ocular muscles that move and rotate the eyes.

Schematically, we can now represent the entire visual system.

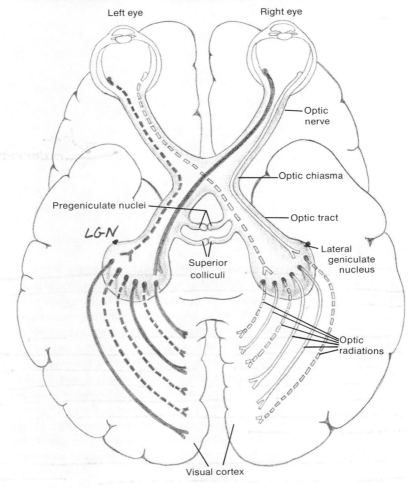

Visual Cortex

Do you recall from Chapter 3 that the visual cortex is located in the occipital lobes, at the back of the brain? The second-order neurons coming from the lateral geniculate nuclei synapse onto third-order neurons located at the rearmost part of the visual cortex. These third-order neurons have short axons that synapse onto another set of neurons located slightly forward of the rearmost part. And these neurons, the fourth-order neurons, in turn synapse onto a final set of neurons. Thus, there are really three groupings of neurons in the visual cortex. Numbers have been assigned by neuroanatomists to various portions of the cortex and the three groupings of neurons in the visual cortex are known as *areas 17, 18,* and *19.*

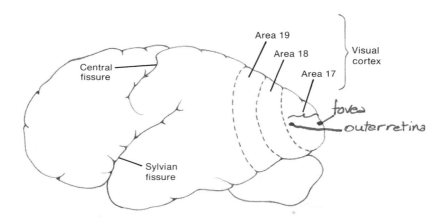

It is in areas 17, 18, and 19 that the information coming from the two eyes is finally combined, and that shape, form, direction, texture, and depth are analyzed. The remainder of this chapter will be devoted to discussing the ways in which the visual system performs its analyses.

Each area collects information from all over the retina. In area 17, the neurons that collect their information from the fovea are located at the rearmost tip of the visual cortex. The outermost edges of the retina send their information to the neurons at the forward edges of area 17, near the border with area 18. The portions of the retina in between the fovea and the edges are represented, systematically, between the rearmost tip and the border with area 18. Areas 18 and 19 are also systematically laid out. You can, in fact, think of each of the areas as a map of the retina. Spots of light that fall side by side on the retina will produce responses in neighboring neurons in each of the three areas. This systematic mapping out of the retina in the visual cortex is called a _retinotopic map._ Each area of the visual cortex has a complete retinotopic map.

The Concepts of Maintained Discharge and the Receptive Field

If an electrode is placed in the optic nerve, a steady stream of action potentials can be recorded, even when no light is shone into the eye. When light is presented, the rate at which the action potentials are produced may increase or may decrease. The rate at which action potentials (nerve impulses) are produced is usually called, simply, the _firing rate._

In darkness, each of the axons in the optic nerve keeps up a slow, steady firing rate. This is called the axon's _maintained discharge._ Why ganglion cell axons should produce action potentials when no light is reaching the eye is largely a mystery. It may be that some of the delicate photochemical molecules isomerize just because of the energy provided by our bodily heat, and that this continuous, slow rate of isomerization eventually produces the maintained discharge. Regardless of how the maintained discharge comes about, it serves as a kind of baseline against which the axon's activity can be compared. When the firing rate increases or decreases from the maintained discharge, the cell has signaled that something has taken place. You may recall that—in Chapter 2, when we were discussing the role of inhibition—we indicated that increases or decreases from a baseline indicate that "something happened." The use of a maintained discharge as a baseline is a common feature of the various sensory systems.

If we record from just one axon in the optic nerve, any light that is large enough to flood the entire retina will create a change in the axon's firing rate. If, however, we use a very tiny spot of light that falls on a very limited region of the retina, the axon will change its firing rate only when the light spot falls on a particular area of the retina. The reason for this will be clear if you think about the structure of the retina: rods and cones located in one area of the retina tend to send their information to intermediate cells located in a limited area. These intermediate cells, in turn, may all send their information to just one ganglion cell (a convergent arrangement). When a spot of light falls on just a few rods and cones, only a few intermediate cells will be affected, and only the ganglion cell that collects its information from those intermediate cells will be affected. This sounds complicated but a sketch may clarify things.

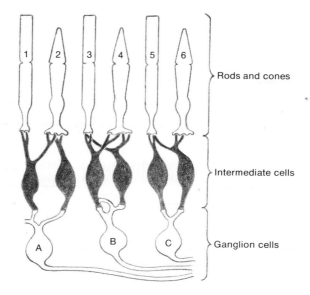

If a light shines only on the receptors marked 1 and 2, only ganglion cell A will be affected. If the light is moved to the right, first ganglion cell B and then C will be affected.

It should now be clear that, if you are recording from a single axon in the optic nerve, a small spot of light will alter the axon's maintained discharge only when it falls within a very small region of the retina. This region on the retina is termed the *receptive field* of the axon.

Each axon will have its own receptive field somewhere on the retina. Two or more axons may have overlapping receptive fields if they collect their information from common receptors or intermediate cells.

The concept of a receptive field is not limited to optic-nerve axons. The neurons of the lateral geniculate nucleus and the visual cortex also have receptive fields. Thus, if an electrode is placed in the visual cortex and a small spot of light is moved across the retina, any individual neuron in the cortex will respond only when the light falls on a particular portion of the retina.

Notice that a receptive field is not a structure or a cell. It is a concept. It describes something about the behavior of a neuron. It defines the area in which a stimulus must be placed if it is going to have an effect on the neuron. We could talk about the receptive fields of neurons that collect information from receptors in the skin. Certainly a neuron that collects its information from receptors in the thumb will not be affected by stimulating the foot. In fact, the neuron may only be affected when a particular portion of the thumb is stimulated. That portion would be the neuron's receptive field.

When you ask the question, "Where should I place this stimulus if I want to affect that neuron?" you are asking, "Where is the neuron's receptive field?"

The Responses of Axons in the Optic Nerve

As we have indicated, all the axons in the optic nerve have a maintained discharge. If the axon increases its firing rate when a light is shone on its receptive field, the neuron is called an *on cell*. When the light first comes on, the firing rate increases but, as the light remains on, the firing rate gradually decreases. When the light is turned off, the firing rate returns to the maintained discharge level.

Neurons whose axons decrease their firing rate when a light is shone on their receptive fields are termed *off cells*. When the light first comes on, the firing rate decreases, and it remains below the maintained discharge level as long as the light is on. When the light goes off, the firing rate increases and then gradually returns to the maintained discharge level.

We can describe the behavior of on and off cells in graphs.

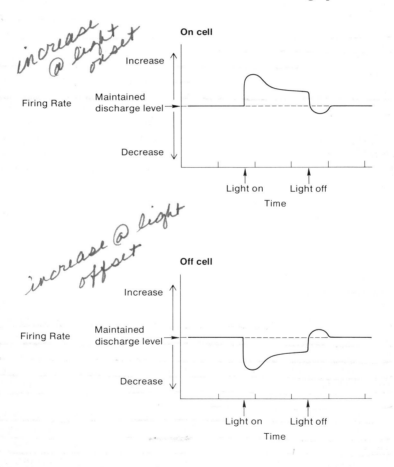

Notice that the cells are named "on" or "off" depending upon whether their firing rates increase at light onset or at light offset.

There are some axons that increase their firing rates at both light onset and light offset. These are termed *on–off cells*, and a graphic description of their behavior can also be given.

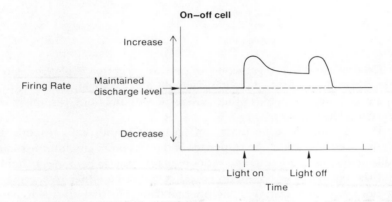

I hope you have noticed that, in all these cases, the cells react most vigorously to *changes* in the light level. Each cell announces light onset and light offset in its own way. What the cells have in common is the fact that the beginnings and endings of light are announced more stridently than is ongoing light or darkness. This should remind you of our earlier discussions of the nervous system's predilection for announcing changes.

The on–off cells reveal their behavior most clearly when a light that is smaller than their receptive fields is shone into the eye. When this very small spot of light falls on one portion of the receptive field, the axon gives only an "on" response or only an "off" response. When the light is moved to another part of the receptive field, the axon gives the opposite response. The two parts of the receptive field have a center–surround arrangement: if the center of the receptive field produces the "on" response, then the surround produces the "off" response, and vice versa.

Because the receptive fields of optic-nerve axons tend to be circular, we can draw four sketches to represent the four kinds of responses.

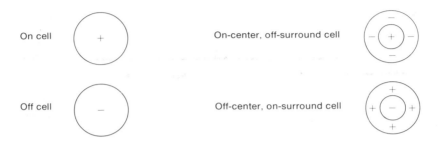

Keep in mind that these sketches portray receptive fields (zones on the retina that activate individual ganglion cell axons), and that the symbols + and − refer to the "on" responses and "off" responses of the ganglion-cell axons.

Why should there be both "on" responses and "off" responses? Think back a bit about the responses of the receptors and intermediate cells in the retina. All rods and cones hyperpolarize in response to light. But the responses of the intermediate cells can be either hyperpolarizations or depolarizations. The intermediate cells that always hyperpolarize or always depolarize, regardless of the wavelength of light, are called the L-units. Imagine that a ganglion cell collects all its information from intermediate cells that are depolarizing L-units. Whenever a light shines on the receptive field, the L-units depolarize, and they activate the ganglion cell. When the light goes off, the L-units return to their resting potential, and the ganglion cell returns to its maintained discharge. Perhaps this is the way an on cell works.

We could make a similar argument about the off cells. Perhaps they collect their information from hyperpolarizing L-units. Each time a light falls on the receptive field, the L-units hyperpolarize and inhibit the ganglion cell. When the light goes off, the L-units return to their resting potential, and the ganglion cell—released from inhibition—produces a burst of action potentials before returning to its maintained discharge.

If these explanations for on and off cells are correct (they are speculations, and it's not clear whether they are correct), how could we account for on–off cells? Well, perhaps they collect their information from both kinds of L-units. Consider the case of an on-center, off-surround cell.

Suppose it collects information from the center of its receptive field via depolarizing L-units, and from the edges of its receptive field via hyperpolarizing L-units. If light falls on the center of the receptive field, the appropriate L-units will depolarize and cause the ganglion cell to increase its firing rate. If light falls on the edges of the receptive field, the appropriate L-units will hyperpolarize and inhibit the ganglion cell. Then when the light goes off, the ganglion cell produces lots of action potentials before settling down to its maintained discharge.

These possible explanations for the responses of the ganglion cells can be schematically represented. In the following sketch, receptor cells, intermediate cells, and the receptive fields of ganglion cells are represented by circles. The H or D within the circle indicates whether the cell hyperpolarizes or depolarizes. The circles representing the ganglion-cell receptive fields are drawn to show the four kinds of responses.

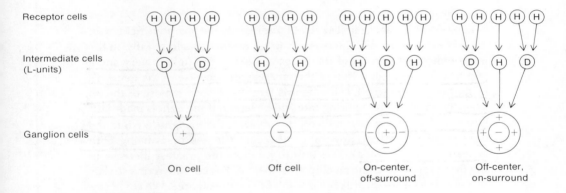

In order to understand why the receptive fields are circular in shape, you need to realize that ganglion cells actually collect their information from a circle of receptors in the retina, rather than from a line of them as indicated in the sketch.

The Receptive Fields of Neurons in the Visual Cortex

A neuron in the visual cortex will respond when a small spot of light falls within its receptive field. The principles are similar to those involved in the receptive fields of ganglion cells. There is, however, an important difference between the receptive fields of neurons in the visual cortex and those of the ganglion cells. The difference has to do with the *shape* of the receptive fields.

Let's begin with neurons in area 17 of the visual cortex. These neurons, remember, are the first ones to receive information coming up from the lateral geniculate nuclei. Many of the neurons in area 17 have receptive fields that are *elongated*. Instead of having the circular shape of ganglion-cell receptive fields, these neurons have ellipsoid-shaped receptive fields. The receptive fields have both on and off areas, and we can draw representations of them as follows.

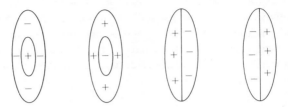

Look carefully at the first sketch. It represents the receptive field of an area-17 neuron that will increase its firing rate when a light falls on the inner elongated portion of its receptive field. If the light is very small and it covers only a portion of the on area, the increase in the neuron's firing rate will be small. If the light is larger and covers more of the on area, the increase in the firing rate will be larger. If the light is made still larger and a portion of it falls on the off area, the firing rate while the light is shining will go down a bit (because the neuron is being both activated and inhibited). The way to produce the greatest increase in the firing rate is to shine an ellipse or "bar" of light on the retina so that it covers the entire on area but doesn't fall on the off area. We could say that the optimum stimulus (the event that will activate the neuron most) is a bar of light of the appropriate width.

Not all area-17 neurons have receptive fields that are vertical. Many have their receptive fields arranged so that the long axis is tilted. For example, we might find area-17 neurons whose receptive fields are all on-center, off-surround, but whose orientations differ.

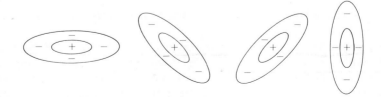

It should be clear that, if you want the neuron to increase its firing rate to the maximum level, the bar of light shone in the eye must be tilted to correspond to the tilt of the on area. Now we can talk about the optimum stimulus as a bar of light of a particular width at a given angle of orientation. Area-17 neurons that respond to such an optimum stimulus are called *simple cells.* With simple cells, if the bar of light is shifted slightly to one side or the other, it will fall on the off area, and the neuron will reduce its firing rate.

But other neurons in area 17 do not reduce their firing rate if the bar of light is shifted. In other words, these neurons have receptive fields that do not contain true off areas. The optimum stimulus for these neurons is still a bar of light of a given width and orientation, but the bar of light can be placed anywhere in the receptive field and the neuron will still increase its firing rate. Area-17 neurons that react this way are called *complex cells.*

In areas 18 and 19, both simple and complex cells are found but, in addition, two new types of receptive field are also present. Because these are even more complicated than the complex cells, they are called *hypercomplex cells.* One type is slightly simpler than the other. The simpler ones are called *lower-order hypercomplex cells;* the more complicated ones are called *higher-order hypercomplex cells.* (Do you have the feeling that the English language is exploding right before your eyes?)

Before we discuss the hypercomplex cells, you need to consider one more aspect of the organization of the visual cortex. As you already know, areas 17, 18, and 19 each have *retinotopic maps;* that is, neurons that collect information from neighboring regions of the retina lie side by side within each area of the visual cortex. Neurons that all collect information from virtually the same region of the retina and whose receptive fields are similar are further grouped together. These neurons tend to be lined up in a column of the cortex, and this kind of grouping is therefore called *columnar organization.* As an example, let's consider those neurons of area 17 that collect information from the fovea. They are all located in one region (the rearmost tip) of area 17. Some of them are simple cells; some are complex cells. All the simple cells that have the same receptive field orientation are arranged in a column extending from the surface of the cortex inward to the depths of the cortex. Simple cells with other orientations are found in neighboring columns. The complex cells are similarly arranged.

Before going any further, take a break. Think carefully and slowly about the receptive fields of the ganglion cells. Go back and reread the discussion of them. Then think about the receptive fields of area-17 neurons. Reread the material on simple cells and complex cells. Think about the fact that each of the areas of the visual cortex is organized according to a retinotopic map and that, within each map, there is an additional columnar organization. Finally, remind yourself that we are going to plunge on into areas 18 and 19 where the hypercomplex cells are found. Please don't rush ahead to the next section without first spending some time reviewing. If you just rush on, it will all soon become gobbledygook.

The Hypercomplex Cells

The optimum stimulus for some of the neurons in areas 18 and 19 is a bar of light of a particular width and a particular orientation, but the *length* of the bar of light is also important. Neurons that react to such stimuli are called the *lower-order hypercomplex cells*. The only difference between complex cells and the lower-order hypercomplex cells is the fact that the lower-order hypercomplex cells require the bar of light to be of a particular length if the neurons are to increase their firing rate to the maximum. The complex cells respond to short and long bars of light equally well; the lower-order hypercomplex cells will respond to one length more than to other lengths.

And, finally, we come to the *higher-order hypercomplex cells*. Their optimum stimulus is a bar of light of a particular width and a particular length, but the bar of light can be at *any orientation* in the receptive field. Regardless of the direction along which the bar falls, higher-order hypercomplex cells respond most to a bar of light of given width and length.

How are the four kinds of receptive fields found in areas 17, 18, and 19 created? Probably the best way to think about this problem is to consider that the simple cells collect their information from neurons having the center-surround arrangement of ganglion-cell receptive fields; the complex cells collect information from the simple cells; the lower-order hypercomplex cells collect from the complex; the higher-order complex cells collect from the lower-order hypercomplex cells.

To see how this might work, imagine that you've made cutouts of sketches of on-center, off-surround receptive fields of ganglion cells. Suppose you made five cutouts. Figure out how you could arrange and overlap the cutouts so that all the on areas lie in a straight line. You would end up with something like the following.

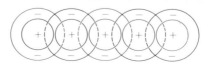

Imagine now that you have a device that collects and pools the information from your cutouts. If you wanted to activate the device as much as possible, you would "push" all the individual on areas. If you wanted to deactivate the device as much as possible, you would make sure not to activate any of the on areas, but you would "push" the off areas. In other words, the optimum stimulus for the device would be a bar that "pushed" all the on areas simultaneously. The bar would have to have a particular width and orientation if you were going to simultaneously "push" all the on areas without "pushing" any of the off areas. If you moved the bar up or down so that it rested on the off areas, you would deactivate the device. In a crude way, the device does what a simple cell does!

When the bar rests over all the on areas, it is also resting on some of the off areas of neighboring cutouts. This may have bothered you a bit but it shouldn't: all we wanted to do was find a stimulus that could activate the device as much as possible. When the bar rests over all the on areas, all the activation that we can manage will occur. Only if the original cutouts were missing their off areas could we produce more activation. But, then, we wouldn't have the off areas above and below.

Obviously, if you had lined up the cutouts vertically or at some intermediate angle, the bar would have to be tilted so that it covered all the on areas.

With all this in mind, you might now think of a simple cell as a neuron that collects its information from a row of neurons with center-surround arrangements to their receptive fields.

Now imagine that you have some cutouts of sketches representing simple cells that all have an elongated on area in the center. How could you arrange these so that they roughly represent the receptive field of a complex cell? Remember that complex cells require a bar of light of a particular orientation and width, but the bar of light can be shifted to any location in the receptive field (there is no true "off" area). You would probably arrange the cutouts so that they were lying side by side, with the off areas overlapping the on areas of neighboring cutouts. This is a pretty good approximation, although the arrangement doesn't work out to be a perfect representation of a complex cell. Nonetheless, it gives you a pretty good idea of how the complex receptive field might be created. Without going into more cutouts, you should at least be able to imagine that the hypercomplex cells might similarly be built upon combinations of complex cells.

More on Receptive Fields

You might be wondering just how far this business of building up more-and-more complicated receptive fields can go. Maybe there are some neurons somewhere in the visual cortex whose optimum stimulus is two bars of light, arranged in the form of a T. And maybe each time you read the capital letter T, those neurons are activated. Maybe there are neurons that are activated only when you read a W or H, or see a square or a particular table top. We could go on and on with this. But no one knows just how complicated receptive fields can be. And it's not easy to find out. There are several million neurons in the visual cortex. And there are countless numbers of shapes and forms that we learn to recognize. Trying to find out precisely which shape in what location at which angle activates any one neuron is a slow, painstaking process. Maybe the best way to view the situation is simply to agree that different neurons are activated by different stimuli, and that any particular stimulus will activate a number of neurons.

There are some intriguing examples of known receptive fields. For example, the receptive fields of the optic nerves of frogs have been studied quite a bit. Some axons in the frog's optic nerve become activated only when a small spot of light is moved erratically in front of the eye. When the spot stops moving, the axon stops responding. Because a frog eats flies only if they are flying (a frog will starve to death if surrounded by immobilized flies), these axons seem to be somehow involved in signaling to the frog that "food is present." For that reason, these axons have been labeled "fly detectors." Other axons in the frog's optic nerve respond whenever a spot of light is first brought into view. Whether the spot moves around or not, these axons stop responding to the spot once it's been visible for a while. They respond again when a new spot is brought into view, and they've been termed "newness detectors."

Monocular and Binocular Responses

The axons in the left optic nerve respond only when the appropriate stimulus appears in the left eye. Obviously, they do not respond to stimuli that appear in the right eye. But what about the neurons in the visual cortex? Will they respond to stimuli that appear only in the left eye or only in the right eye?

Remember that at the optic chiasma, about half the axons from each optic nerve cross over to the other side of the brain. Each side of areas

17, 18, and 19 receives information that originated in both eyes. Most of the neurons in these areas respond when the appropriate stimulus appears in either the left eye or the right eye.

The axons of the optic nerve give only *monocular* ("mono-" meaning one; "-ocular" meaning eye) *responses.* That is, they collect their information from only one eye, and therefore they react only to stimuli in that eye. The vast majority of the neurons in the visual cortex give *binocular* ("bi-" meaning two) *responses.* That is, they collect their information from both eyes, and therefore they react to stimuli in either eye.

Summary

In order to summarize the information about the structure of the visual system, you should draw a sketch of it. Be sure to include the *optic nerves, optic chiasma, optic tracts, lateral geniculate nuclei, optic radiations,* and *visual cortex* (and don't forget the *pregeniculate nuclei* and the *superior colliculi*). As you look at your sketch, think about what happens at each location. Make sure that, when you think about the optic nerve and the visual cortex, you describe for yourself what a *maintained discharge* is. Describe for yourself what has to be done to get the *firing rate* to increase or decrease from the maintained discharge. Remember that each neuron will have its own *receptive field,* and that there are four kinds of ganglion-cell receptive fields (*on cell; off cell; on-center, off-surround cell; off-center, on-surround cell*) and four kinds of visual-cortex receptive fields (*simple cell; complex cell; lower-order hypercomplex cell; higher-order hypercomplex cell*). Each area of the visual cortex is organized according to a *retinotopic map*. In addition, within each location of a retinotopic map, there is *columnar organization* in which neurons with similar receptive fields are arranged in a column. And be certain you understand all the italicized terms in this paragraph.

An Addendum: The Compound Eye

Many arthropods (animals that have a hard exoskeleton and jointed limbs) have eyes that differ markedly from our eyes. Their eyes are made up of clusters of light-sensing units. Each unit contains its own lens, several receptor cells, and a neural cell that collects information from the receptor cells and sends it to the brain. Each complete unit is called an *ommatidium* (plural, ommatidia); eyes that are made up of ommatidia are called *compound eyes.* The compound eyes of the horseshoe crab, *Limulus polyphemus,* have been studied extensively, and they have provided a considerable amount of information about the nature of vision.

The Structure of Ommatidia

Each of the two compound eyes of *Limulus* contains several hundred ommatidia. Each individual ommatidium is a rather long and narrow structure. The lenses of the ommatidia are embedded in the animal's exoskeleton. The receptor cells are located underneath the lenses.

Let's take a look at a single ommatidium. Looked at from the side, we can see the lens, some of the receptor cells, and the neural cell.

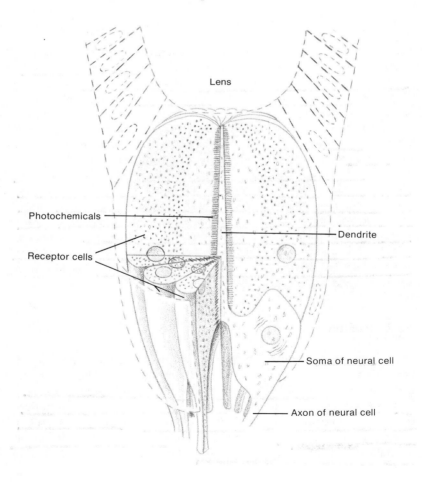

Lens

Photochemicals

Dendrite

Receptor cells

Soma of neural cell

Axon of neural cell

The receptor cells of *Limulus* are called *retinular cells*. Each retinular cell is long and wedge-shaped. An ommatidium may contain as many as 12 retinular cells, arranged in a circle around the dendrite of the neural cell. Thus, if we made a cross-section of an ommatidium, below the lens, we'd see the following.

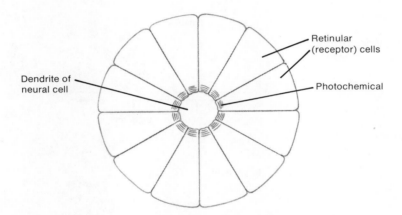

Dendrite of neural cell

Retinular (receptor) cells

Photochemical

   Each retinular cell contains photochemicals that are located along the length of the cell, at the edge of the cell closest to the dendrite. Because the photochemicals are found along the length of the relatively long retinular cells, the lens that caps each ommatidium need not focus light at one particular location along the length of the ommatidium. Thus, unlike our eye, *Limulus* does not need a mechanism to perform accommodation. The lens does not change shape; it is a rigid structure.
   The neural cell of the ommatidium is called the *eccentric cell*. Its dendrite extends upward through the central region of the ommatidium. Its soma lies near the base of the ommatidium, and the eccentric cell's axon carries information to the brain. The eccentric-cell axons of all the ommatidia that form a compound eye travel together, as a bundle, to the brain. This collection of eccentric cell axons is the *Limulus'* optic nerve.

The Function of Ommatidia

Electrodes can be placed in the optic nerve of *Limulus* so that the action potentials of individual eccentric cells can be recorded. Eccentric-cell axons do not have a maintained discharge; when the ommatidia are in complete darkness, there are no action potentials. When light shines on an ommatidium, there is a brief delay, called the *latency*, before its eccentric-cell axon begins to produce action potentials. As long as the light remains on, action potentials are produced, although the firing rate gradually declines during the first few seconds of illumination. We can graph the axon's activity as follows.

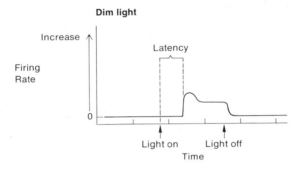

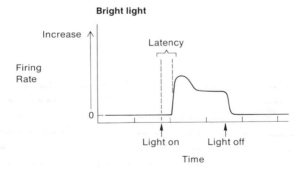

If the light is made brighter, the latency is reduced and the firing rate increases. If a dim light that remains on for 1 second produces a total of 5 action potentials, a brighter light that also remains on for 1 second might produce 10 or 15 action potentials.

Each ommatidium influences all the neighboring ommatidia in an inhibitory fashion. The inhibition occurs via synapses between branches of each eccentric cell's axon and the eccentric-cell axons of its neighbors. We can schematically represent three ommatidia and their inhibitory lateral interconnections as follows.

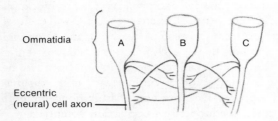

Ommatidia

Eccentric
(neural) cell axon

The negative signs in the sketch signify that the synapses are inhibitory.

Suppose we place three microelectrodes so that each one records the activity of one of the eccentric-cell axons. If we shine a one-second, moderately bright light only on ommatidium A, we might record 10 action potentials from its eccentric-cell axon, but the other two axons would not produce any action potentials. Similarly, if the same light shines only on ommatidium B, its eccentric-cell axon will produce 10 action potentials, but neither of the other two axons will produce action potentials. If we shine the same light, at the same time, on ommatidia A and B, both of their axons will produce action potentials. However, each axon will produce fewer action potentials than it did before. Perhaps now each axon will produce only 7 action potentials rather than 10. What has happened is that each eccentric-cell axon has inhibited the other axon.

The brighter the light that shines on an ommatidium, the more action potentials its eccentric-cell axon will produce, and the more that axon will inhibit its neighbors. If we allow our original light to shine on ommatidium A but we simultaneously shine a brighter light on ommatidium B, the eccentric-cell axon of ommatidium A will produce fewer than 7 action potentials. This demonstrates the first principle of the mutual, lateral inhibition: the amount of inhibition sent out from each ommatidium varies directly with the intensity of light shining on that ommatidium.

If we shine our original, one-second light only on ommatidium C, its eccentric-cell axon may produce 10 action potentials. If we simultaneously shine the light on only A and C, neither axon will produce 10 action potentials. Now they may each produce 8. Notice that A and C mutually inhibit each other less than A and B. In fact, this demonstrates the second principle of lateral inhibition: the amount of inhibition varies inversely with the distance between ommatidia.

Suppose we shine the light on all three ommatidia. What will happen? Each eccentric cell axon will receive inhibition from the other two axons. The eccentric cell axons of A and C will each receive quite a bit of inhibition from the axon of nearby B, and some inhibition from each other. Perhaps they'll each produce 6 action potentials. But what about the axon of B? It will receive inhibition from two nearby axons. Because the amount of inhibition increases as the distance decreases, the axon of B will receive quite a bit of inhibition from both A and C. It may, as a result, produce only 4 or 5 action potentials.

The Mach Band

Suppose we arrange two lights, one fairly dim and one fairly intense, so that each light shines on all the ommatidia in one half of the compound eye. If the left half of the compound eye is illuminated by the dim light, and the right half is illuminated by the intense light, we could graphically represent the arrangement as follows.

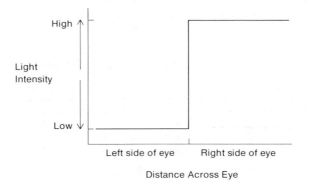

Distance Across Eye

Notice that, across each half of the compound eye, the light is of a uniform intensity. At the middle, there is a sudden change in the illumination. How will the eccentric-cell axons of all the ommatidia react?

You'll need to keep in mind the principles of lateral inhibition: the brighter the light falling on an ommatidium, the more its eccentric-cell axon will inhibit all the other axons—and, the closer ommatidia are to each other, the greater the amount of inhibition will be.

Let's see what happens to just a few of the ommatidia. Looked at from above the eye, we'd have the following situation.

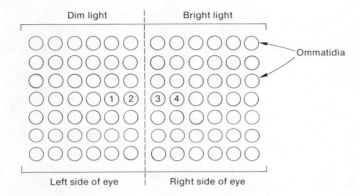

Consider the ommatidium marked 1, which is illuminated by the dim light. It will receive a moderate amount of inhibition from all its dimly illuminated neighbors and some inhibition from the more distant, brightly illuminated ommatidia. What about ommatidium 2? It will also receive a moderate amount of inhibition from its dimly illuminated neighbors. But notice that some of the brightly illuminated ommatidia are right nearby. Because they are brightly illuminated and nearby, they will strongly inhibit ommatidium 2. The result will be that ommatidium 2 will produce fewer action potentials than ommatidium 1.

What about ommatidium 4, which is illuminated by the intense light? It will receive a great deal of inhibition from its brightly illuminated neighbors and a small amount of inhibition from the more distant, dimly illuminated ommatidia. Now consider ommatidium 3. It will receive less inhibition because some of its immediate neighbors are only dimly illuminated. Yet it is being illuminated by bright light. It will produce many action poentials.

We can now see that ommatidium 1 will produce relatively few action potentials but ommatidium 2 will produce even fewer. Ommatidium 4 will produce many action potentials but ommatidium 3 will produce even more. All of the ommatidia of the four rows will be similarly affected. The net result will be that the information sent to the *Limulus* brain will not be "left half uniformly dim and right half uniformly bright"; rather it will be "left half dim with a very dim strip toward the middle of the eye, and right half bright with a very bright strip toward the middle of the eye." We can represent the original light arrangement and the information sent to the brain on one graph.

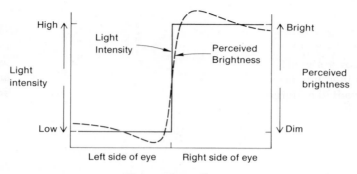

One way to describe the result is to say that the edge or contour between the dim and bright sides has been enhanced. This effect is called the *Mach* (pronounced "mock") *band*. In *Limulus*, the Mach-band effect occurs because of the nature of the lateral inhibitions. The important point is that, although we don't have a simple arrangement for lateral inhibition, we too see Mach bands. If you look closely at the contour between a sheet of bright, white paper and a sheet of black paper, you'll be able to detect the Mach band. And if you think about it, you should recognize that the Mach band effect is yet another example of the way in which we (and the horseshoe crab) are built to notice changes in stimulation rather than constant and uniform stimulation.

Recommended Readings

The following articles will help you understand the functioning of the visual system.

Hubel, D. H. "The Visual Cortex of the Brain," *Sci. Amer.,* Nov. 1963 (Offprint #168).

Lettvin, J. Y., H. R. Maturana, W. S. McCulloch, and W. H. Pitts. "What the Frog's Eye Tells the Frog's Brain," *Proc. Inst. Radio Engr.,* 1959, **47:** 1940–1951.

Michael, C. R.   "Retinal Processing of Visual Images," *Sci. Amer.*, May 1969 (Offprint #1143).

Pettigrew, J. D.   "The Neurophysiology of Binocular Vision," *Sci. Amer.*, Aug. 1972 (Offprint #1255).

For more information about *Limulus,* see the following articles.

Miller, W. H., F. Ratliff, and H. K. Hartline.   "How Cells Receive Stimuli," *Sci. Amer.*, Sept. 1961 (Offprint #99).

Ratliff, F. "Contour and Contrast," *Sci Amer.*, June 1972 (Offprint #543).

7

Color Vision

We've already made note of the fact that there are three different photochemicals found in cones. These photochemicals form the basis for color vision. The lateral geniculate nuclei analyze the information that is available from the cone photochemicals. Thus, our ability to see colors depends on the proper functioning of the area in the thalamus devoted to vision, as well as on the proper functioning of the photochemicals.

Cone Photochemicals

The three cone photochemicals differ in their sensitivities to different wavelengths of light. We've already discussed one method of determining their sensitivities: the hyperpolarizations of individual cones can be recorded when lights of different wavelengths are shone on the cones. This particular method indicates that, while the three kinds of cones all hyperpolarize in response to many different wavelengths, each kind of cone responds maximally to one particular region of the spectrum. The wavelength that produces the greatest response is called the λ_{max} (pronounced "lambda max"), and the three kinds of cones have λ_{max} of 440 nm, 540 nm, and 570 nm, respectively.

There is a more direct method of examining the cone photochemicals themselves. Rather than measuring the responses of cones, we can look at the ability of the photochemicals to absorb different wavelengths of light.

Any pigment absorbs light. Suppose you look through glass that is tinted blue. When the light from the sun or a light bulb passes through the glass, many wavelengths are absorbed by the pigment in the glass. The pigment does not absorb lights in the blue region of the spectrum; these reach your eye and, when you look through the glass, everything appears bluish. If you wanted to determine precisely which wavelengths the pigment absorbs, you could measure the difference between the light that enters the glass (the incident light) and the light that emerges from the glass.

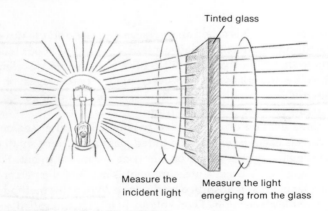

Tinted glass

Measure the incident light

Measure the light emerging from the glass

If the incident light is coming from an ordinary light bulb, it contains a mixture of wavelengths (that is, it is white light). The light that emerges from the glass contains only a few of the original wavelengths; the remainder have been absorbed by the pigment in the glass. To determine the λ_{max} of the pigment, white light would not be used.

Instead, we would use a series of lights, each of which contains just one wavelength. Such lights are called *monochromatic* ("mono-" meaning one; "-chromatic" meaning color) lights. We might begin with a monochromatic light of 400 nm; we would measure the percentage of the incident 400 nm light that is absorbed by the glass. Then we might use a 450 nm light—and so on, through the spectrum. When we finished, we would know how readily the pigment absorbs wavelengths throughout the spectrum, and we could easily graph the results.

Absorption Spectrum

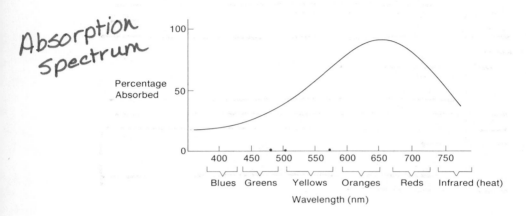

This kind of graph is called an *absorption spectrum*, and the wavelength associated with the maximum absorption is the λ_{max}. For our blue glass, the graph shows us that very little blue light (short wavelength) is absorbed by the glass. Progressively higher percentages of longer wavelengths are absorbed, and the λ_{max} is in the orange-red (long-wavelength) portion of the spectrum.

The same method can be applied to cones. The outer segment of a single cone is used in place of the tinted glass and a very small spot of monochromatic light is shone on the cone's outer segment. For each incident light that is used, a measurement is made of the percentage of that wavelength that is absorbed by the cone. When this method is used to measure the absorption of cone photochemicals, it is called *microspectrophotometry* ("micro-" meaning small; "-spectro-" meaning the spectrum; "-photometry" meaning light measurement—that is, the measurement of small spots of different wavelengths of light).

When microspectrophotometry is used to study the cones in our eyes, three different absorption spectra are found. One set of cones has an absorption spectrum with a λ_{max} of 440 nm; a second set has an absorption spectrum with a λ_{max} of 540 nm; the third set has an absorption spectrum with a λ_{max} of 570 nm.

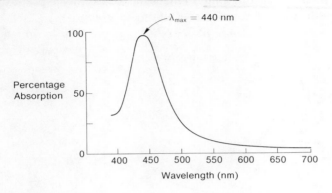

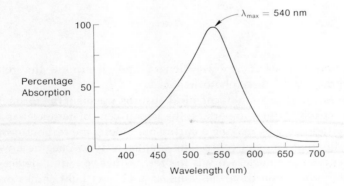

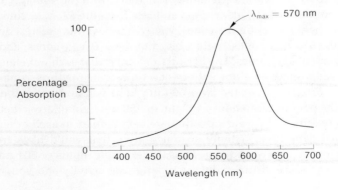

Pay particular attention to the fact that each kind of cone photo-chemical absorbs wavelengths throughout the spectrum. If a light of 500 nm is shone in the eye, all the photochemicals will absorb some of the light; the 540 λ_{max} photochemical will absorb more than the others, but all three will absorb some. Perhaps the easiest way to portray this is to place the three absorption spectra on one graph.

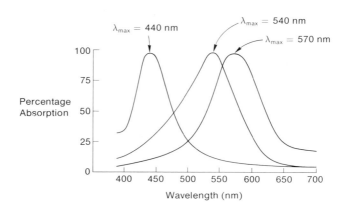

Now you can select any wavelength and determine the relative absorption by the three photochemicals.

The fact that each photochemical absorbs wavelengths throughout the spectrum is quite important; the lateral geniculate nuclei analyze color information by making comparisons among the responses of the three different kinds of cones. The simplest way to imagine how the lateral geniculate nuclei work is to pretend that you are a device that collects information from the cones. If a 420 nm light shines on the cones, you will receive a great deal of activity from the 440 λ_{max} cones, less from the 540 λ_{max} cones, and still less from the 570λ_{max} cones. If a 550 nm light shines on the cones, you will receive the greatest activity from the 540 λ_{max} cones, quite a bit from the 570 λ_{max} cones, and little from the 440 λ_{max} cones. The important point is that each wavelength of light will produce a unique pattern of activity from the three cones. The pattern of activity created by a 600 nm light will always be different from the pattern created by a 400 nm or 450 nm light or any other light in the spectrum. Wavelengths that are very similar to each other may produce patterns of activity so much alike that you'd have trouble distinguishing between them. Thus, for example, lights of 501 nm and 502 nm produce virtually the same pattern of activity and you, as the collecting device, might not be able to tell them apart. However, with this exception, lights of different wavelengths will produce patterns of activity so different that you can tell which wavelength of light is shining on the cones just by examining the pattern of activity of the cones (and never looking at the light itself).

Imagine what would happen if we had only one kind of photochemical. Suppose we measured its absorption spectrum and discovered it had a λ_{max} of 500 nm.

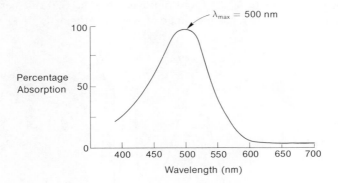

If you were the collecting device, you would receive information only from the receptors containing this photochemical. A light of 400 nm would certainly produce less activity than a light of 500 nm, as long as *the lights were equally intense*. But what would happen if the 400 nm light were quite intense and the 500 nm light were dim? Because the photochemical is affected most by 500 nm lights, even a dim 500 nm light will produce some activity; because the photochemical is moderately affected by 400 nm lights, an intense 400 nm light will produce quite a bit of activity. In fact, if we adjusted the intensities of the two lights correctly, the 400 nm and 500 nm lights would produce exactly the same amount of activity. You, as the collection device, would have no way of distinguishing between the effects of the two lights. And any wavelength of light could be made to produce exactly the same amount of activity as any other wavelength, just by adjusting the intensities. You would be unable to determine which wavelength of light was producing the activity.

What we've described is the way rods work. Rhodopsin has a λ_{max} of 500nm, and its absorption spectrum is the one shown in the preceding graph. Rods do not signal color; any wavelength of light can produce an effect on rods that is identical to the effect produced by any other wavelength, when the intensities of the lights are correctly adjusted.

It should be clear now that, in order to distinguish among wavelengths (that is, to see color), there must be more than one photochemical involved. But, most importantly, the absorption spectra of the photochemicals must overlap each other. To understand why, imagine again that you are the collection device. Suppose we had three photochemicals, with λ_{max} of 440 nm, 540 nm, and 570 nm—each of which absorbed only a narrow range of wavelengths.

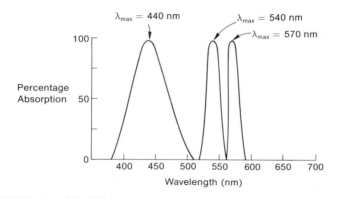

A light of 400 nm would produce activity in only one kind of cone. If you were the collection device, you would never confuse a 400 nm light with a 530 nm or a 580 nm. Each light would produce activity in only one kind of cone, no matter how bright or dim the light was. You, as the collection device, could certainly tell the differences among short, medium, and long wavelengths. However, would you be able to tell the difference between 420 nm, 440 nm, and 460 nm lights? All of the lights would produce activity in the same kind of cone and, if the intensities of the lights were properly adjusted, the lights would all produce the same amount of activity. The best you could do would be to identify which third of the spectrum the lights were in.

When the absorption spectra overlap each other, you can do a great deal more. Because different wavelengths will produce different patterns of activity, you'll be able to identify many different wavelengths on the basis of their effects on the three kinds of cones.

What we've been describing is actually a theme that applies to all sensory systems: we analyze and interpret stimuli on the basis of the patterns of activity they produce in the nervous system. Any individual stimulus affects many receptor cells and neurons in different ways and to varying degrees. We do not rely on any one receptor cell or neuron as the sole or primary source of information about a stimulus; instead we make comparisons among the receptor cells and neurons. As you consider this, it may occur to you that the various kinds of receptive fields we described in Chapter 6 really represent comparisons being performed by cells. On–off cells, for example, compare the relative intensity of stimulation falling on their on and off areas, and they respond accordingly. Similarly, what is behind the Mach-band effect is a comparison of what is occurring in various ommatidia. You may want to be on the lookout for other examples of cases in which the *pattern* of activity created by a stimulus determines our perception of the stimulus.

The Analysis of Color Information

The information from the three kinds of cones is carried via the C-units in the intermediate layer of the retina (if you recall, those are the units that hyperpolarize in response to some wavelengths and depolarize in response to others) to the ganglion cells. The ganglion cells send the information to the *lateral geniculate nuclei* (abbreviated *LGN*) of the thalamus. Let's concentrate on the LGN.

   Neurons in the LGN have receptive fields with a center–surround arrangement. Some of the receptive fields are identical to those of the ganglion cells; they have an on-center and off-surround, or vice versa. But the overwhelming majority of the LGN neurons have receptive fields that are color-coded. They may have an on-center that is activated only by red (long-wavelength) lights and an off-surround that is activated only by green (moderate-wavelength) lights. Or the center may be red-off and the surround be green-on. There are actually four kinds of receptive fields that react to reds and greens.

There are four other kinds of receptive fields that are color-coded. These respond to yellow and blues.

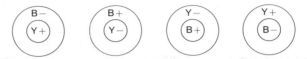

These eight kinds of receptive fields belong to LGN neurons that, as a group, are called the *opponent cells* (because they react in opposite or *opponent* ways to different wavelengths of light). The LGN neurons that aren't color-coded but that have plain on–off, center–surround arrangements are called the *nonopponent cells* (because they react to all wavelengths of light in the same way).

The opponent cells are the ones that collect information from the C-units—which, in turn, get their information from the cones. The information that goes to the four kinds of red–green opponent cells originates in the cones that have λ_{max} of 540 nm and 570 nm. The information for the yellow–blue system originates in the 440 nm and 570 nm cones. A diagrammatic sketch of the information flow might look as follows.

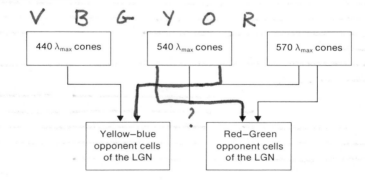

The opponent cells perform comparisons among the three kinds of cones. In effect, they compare the activity produced in the cones by different wavelengths of light, and they serve as the collecting device we mentioned earlier.

Trichromatic and Dichromatic Theories

Historically there has been a debate between proponents of two theories of color vision. One camp argued that normal color vision depends upon having three kinds of color receptors. The theory was first proposed by Thomas Young and later revised by Hermann von Helmholtz, both of whom lived long before any of the microspec-trophotometry or electrical recordings had been performed. Their theory, called the *Young–Helmholtz trichromatic* ("tri-" meaning three; "-chromatic" meaning color) *theory,* postulated that there is one receptor especially sensitive to red, a second most sensitive to green, and a third most sensitive to blue.

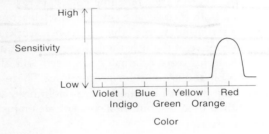

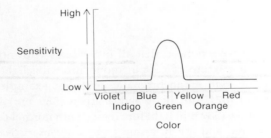

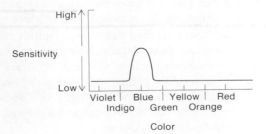

The trichromatic theory proposed that all our color perceptions come about as a result of the relative amount of activity produced by these three kinds of color receptors.

The other theory, proposed by Ewald Hering at about the same time that Helmholtz was revising the trichromatic theory, suggested that normal color vision required having two "color elements." One element was thought to be responsive to reds and greens, the other responsive to yellows and blues. Each element could be "built up" by one of the colors and "broken down" by the other. (A third, black–white element was proposed to account for night vision.) Because the theory postulated two color elements, it's called the *Hering dichromatic* ("di-" meaning two; "-chromatic" meaning color) *theory.*

As we now know, both theories are correct. The trichromatic theory is a fairly accurate representation of the way cones work; the dichromatic theory is descriptive of the way the LGN works. But understanding why the two theories were originally proposed will allow you to understand quite a bit about our color preceptions. There were many bits of evidence brought forth by the Young–Helmholtz and Hering camps to support their theories, but we'll concentrate on just two areas: color mixtures and afterimages.

Color Mixtures

Young and Helmholtz noticed that all individuals with normal color vision perceive a mixture of certain monochromatic lights as being identical to a different monochromatic light. For example, an equal mixture of a red (671 nm) light and a green (536 nm) light looks identical to a yellow (589 nm) light for anyone with normal color vision. The mixture of red and green is said to be a *metameric match* for the yellow light. Not all monochromatic lights can be metamerically matched by mixing just two lights together. However, any monochromatic light can be metamerically matched by a mixture of *three* other lights. It was this fact that intrigued Young and Helmholtz.

Before we go on with any more details about color mixture, we need to clarify what happens when lights of different colors are mixed. You probably know that if you mix yellow and blue paint, you get green paint. However, if you mix yellow and blue light, you do not get green light. (Just ask anyone who has done theatrical lighting!) Obviously, paints and lights don't work the same way.

Let's take the case of paints first. Yellow paint contains a pigment that absorbs all wavelengths except those in the yellow region of the spectrum. Wavelengths in the yellow region are reflected from the paint and, when you look at something painted yellow, only those wavelengths reach your eye. Blue paint contains a pigment that reflects light in the blue region of the spectrum, absorbing all others. We can represent yellow and blue paint as follows.

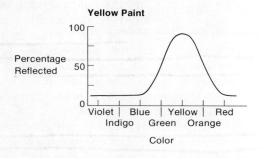

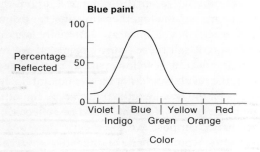

If we place the graphs together, we can see why a mixture of yellow and blue paints yields green paint.

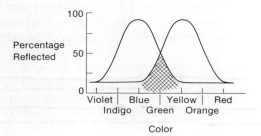

The yellow paint most readily reflects light in the yellow region (that is, it absorbs the light above and below the yellow region); the blue paint most readily reflects light in the blue region (that is, it absorbs the light above and below the blue region). The only portion of the spectrum that is significantly reflected by *both* paints is the green region, represented by the cross-hatched area in the graph. One way to understand the mixture of paints is to realize that the yellow paint absorbs some of the light reflected by the blue paint, and the blue paint absorbs some of the light reflected by the yellow paint. In a sense, each paint subtracts some of the light reflected by the other paint. The light that is not completely absorbed by either paint is the resulting color we see. This kind of process is called *subtractive mixture.*

The results of subtractive mixture depend upon the reflecting properties of the paints we mix together. Imagine, for example, that we have paints that each reflect only an extremely narrow range of wavelengths. We might call these "pure" paints. If we mix a "pure" yellow (a paint that reflects *only* yellow) with a "pure" blue (a paint that reflects *only* blue), the result would not be green paint. Instead, because each paint absorbs all the wavelengths reflected by the other paint, the result would be black paint! (No light would be reflected.)

On the other hand, suppose we have very "impure" paints. The results of their mixture would depend on the range of wavelengths each reflects. Actually, a typical paint reflects a fairly wide range of wavelengths. Further, a paint may reflect wavelengths that are at some distance from each other in the spectrum, while it absorbs the intermediate wavelengths. (The graph of its reflected light spectrum would have two distinct "peaks.") This brief discussion should convince you that predicting the outcome of subtractive mixture requires thorough knowledge of the reflecting properties of the particular paints being mixed.

When a beam of yellow light crosses a beam of blue light, no subtraction occurs. There is nothing in either beam of light to absorb any of the light in the other beam. Instead, the lights are added together. This kind of process is called *additive mixture,* and we can represent it graphically.

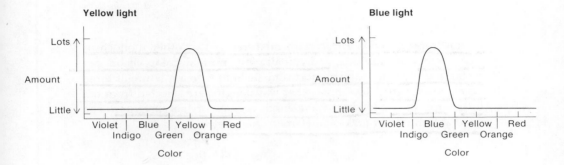

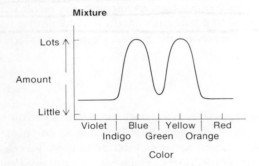

The result of mixing two lights is that all the wavelengths found in each of the original beams will be present.

Because in subtractive mixture we are taking away some of the light in the original components, the mixture will not be as bright as the originals. In additive mixture, we are summing up the original components, and the mixture will be brighter than either of the original lights.

Color Blindness

As we've said, Young and Helmholtz noticed that individuals with normal color vision can form metameric matches between some monochromatic lights and certain mixtures of two other monochromatic lights. In addition, individuals with normal color vision can metamerically match any monochromatic light with a mixture of three other wavelengths. The three other wavelengths are selected from the long, moderate, and short wavelength regions of the spectrum. The general formula for making metameric matches is

$$a(\lambda_1) + b(\lambda_2) = c(\lambda_3) + d(\lambda_4).$$

In other words, if some amount of a light of one wavelength is added to some amount of light of another wavelength, the result will be a light that looks identical to a particular mixture of two other wavelengths. Notice that we could rewrite the general formula in a slightly different form:

$$a(\lambda_1) + b(\lambda_2) - c(\lambda_3) = d(\lambda_4).$$

Although it isn't possible to subtract one monochromatic light from a mixture of two others, this version of the formula emphasizes the idea that normal color vision requires a mixture of three wavelengths for a metameric match (as the Young–Helmholtz theory predicts). The first version of the formula emphasizes the idea that normal color vision requires mixtures of pairs of wavelengths for a metameric match (as the Hering theory predicts). In either case, the ability of someone with normal color vision to make metameric matches provides a good reference for understanding various forms of color blindness.

Some individuals require a larger amount of one of the wavelengths if they are to make metameric matches. These individuals are said to have a "color weakness." Presumably, they possess the usual three kinds of cones but one of the cone types doesn't operate properly or is underrepresented. If the 570 nm λ_{max} cones are malfunctioning, the individual will require a greater amount of the long-wavelength light than someone with normal color vision. If the 540 nm λ_{max} cones are involved, a greater amount of the moderate-wavelength light is needed—and, if the 440 nm λ_{max} cones are at fault, more of the shorter-wavelength light is needed.

Individuals with normal color vision are called *trichromats*, reflecting the fact that they have three kinds of cones ("tri-" meaning three). Individuals with a color weakness are called *anomalous trichromats* ("anomalous" meaning abnormal), indicating that, although they have three kinds of cones, one kind is not operating properly.

Some individuals possess only two kinds of cones. They are called *dichromats* ("di-" meaning two), and they can form a metameric match to any wavelength by mixing together just two other wavelengths. If the individual is missing the 570 nm λ_{max} cones, the long wavelengths will all look very much alike. Shades of red and orange will not appear different from each other. Because of this, the individual is said to be "red blind." If the 540 nm λ_{max} cones are missing, shades of green and blue will look alike. The individual is said to be "green blind." These conditions are relatively common (especially among men), and often they are both referred to as "red–green color blindness." Because both the 570 nm and 540 nm cones send their information to the red–green opponent cells in the LGN, both red and green perceptions will suffer if either kind of cone is missing. However, depending upon which kind of cone is lost, the person will have more trouble distinguishing among wavelengths in either the long or moderate wavelength portions of the spectrum. Remember that the 570 nm cones also send information to the yellow–blue opponent cells in the LGN. Therefore, the absence of the 570 nm λ_{max} cones will actually produce deficits in the perception of virtually all wavelengths.

There is a third type of dichromacy that is relatively rare. It involves the absence of the 440 nm λ_{max} cones; individuals who have this condition are unable to distinguish among yellows, yellow-oranges, and yellow-greens.

On occasions, individuals are found who have only a single cone type. They are called *monochromats* ("mono-" meaning one). Because they do not have any basis on which to compare different wavelengths of light, they can match any wavelength with any other wavelength by adjusting the intensities of the lights. Their vision during the day is similar to our night vision: everything is seen in shades of gray. They are the only individuals who truly deserve to be called "color blind." (Dichromats are color deficient. They can't see as many colors as a trichromat, but they do see colors.)

Afterimages

If you stare at a bright patch of red for a while, when you look away you will see a patch of green, and vice versa. Similarly, staring at a bright patch of yellow produces an *afterimage* of blue, and vice versa. These effects were noticed by Hering, and they suggested to him that our color vision is built on a double dichromatic system (that is, a red–green mechanism and a yellow–blue mechanism).

Let's see if—given the information you have about cones, C-units, and the LGN—we can figure out why these afterimages occur.

If you stare at a bright patch of red, the cones containing the 570 nm λ_{max} will be most affected. The photochemical will absorb quite a bit of light, and it will be bleached. The cones will hyperpolarize, and this hyperpolarization will produce activity in C-units. Some of the C-units will hyperpolarize, while others will depolarize. The ganglion cells, in turn, will either increase or decrease their firing rates (depending upon whether they are on, off, or on–off cells). Opponent cells in the LGN will either increase or decrease their firing rates (depending upon whether they have a red-on or red-off area). When you look away from the red patch (the simplest situation would be one in which you just close your eyes after staring at the red patch for a while), the cones and C-units return to their resting potential, and the ganglion cells and opponent cells return to their maintained discharge.

Part of the reason for afterimages has to do with the similarity between what happens when a red light goes off and what happens when a green light comes on. When you look away from the red patch, for example, any opponent cell in the LGN that had increased its firing rate will now reduce its firing rate. That same opponent cell also reduces its firing rate when a green light comes on. Any opponent cell in the LGN that had decreased its firing rate in response to red will increase its firing rate when red goes off. And that opponent cell would also increase its firing rate when green comes on. Let's see if we can show this diagramatically.

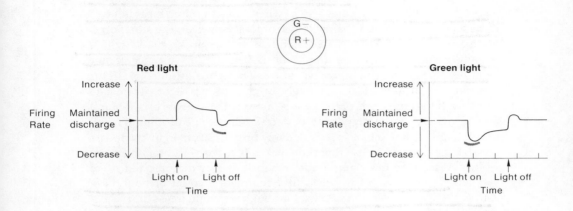

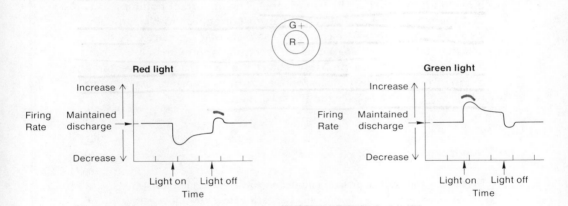

Notice that the *offset* of a red light produces a decrease in the firing rate of the red-on, green-off opponent cell. The *onset* of a green light also produces a decrease. For the red-off, green-on opponent cell, the *offset* of a red light and the *onset* of a green light both produce an increase in the firing rate.

At least part of the reason for afterimages has to do with the fact that individual neurons in the LGN signal two different events in the same way. It shouldn't be surprising for us to discover that we confuse the two events, and we perceive what is actually the offset of one light as the apparent onset of another.

A Final Word on Color Perception

As you already know, when the wavelength of light is changed, we perceive a change in color—and, when the amplitude of light is changed, we perceive a change in brightness. However, the situation is actually a bit more complicated than that. If a monochromatic light is made more intense (if its amplitude is increased), we perceive not only an increase in brightness; we also see a slight shift in color. If, for example, you look at a moderately bright 565 nm light, it appears yellow. If the amplitude of the light is increased, it appears brighter and more orange. If the amplitude is decreased, it appears dimmer and yellow-green. If you look at a moderately bright 420 nm light, it appears violet. An increase in its amplitude makes it appear brighter and more blue. A decrease in its amplitude makes it appear dimmer and more violet. No one has yet worked out a complete account of how these *amplitude-induced color changes* occur (although we might guess that, as the amplitude of a monochromatic light changes, the relative effects on the three kinds of cones might also change). The important point for us is that there are three wavelengths that do not appear to change color when their amplitudes are changed. The facts that there are only three and that they are well-spaced in the spectrum (approximately 572 nm, 503 nm, and 478 nm) probably reflect the fact that we have three different cone photochemicals whose absorption spectra overlap but whose λ_{max} are well-spaced in the spectrum.

Summary

Make sure you can understand and define all the italicized terms.

There are three cone photochemicals, each with its own *absorption spectrum* and λ_{max}. The ability of each photochemical to absorb *monochromatic light* can be studied by using *microspectrophotometry* or by recording the hyperpolarizations of the cones. Both methods indicate that each of the photochemicals is affected by a wide range of wavelengths, and that any particular wavelength will affect all three photochemicals to varying degrees.

Visual information is sent, by the intermediate and ganglion cells, to the *lateral geniculate nuclei (LGN)*. There the *nonopponent cells* analyze information about brightness, while the *opponent cells* analyze information about color. The opponent cells are of eight varieties; four have red–green receptive fields, and four have yellow–blue receptive fields.

Because individuals with normal color vision have three kinds of cones, they are called *trichromats*. They can form *metameric matches* by mixing three wavelengths of light. Individuals who are *anomalous trichromats* require a greater than normal amount of one of the three wavelengths. *Dichromats* can form metameric matches by mixing just two wavelengths, and *monochromats* perceive any two wavelengths as being the same when the intensities are correctly adjusted.

Both the *Young—Helmholtz trichromatic theory* and the *Hering dichromatic theory* find support in the nature of metameric matches. (Remember that, when lights are mixed, they form *additive mixtures,* while paints form *subtractive mixtures.* As you consider additive and subtractive mixtures, see if you can explain this fact: when many lights of different wavelengths are combined, we see white; but when many paints of different colors are combined, we see black.) The dichromatic theory finds additional support from the nature of *afterimages,* while the trichromatic theory gets support from the nature of *amplitude-induced color changes.* In fact, both theories are correct. The trichromatic theory describes the functioning of the cones, while the dichromatic theory describes the functioning of the LGN.

Recommended Readings

For more on the general nature of color vision, try this book.

Alpern, M., M. Lawrence, and D. Wolsk. *Sensory Processes.* Brooks/Cole, 1967. (Chapter 2.)

For more advanced and specific information, you may wish to look at the following somewhat difficult articles in the *Cold Spring Harbor Symposia on Quantitative Biology, Vol. XXX: Sensory Receptors* (1965).

DeValois, R. L. "Analysis and Coding of Color Vision in the Primate Visual System," pp. 567–580.

Tomita, T. "Electrophysiological Study of the Mechanisms Subserving Color Coding in the Fish Retina," pp. 559–566.

Wald, G., and P. Brown. "Human Color Vision and Color Blindness," pp. 345–362.

There were two Offprints listed among the Recommended Readings for Chapter 5 that are especially helpful for understanding color vision.

MacNichol, E. F. "Three-Pigment Color Vision," *Sci. Amer.,* Dec. 1964 (Offprint #197).

Rushton, W. A. H. "Visual Pigments in Man," *Sci. Amer.,* Nov. 1962 (Offprint #139).

8

Visual Perception

Our visual perceptions are not simply the results of the visual events themselves. We modify, change, compare, analyze, and interpret visual information. One of the most basic questions that can be asked about our visual perceptions is how accurately they correspond to the visual stimuli: to what degree do our perceptions reflect the actual, physical, visual events out there in the world?

One way to answer the question is to examine our visual *thresholds:* how bright does a light have to be before we can see it? How different do two lights have to be before we can tell that they're different? When we pose questions about our visual thresholds, we're essentially asking what the limits of our visual perceptions are. Thresholds are measurements of our sensitivity. If we are very sensitive to a light, our threshold is low. If we are relatively insensitive to a light, our threshold is high.

Another way to assess the degree to which our perceptions accurately reflect visual events is to examine the ways in which we interpret fairly complicated visual information. When we look off into the distance, how do we interpret all the information (the sizes of objects, their shapes, their relationships to each other, etc.) in the scene? When we look at a complicated sketch, how do we abstract meaning from all the lines in the sketch? When we pose these kinds of questions, we're asking what biases we have and how the visual system analyzes information.

Actually, the study of visual perception is vast and enormously detailed. We'll discuss just a few topics in visual perception.

Dark and Light Adaptation

Let's begin with a discussion of how our visual thresholds change as we become accustomed to the light level in a room.

Imagine what happens when you walk into a darkened theatre on a bright day. Initially, you have great trouble seeing. After a while, more and more of the theatre becomes visible. At first, you can make out lighted signs or aisle lights. Later, the shapes of seats, people, and objects in the theatre can be seen. The process of becoming adjusted to the darkened situation is called *dark adaptation.* There are several steps involved in dark adaptation. The first is one you already know about: the pupils widen to allow more of the available light to enter the eyes. But there are far more complicated changes that take place. In order to study them, we can arrange a situation more controlled than walking into a darkened theatre.

Suppose you are placed in a well-lighted room for about 30 minutes. Then, all the room lights are turned off. You are told to look straight ahead and to tell the experimenter when you first notice that a light has been turned on. The experimenter first turns on a very dim light (so dim that you can't see it) and then gradually makes it brighter. When you indicate that you can see the light, the experimenter makes note of its intensity.

Try to figure out what would happen if you were allowed to sit in the dark for different periods of time before the experimenter turned on the light.

If you had been sitting in the dark for a very short period of time, the light would have to be made relatively bright before you noticed it. If you had been in the dark for a relatively long period of time, the light wouldn't have to be nearly as bright for you to notice it. One way to express this is to say that your threshold goes down as you sit in the darkened room.

Suppose we tested you after 1 minute, 2 minutes, 3, 4, 5 minutes, and so in the darkened room. We would end up with a series of measurements of your threshold and, plotted on a graph, we would get what's called the *dark-adaptation curve.*

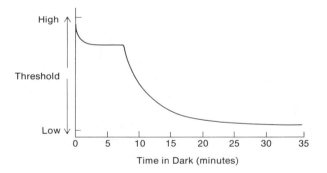

Notice that the thresholds don't decline smoothly. Within the first 6 or 7 minutes, your threshold declines gradually. Then there is a sharp decline. Finally, after about 25 minutes, the threshold reaches a low level that does not substantially change thereafter.

Let me give you some additional information and then see if you can figure out why there seems to be a sudden shift after 7 or 8 minutes.

If we run exactly the same experiment except that we make sure that the light falls only on the foveas or only on the periphery of the retinas, we'd get the following results.

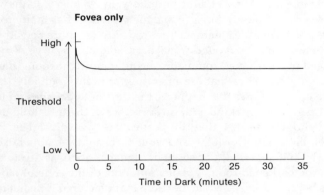

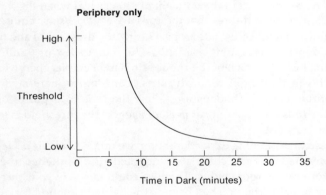

When the light shines only on the fovea, there is only an initial and small decline in the threshold. It's as if we just extended the first part of the dark-adaptation curve and we never got the second part, the rapidly declining part, of the curve. When the light shines only on the periphery, there is a rapid decline in the threshold after a short, initial period during which the threshold is infinitely high (we can't see any light, no matter how intense it is). It's as if we skipped the first part of the dark-adaptation curve and went right to the second part after a few minutes.

Think about the fovea and the periphery. In what way do they differ? The fovea contains only cones, while the periphery has many rods and relatively few cones. Remember that rods are far more sensitive than cones. Now, think about our original dark-adaptation curve. When you are placed in a darkened room after being in a bright room, the cones are the only receptors that are operating at first. Gradually the rods begin to operate. Once that happens, the threshold declines rapidly. So the first part of the dark-adaptation curve, when the threshold declines only slightly, indicates that the cones are active. Cones need a considerable amount of light, and your threshold remains fairly high during this initial period. The slight decline that occurs is due to the fact that, in the darkened room, smaller amounts of the cone photochemicals are being bleached, while more are manufactured. The net result is that gradually more of the cone photochemicals are ready to absorb light. The second part of the dark adaptation curve, when the threshold declines sharply, indicates that the rods are active. Rods require much less light, and your threshold drops. During the drop, more and more of the rhodopsin is becoming available. The rods took 7 or 8 minutes to get going because much of the rhodopsin had been bleached when you were still in the bright room. It takes that long to manufacture and reconstitute enough rhodopsin to allow the rods to begin to operate. Once the rods are operating at peak efficiency, the threshold is low and remains constant.

Instead of examining dark adaptation, we might study *light adaptation:* once you had become completely adapted to a darkened room, we could turn on the room lights. Then we could measure your thresholds to a spot of light after you had been in the lighted situation for different lengths of time (this is a similar to what happens when you come out of a darkened theatre on a bright day). Initially, your threshold will be quite low. Within minutes, the threshold will increase and reach a steady level. Again, several things are involved. First, the pupils narrow to cut down on the amount of available light that enters the eye. Within seconds, the rods stop operating (most of the rhodopsin gets bleached very rapidly). The cones become active. Quite a bit of the cone photochemicals is bleached initially. Gradually, the bleaching of cone photochemicals and the manufacturing (or reconstituting) of them reach a balance. Your threshold remains steady.

There is an initial rapid increase in the *light-adaptation curve,* representing the changeover from rods to cones. This is followed by a more gradual increase, representing the bleaching of cone photochemicals. Finally, the threshold reaches a steady level.

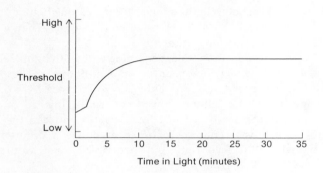

Notice that light adaptation is a faster process than dark adaptation; it takes only about 10 minutes of light adaptation to reach the steady threshold level. It requires about 25 or 30 minutes of dark adaptation to reach the steady threshold level.

Difference Thresholds

Instead of studying the way in which thresholds change when the light level changes, we could examine our ability to detect the differences between two lights once we're accustomed to the light level in a room. Suppose you're seated in a moderately well-lighted room. Once you've adapted to the room light, you're asked to look at two spots of light lying side by side and to indicate when the two spots first appear to differ in their brightnesses. The experimenter initially makes the two spots equal in intensity and then gradually increases the intensity of one. When you indicate that the two spots of light look different, the experimenter makes note of the difference in their intensities. The smallest difference you can detect is called your *difference threshold.*

Imagine that we begin with the two spots of light set at an arbitrary intensity; we could set them both at light level 5 (the light-level numbers we're going to use are arbitrary). One light is left at level 5 and the other is gradually increased. Perhaps when it is at level 6, you first notice that the two lights look different.

Now we could set both lights at level 10. When one light is increased to level 11, the two lights still appear to be the same. When it reaches level 12, the two lights look different.

Let's repeat this one more time, beginning with both lights set at level 20. Now the two lights will appear the same until one reaches level 24.

Notice that in every case, one light had to increase by a particular percentage before the difference was noticeable. Instead of figuring out the percentage, we could just form a ratio between the amount of change (that was required in order to notice a difference) and the original light level. In our examples, we would have: 1/5, 2/10(=1/5), 4/20(=1/5).

The constant ratio of the difference threshold was discovered long ago by Ernst Weber (the "W" is pronounced "V"). He stated it in a general form:

$$\frac{\Delta I}{I} = k.$$

where ΔI = the required amount of change;
$\quad I$ = the original intensity; and
$\quad k$ = constant.

The equation has come to be called *Weber's Law.* We can plot Weber's Law on a graph.

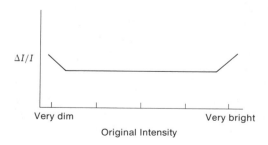

$\Delta I / I$

Very dim   Very bright

Original Intensity

Where the graph is flat, $\Delta I/I = k$. Notice that, when the original intensity is very low or very high, the graph is no longer flat. At these extremes, the two lights would have to differ by more than 1/5 for us to notice the difference. But over the broad, middle range of intensities, Weber's Law is correct.

Weber's Law describes our difference thresholds in a wide variety of situations. Suppose I had several animals, each of which had the remarkable ability to lengthen when given the command to grow. Let's begin with my 6-inch-long earthworm; it lengthens on command and perhaps when it reaches 8 inches, we first notice that it appears longer. Now I bring out my dachshund. It is originally 36 inches long. When it lengthens to 48 inches, we first notice a difference. Finally, there is an alligator whose original length is 96 inches. When it reaches 128 inches, we notice a difference. In these examples, we are dealing with a difference threshold for length instead of intensity. Still, Weber's Law is correct: $\Delta L/L = 1/3$. If we were dealing with extremely small or extremely large animals, they would have to increase their length by more than one-third for us to notice the difference. But, for animals of medium length, an increase of one-third of the original body length is all we would need.

Weber's Law accurately reflects our difference thresholds to two tones of different loudnesses. (If one tone is set at loudness level 6, perhaps we notice a difference when the other tone is at level 7. If this is the case, at what loudness level must the second tone be set when the first tone is at level 12, or then at level 24, if we are to notice the difference?) It also reflects our ability to tell the difference between two weights resting on the hand. (Suppose I found that $\Delta W/W = 1/10$. If I rest a 100 gram weight on your hand, how heavy do I have to make the second weight for you to notice the difference?) Each situation will have its own value for the constant. (In fact, different people in the same situation may have different constants. My constant for the different threshold to the temperatures of objects resting on my hand may be 2/15; yours may be 2/13.) But, in each situation, Weber's Law will hold true over the middle range of stimuli.

Additional Laws

Let's go back to our original difference-threshold experiment dealing with two lights of different intensities. We found that, if one light was at level 5, the other light had to reach level 6 before we noticed the difference. Suppose we now start with both lights set at level 6; how much do we need to increase one light before we'll notice a difference?

We know that

$$\frac{\Delta I}{I} = k, \qquad \text{and} \qquad \frac{1}{5} = k,$$

so

$$\frac{\Delta I}{6} = \frac{1}{5}.$$

Therefore,
$$\Delta I = 1.2.$$

We'll need to increase one light to level 7.2 if we are to notice that it's different from a light at level 6.

Suppose we start with both lights set at level 7.2; calculate the ΔI needed to notice the difference between the lights.

$$\frac{\Delta I}{7.2} = \frac{1}{5};$$

therefore,
$$\Delta I = 1.44.$$

We'll need to increase one light to level 8.64 if we are to notice that it's different from a light at level 7.2.

We could go on and on with this ascending series, and that is exactly what was done by an individual named Gustav Fechner (pronounced "fek'-ner"). Furthermore, he decided that each ΔI jump is just like every other ΔI jump. Each ΔI jump in the series represents one difference-threshold unit, and Fechner argued that the difference between light levels 5 and 6 "felt the same" as the difference between levels 6 and 7.2, or that between 7.2 and 8.64. He called each of these jumps a "sensation" unit or level. So we could say that, at the first sensation level, the light had to reach level 6; for the second sensation level, the light had to reach level 7.2; and for the third sensation level, 8.64. And we can draw a graph to represent all this.

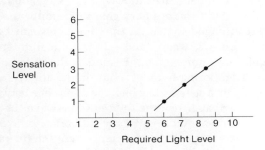

Notice that, as the sensation level increases in equal steps, the required light intensity increases by bigger and bigger steps. (At the first sensation level, we required light level 6 and, at the second sensation level, we needed a 7.2 light. That's a difference of 1.2. But the difference in the required light intensity between the second and third sensation levels is 1.44.) In fact, the required light intensities grow so rapidly that, if we continued the series, the graph would look as follows.

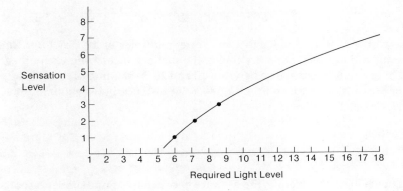

Fechner looked at that and realized that there was a simple way to keep the curve from climbing off the graph paper. He replotted the graph using a logarithmic scale for the required light intensity.

If you're unfamiliar (or uncomfortable) with logarithms, don't panic. Let's use a simple, nonmathematical way of thinking about logarithms. First of all, think about the ordinary counting numbers: 1, 2, 3, 4, 5, 6. . . . They're arranged so that the difference between 1 and 2 is the same as the difference between 3 and 4. In fact, the difference between any two neighboring numbers is the same as the difference between any other two neighboring numbers. But things don't *have* to be that way. We could set up a scheme in which the difference between the first two numbers was greater than the difference between the second and third numbers. And we could make the difference between any two succeeding numbers less than the difference between the previous two numbers. That's exactly what a logarithmic scale does.

We can represent the ordinary counting numbers and the logarithmic scale as follows.

Counting numbers

Logarithmic scale

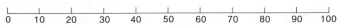

Notice that, on the logarithmic scale, multiples of 10 that form the same ratio to each other are found at equal distances from each other. For example, the distance between 10 and 20 is the same as the distance between 20 and 40, and the same as the distance between 40 and 80. Notice that

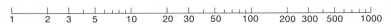

$$\frac{10}{20} = \frac{20}{40} = \frac{40}{80} = \frac{1}{2}.$$

On the logarithmic scale, the distance between two numbers represents their ratio (obtained by division). On the usual graph scale (called an arithmetic scale), the distance between two numbers represents their difference (obtained by subtraction). In effect, the logarithmic scale simply stretches out the lower-value parts of the scale and squeezes together the higher-value parts of the scale. It makes it much easier to show a wide range of values on a single graph—and sometimes (as in this case) it simplifies the nature of the curve.

Fechner used the logarithmic scale on the horizontal axis of his graph and came up with the following.

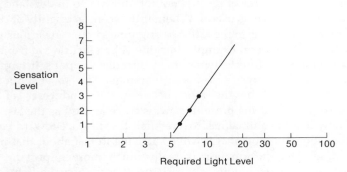

Not only does a logarithmic scale keep the curve from going off the graph; it also changes the curved line into a straight line. And this allowed Fechner to say that the sensation level is proportional to the logarithm of the light's intensity. As the sensation level increases steadily, the logarithm of the required light level also increases steadily. The rate at which the logarithm of the light increases is indicated in the graph by the slope (or angle) of the line. Fechner summarized all this in a single equation, which is usually referred to as *Fechner's Law:*

$$S = k \log I$$

where S = sensation level;
$\quad \log I$ = logarithm of the required light level; and
$\qquad k$ = slope.

It turns out that the k in Weber's Law is the same as the k in Fechner's equation. And it turns out that Weber and Fechner were describing the same process. Weber found that our difference threshold was always the same fraction of the original stimulus in any particular experiment. Fechner declared that the intensity of our sensations was always proportional to the logarithm of the intensity of the stimuli in any particular situation.

What's interesting about Fechner's Law is that it seems to suggest that our sensory systems may operate on a logarithmic scale. It seems to indicate that our sensory systems are designed to weigh more heavily the ratios between stimulus intensities, rather than the differences between stimulus intensities. It is not too difficult to understand why such a sensory system is useful. Whether the scene is brightly or dimly lit, our main interest is in the ratios of brightness between various parts of the scene. As another example, imagine yourself sitting in front of a fire, surrounded by forests, without any effective weapons, listening to the growls of a large and hungry animal. The most important information would be the ratio between the loudnesses of two successive growls. If the present growl is twice as loud as the last one, you know that the animal has covered half the distance toward you in that time. So you know that it will be arriving in just about that much more time! That information is really much more important than estimating the actual loudness of each growl or the actual difference in loudness of two growls.

It is not certain that our sensory systems operate on a logarithmic scale, but it is a possibility. However, there has been an important debate on this issue. It will be easier to understand the debate if we go back and re-emphasize Fechner's basic assumption: he declared that each ΔI jump is just like every other ΔI jump. Thus, as far as he was concerned, going from one sensation level to the next "feels the same" as going from any other sensation level to the next. He never proved this; he simply assumed it.

In the 1950s, a researcher named S. S. Stevens decided to test Fechner's assumption. He began by showing individuals a moderately intense light and telling them that they should assign it a value of 100. Then he showed the individuals various lights, ranging from ones that were substantially less intense than the moderate light to ones that were substantially more intense than the moderate light. Each time the individuals saw a light, they were asked to assign it a value which they felt expressed its brightness relative to the moderate light. For example, if a light appeared to be half as bright as the moderate light, the individuals would assign it a value of 50; if it appeared to be twice as bright, the assigned value would be 200. Stevens recorded the actual (physical) intensity levels of the lights and the values that were assigned. He found that individuals differ somewhat in the values they assign. However, he computed the average values and graphed them as follows.

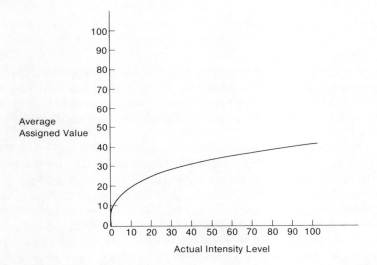

If Fechner's assumption were correct, we should be able to replot that graph using a logarithmic scale for the horizontal axis and come up with a straight line. Remember that, in a logarithmic scale, numbers that stand in a particular ratio to each other are equally distant from each other. In other words, the distance between light levels 10 and 20 would be the same as the distance between light levels 20 and 40, or that between 40 and 80. Instead of replotting the graph, let's just draw up a table that contains these light levels and the values they were assigned.

Light Level	Assigned Value
10	20
20	25
40	31
80	39

If Fechner's assumption were correct, we should find that light levels standing in the same ratio to each other produce assigned values equidistant from each other. But they do not! The difference between the assigned values for levels 10 and 20 is 5; the difference between the assigned values for levels 20 and 40 is 6; the difference between the assigned values for levels 40 and 80 is 8. If we had replotted the graph using a logarithmic scale on the horizontal axis, we would still have a curved line.

Is there any way to replot the graph and produce a straight line? The answer is, yes. What we would need to do is use logarithmic scales on both the horizontal axis and the vertical axis. If you look once again at the table, you'll see why. The asssigned values stand in a particular relationship to each other. There is a 25 percent difference between the assigned values for levels 10 and 20, for levels 20 and 40, and for levels 40 and 80. In other words, these assigned values are not equidistant from each other, but they stand in the same ratio to each other.

Stevens concluded that it is the logarithm of a sensation that is proportional to the logarithm of the stimulus intensity. (Remember that Fechner believed that it is sensation that is proportional to the logarithm of the stimulus.) Stevens formulated an equation to summarize his findings:

$$\log S = b \log I + \log k,$$

where $\log S$ = logarithm of the sensation (logarithm of the assigned values);

$\log I$ = logarithm of the stimulus (logarithm of the actual intensity);

b = slope; and

$\log k$ = a constant, indicating the point on the graph where the straight line originates (the intercept).

A graph that uses logarithmic scales on both axes has the following appearance. (In this case, the value of $\log k$ is such that the average assigned values in the following graph are one-tenth of what they were in the previous graph).

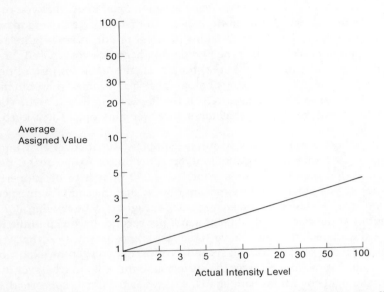

The equation is usually written in a different but mathematically equivalent form:

$$S = kI^b,$$

where S = sensation;
 I = intensity;
 b = exponent; and
 k = a constant.

When the equation is written in this form, we can see why it's appropriate to say that sensation is proportional to the intensity raised to a particular power (or exponent). And it should seem logical to you that these formulations are called the *Stevens Power Law*.

In many situations, the Stevens Power Law best describes our perceptions: equal stimulus ratios produce equal sensation ratios. In some situations, Fechner's Law is the best description: equal stimulus ratios produce equal sensations. In all situations, we perceive stimuli in relationship to each other, rather than in terms of their absolute physical magnitude.

Trading Ratios

If you've had much experience using a camera, you know that you can change the exposure time on the camera so that the correct amount of light reaches the film. If you're taking photographs on a very bright day, you want to make sure that the film doesn't become overexposed. You set the exposure time so that the shutter remains open for just a brief period of time. If you're taking photographs on an overcast day or in the evening, you want to make sure that the film isn't underexposed. You set the exposure time so that the shutter remains open for a longer period of time.

Let's take a hypothetical example. Suppose we discover that on a bright day, light is arriving at the shutter at the rate of 10,000 quanta per second. If your film requires a total of 2,000 quanta to be properly exposed, you would set the exposure time so that the shutter remained open for 1/5 second. But on an overcast day, light may be arriving at the shutter at the rate of only 4,000 quanta per second. If you continue to use the same film, you'll have to set the exposure time so that the shutter remains open for 1/2 second. Notice that you set the exposure time so that the film receives the correct amount of light, whatever the general light conditions happen to be. As far as the film is concerned, it makes no difference whether it receives 2,000 quanta spread over 1/5 second or 1/2 second. What's important is that the total number of quanta is 2,000. We can express this in a simple equation:

$$I \times t = k,$$

where I = intensity;
t = time; and
k = constant.

One way to describe this is to say that the intensity and the time can be "traded off" against each other: when the intensity is increased, time should be decreased, and vice versa. As long as their product remains constant, the film will receive the same total amount of light.

The same relationship occurs in the visual system. If you look at a bright light for only a very brief period of time, it will appear to be equal in brightness to a dimmer light that you look at for a longer period of time. This trading ratio is called the *Bunsen–Roscoe Law*. In the visual system, there is a limit to the length of time over which the Bunsen–Roscoe Law holds true. It's as if the visual system totals up the number of quanta it receives within 0.1 second periods. Imagine that the visual system has a series of counters. One counter totals up the number of quanta received in the first 0.1 second period; the second totals up the number of quanta received in the next 0.1 second; and so on. If during the first 0.1 second period, you had been looking at a bright light and, during the second 0.1 second, you had been looking at a dim light, the first counter will have a larger total than the second. You could arrange things so that the counters will have the same totals by looking at the bright light for less than 0.1 second.

One way to describe what's going on is to say that the visual system is designed to measure the total amount of light energy it receives within each 0.1 second period, and that we judge the brightness of a light on the basis of this total. We can represent this in graph form.

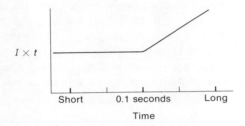

$I \times t$

Short   0.1 seconds   Long

Time

Where the graph is flat, the Bunsen–Roscoe Law is correct: intensity and time can be traded off against each other to produce the same total effect. For exposure times longer than 0.1 second, the law no longer holds. Let's try an example.

Suppose we have three different lights. Light A delivers 50,000 quanta in one second. Light B delivers 5,000 quanta in one second. Light C delivers 500 quanta in one second. Let's turn on light B for 0.1 second. It will deliver 500 quanta in that time period. How could you make light A look equal in brightness to light B? You'd turn on light A for just 0.01 second. That's the Bunsen–Roscoe Law:

$$\text{light A:} \quad 50{,}000 \times 0.01 = 500;$$
$$\text{light B:} \quad 5{,}000 \times 0.1 = 500.$$

But what about light C? It delivers 500 quanta in one second. If the Bunsen–Roscoe Law could be applied to light C, we would expect that, when light C was left on for 1 second, it would appear as bright as light

A left on for 0.01 second and light B left on for 0.1 second. But it does not. The Bunsen–Roscoe Law only applies to lights that are exposed for no more than 0.1 second. In order to make light C appear the same brightness as the other lights, its total energy ($I \times t$) must be greater than 500. We would have to increase either the intensity or the time or both to make that light appear equal to the others.

There is another trading ratio we need to consider. It involves the size or area of illumination rather than the exposure time. Suppose we have two lights that produce different areas of illumination. One light is small, and perhaps it produces a visual image of only 2 minutes on the retina (remember we discussed the size of a visual image in terms of degrees, minutes, and seconds). The second light is larger, and perhaps it produces a visual image of 5 minutes. If we leave both lights on for the same amount of time, how could we make them appear equally bright? We'd have to make the smaller light more intense so that it delivered more quanta per unit area of its image. Again, let's try an example.

Imagine that the larger light produces, in a given period of time, 10 quanta in each minute of its 5 minute image. The retina will receive a total of 50 quanta. If we wanted the smaller light to produce the same total number of quanta in the same time period, it would have to produce 25 quanta in each minute of its 2 minute image. We can state this principle in another simple equation:

$$I \times a = k,$$

where I = intensity;
$\quad a$ = area; and
$\quad k$ = constant.

The relationship expressed by the equation is usually called *Ricco's Law*, and it too has an upper limit. Ricco's Law holds true only for lights that produce an image of 10 minutes or less. Again, we can represent this in graph form.

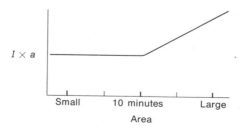

It's as if the visual system adds up the total number of quanta received in an area of 10 minutes or less, and we judge the brightness of a light on the basis of this total.

We can summarize both the Bunsen–Roscoe Law and Ricco's Law by saying that the visual system computes the total energy (the number of quanta received per unit area per unit time) it receives within each 0.1 second period over each 10 minute area, and we judge the brightness of lights on the basis of the total energy received.

The Absolute Threshold

Armed with all this information, we ought to be able to figure out what situation would be best for studying the minimum amount of light needed for seeing under perfect viewing conditions. The minimum amount of light required under ideal viewing conditions is called the *absolute threshold.*

Let's see if we can decide what the ideal viewing conditions are.

1. Should the individual be dark adapted or light adapted?

    Because we are more sensitive when we are dark adapted, we would want the individual to be dark adapted. Because complete dark adaptation takes about 25 or 30 minutes, we'll have the individual sit in a completely dark room for 30 minutes before trying to measure the absolute threshold.

2. Should the individual look directly toward the test light or off to one side?

    Because the more sensitive rods are found in the greatest abundance in the periphery of the retina, we'll have the individual look toward one side of the test light. Then the image of the test light will fall on the rod-rich portion of the retina and not on the cone-rich fovea.

3. What wavelength should we make the test light?

    Because the rods are most sensitive to lights in the blue-green region of the spectrum, we'll use a test light that is blue-green (around 500 nm).

4. How long should the test light remain on?

    Because we want to be sure that we'll be working under optimal conditions, we should make sure that the duration of the test light is within the range covered by the Bunsen–Roscoe Law.

We will therefore have the test light remain on for less than 0.1 second. We could make the duration of the test light well below this limit, perhaps only 0.001 second.

5. How large an area should the image of the test light cover?
    Because we want optimal conditions, we should make sure the area is within the range covered by Ricco's Law. Therefore, we'll make the test light 10 minutes.

Finally, let's allow the individual to turn on the test light rather than having the experimenter decide when the test light comes on. If the individual can control the onset of the test light, the test light will come on only when the individual is prepared and concentrating completely. If the experimenter controls the test light, the light may come on while the individual's attention is wandering.

A group of three experimenters (Hecht, Shlaer, and Pirenne) set up these conditions. The test light was very dim at the start and was made slightly brighter each time it was turned on. Each individual was asked, after each test-light exposure, whether he saw anything. And each individual was tested several times. After all the tests had been made, it was found that none of the individuals ever reported seeing the very dimmest test light. Sometimes the individuals reported that they could see the next brightest test light. More often, they reported seeing a brighter test light. We can summarize the results in the following way.

Light Level	Percentage of times individuals reported seeing the light
1 (dimmest)	0%
2	25%
3	50%
4	60%
5	75%
6	85%
7 (brightest)	100%

Remember that we're trying to find out the minimum amount of light required for seeing. Well, given the results, what's the minimum amount? Is it light level 2? Some individuals sometimes reported seeing that light. But maybe they really didn't see the test light. The individuals were sitting in a dark room and they knew they were supposed to see a light, sooner or later. Maybe they just "guessed" they saw a light. Well, how about light level 3? At that level, the individuals reported seeing the test light half the time. But they still might have been "guessing." After all, they could only say "yes, I saw something" or "no, I didn't see anything." If they just guessed "yes" and "no," we'd expect to get a 50/50 split between the yesses and noes. Well, how about light level 7? At that level, everyone always reported seeing the test light. But if we want to figure out the *minimum* level required for seeing, we probably want something that is not seen every time by everybody. We probably want to select a light level that individuals report seeing between 50% and 100% of the time. By convention, the 60% level is the one that is chosen as the absolute threshold level.

Now we know that light level 4 is the one we want to study. When a photocell was used to measure the total energy that the individuals received from light level 4, it was found that, on the average, 100 quanta of light were received. We can now say that the absolute threshold is 100 quanta arriving at the eye of the individual.

Hecht, Shlaer, and Pirenne didn't stop there. They wanted to figure out how many quanta must be absorbed by the rods in order for the individual to report seeing the light. The figure of 100 quanta is the number of quanta that must arrive at the cornea. But how much of the light that arrives at the cornea ever gets to the rods? A few quanta are reflected by the cornea; many more are absorbed by the aqueous humor, the lens, and the vitreous humor; more are absorbed by the pigment and blood vessels in the choroid layer. In fact, of the original 100 quanta, only between 5 and 14 end up being absorbed by rods! Now we can say that the absolute threshold is 5 to 14 quanta being absorbed by rods.

Let's go a step further. What are the chances that any one rod has to absorb more than one quantum in order to be activated? Hecht, Shlaer, and Pirenne reported that, on the average, the area of the retina on which the image of the test light fell contains 500 rods (that is, in an area of 10 minutes of retina located off to one side of the fovea, there are about 500 rods). Because only 5 to 14 quanta reached the area, it's extremely unlikely that any one of the 500 rods absorbed more than one quantum.

It is strongly suspected that each quantum of light isomerizes a single rhodopsin molecule. Now we can say that, under ideal viewing conditions, only 5 to 14 rods need to have one of their rhodopsin molecules isomerized in order for us to notice that a light is on. Because one quantum is the smallest possible amount of light, we really have amazingly sensitive visual systems. In fact, if our visual systems were any more sensitive, we'd have problems: imagine what would happen if we thought a light had gone on every time any single molecule of rhodopsin anywhere in the retina was bleached. We'd constantly see "light" because rhodopsin molecules can be affected by the energy available from body heat. (As it is, we tend to see some patterns of light when we're in a completely dark room. This so-called "dark light" would be far more intense and distracting if we didn't require at least 5 to 14 isomerized rhodopsin molecules before perceiving light.)

Many researchers have found that, whenever the visual threshold is measured, the results always turn out to be similar to the ones we've described: as the light level is gradually increased, a larger and larger percentage of the individuals reports seeing the light. It is somewhat curious that individuals do not all report seeing the same light level. Perhaps there are individual differences in sensitivity. What is more curious is the fact that any one individual who is repeatedly tested sometimes reports seeing the light when it is at a particular level and sometimes reports not seeing the light when it's at the same level. We said before that this variability might be due to "guessing." That seems reasonable enough. After all, it's hard to be sure of what you saw or didn't see if you're sitting in the dark, trying to concentrate, remembering where to look, and searching for a tiny, brief, dim spot of light. But Hecht, Shlaer, and Pireene suggested that maybe the problem isn't "guessing" or having the individual's attention wander. They suggested that the variability was related to the nature of light, not to the nature of people. You'll need to read the next section slowly and carefully to understand what Hecht, Shlaer, and Pirenne discovered.

The Poisson Distributions

Remember that we said that, when individuals looked at light level 4, 100 quanta were received at the cornea *on the average.* If light level 4 is repeatedly tested with a photocell, most of the time 100 quanta are received by the photocell. But sometimes fewer or more than 100 quanta are received, even though we always turn on the same light for the same amount of time and it always illuminates the same area. The likelihood that the photocell receives a particular number of quanta each time the light is turned on is best shown in a graph.

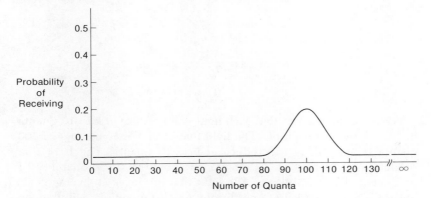

Notice that it's quite likely that 100 quanta will be received. It's somewhat less likely that 90 or 110 quanta will be received. And it's even less likely that 70 or 130 quanta will be received. But if we keep testing the light that, on the average, produces 100 quanta, it will sometimes produce fewer or more than 100 quanta. It will even produce 0 quanta or 200 quanta sometimes, although we may have to do an awful lot of testing before we come across one of these unlikely instances.

Suppose we wanted to know how likely it is that the next time we turn on the light, it will produce *100 or more* quanta. How would you figure out the odds that the light will produce *at least* 100 quanta? Because half the curve is above 100 quanta, we'd guess that the odds are about 1 out of 2, or a probability of about 0.5. What are the odds that the light will produce at least 50 quanta? Because about three-fourths of the curve is above 50, we'd guess that the odds were around 3 out of 4, or a probability of about 0.75.

All lights behave in this way. We can figure out the average number of quanta a light will produce, but the light will sometimes produce more or fewer than its average. The production of quanta is probabilistic.

Suppose we have a light that, on the average, produces 10 quanta, and another that produces 2 quanta on the average. Let's add their probability distributions to the graph for the 100 quanta light.

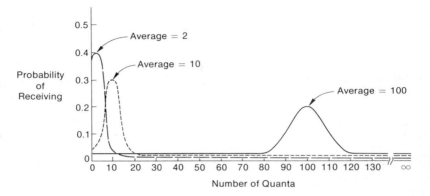

What are the chances that each light will produce *at least* 10 quanta the next time we turn it on? The light that produces an average of 100 quanta is very likely to produce *at least* 10 quanta. The light that produces an average of 10 quanta has about a 0.5 probability of producing *at least* 10 quanta. The light that produces an average of 2 quanta is not very likely to produce *at least* 10 quanta (it will happen sometimes but not very often). We can represent this in a simple graph. (We're going to use a logarithmic scale on the horizontal axis for the next series of graphs.)

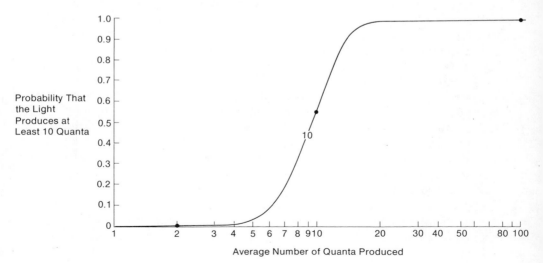

The number 10 on the curve indicates the minimum number of quanta we want to have produced.

What are the chances that each light will produce *at least* 5 quanta the next time we turn it on?

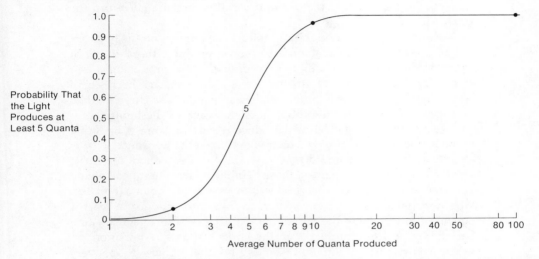

We could calculate the probability that any light that produces an average number of quanta will produce at least a particular number of quanta the next time we turn it on. And we'd end up with a family of curves, with each curve representing a different minimum number of quanta.

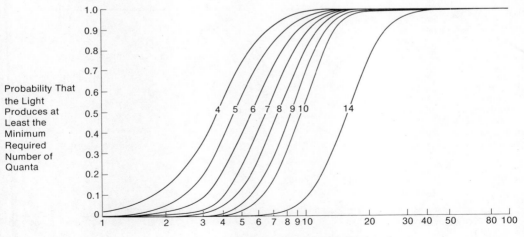

These curves are called the *Poisson* (pronounced "pwah-sone' ") *probability distributions.* I know that the graph may look confusing. It really isn't all that complicated, but you need to keep reminding yourself what it means (don't get lost now that we're almost at the finale!). First, go back to the beginning of this section and reread the material.

Now let's examine the graph carefully. Each number on the horizontal axis refers to a light that, on the average, produces that number of quanta. The vertical axis indicates the probability of producing *at least* the minimum number of quanta we're interested in. Each curve represents a different minimum number of quanta. The curve marked 4, for example, shows the probabilities that each of the lights represented on the horizontal axis will produce at least 4 quanta. A light that produces an average of only 2 quanta (find 2 on the horizontal axis) is relatively unlikely to produce at least 4 quanta (see where the curve marked 4 crosses an imaginary line extending up from number 2 on the horizontal axis?). A light that produces an average of 3 quanta (find 3 on the horizontal axis) is somewhat more likely to produce at least 4 quanta (notice where the curve marked 4 crosses an imaginary line extending up from number 3 on the horizontal axis). And so on.

Each curve has a different slope. And that proves to be very important because Hecht, Shlaer, and Pirenne wanted to make a precise comparison between the results of their absolute threshold experiment and the Poisson probability distributions. They organized the results of their experiment in graph form, listing the average number of quanta arriving at the rods on the horizontal axis.

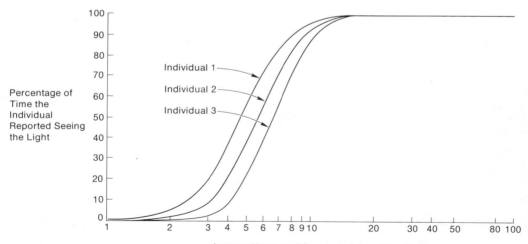

Then they compared their graphed results with the Poisson probability distributions. They found that the graphed results for one individual in their experiment perfectly matched the Poisson distribution for a curve of 5; a second individual's results perfectly matched the curve of 6; the third individual's results perfectly matched the Poisson curve of 7. (The individuals were—as you might have guessed— Pirenne, Hecht, and Shlaer.) What does all this mean? It means that Pirenne always reported seeing the light if at least 5 quanta reached his rods. Hecht always reported seeing the light if at least 6 quanta reached his rods. And Shlaer always reported seeing the light if at least 7 quanta reached his rods. The only reason they sometimes said yes, they could see the light, and sometimes said no, they could not, when the same light was repeatedly shown to them is that the light didn't always produce enough quanta. Even if the light produced 100 quanta on the average (and only 5 to 14 of them reached the rods), sometimes it produced fewer than 100 quanta (and, consequently, fewer would reach the rods). If the light produced enough quanta so that 5 (for Pirenne) or 6 (for Hecht) or 7 (for Shlaer) reached the rods, the answer was always "yes, I see a light." And the three experimenters concluded that the variability that's found when the visual threshold is measured is due to the nature of light. They suggested that the variability does not indicate that people are "guessing" or are having trouble maintaining their concentration. The problem is that the same light repeatedly turned on in the same way for the same amount of time produces different numbers of quanta. At least under the ideal viewing conditions of the experiment, our visual system behaves as if it were an infallible light detector, but the light doesn't always provide the same number of quanta for us. This is really a remarkable and stunning idea; it implies that, at least under certain circumstances, our responses to the physical world vary only because the physical world varies!

Depth Perception

Let's deal with an example of our ability to interpret complicated stimuli. Put simply, we can ask how it's possible for us to see things in three dimensions when the retina really has only two dimensions. (The receptor layer of the retina is only one cell thick. It has no depth, yet we see in depth.)

There are two categories of information we use to see things in depth: the information that's available when we look out at the world through just one eye (the *monocular cues* to depth perception), and the information we receive when we use both eyes (the *binocular cues* to depth perception).

Close one eye and look out through a window or across a room. Notice that objects still appear in depth. As you look with just one eye, try to figure out how you can tell that some objects are closer to you than others. Let me give you one example, and then spend a few minutes thinking about the problem: we use the *relative size* of objects as a cue to their distance from us. Nearby objects appear larger than more distant objects of the same physical size.

After you've spent some time thinking about monocular cues, consider the following list.

Monocular Cues to Depth Perception

1. *Relative size:* nearby objects appear larger than more distant objects of the same size.

2. *Interposition:* nearby objects appear to cut off the view of more distant objects.

3. *Details:* we can discern the details of nearby objects better than the details of distant objects.

4. *Height in the horizontal plane:* more distant objects appear to be "higher up" than nearby objects. (Think about looking out over a broad area of sand or grass or concrete. As you look off into the distance, the ground appears higher in the horizontal plane.)

5. *Geometric perspective:* parallel contours seem to converge in the distance.

There are other monocular cues, but this list should give you a good idea of the kinds of information about depth that are available to us.

Now consider how your ability to see things in depth improves when you use both eyes instead of just one. (The advantage of binocular cues is obvious when you do detailed, intricate, close work. Just try to thread a needle or hammer a nail when you keep only one eye open.) Spend a few minutes thinking about what information, in addition to the monocular cues, is available when you use both eyes.

Binocular Cues to Depth Perception

1. *Convergence:*   when you look at the tip of your own nose and then look off into the distance, you contract different extraocular muscles. These muscles send information to the brain, and they supply some cues about the distance of an object. When you look at nearby objects in the direct line of sight (such as the tip of your nose), the extraocular muscles that pull the eyes toward the nose are strongly contracted. If you then look at a distant object in the direct line of sight, the extraocular muscles that pull the eyes outward, toward the temples, are contracted. The contractions of the muscles line up the eyes so that the image of the object falls on the foveas of both eyes. But this process of correctly lining up the eyes (called *convergence*) also supplies some information about the relative distance of the object.

2. *Stereoscopic vision:*   our eyes are separated from each other, and each eye receives a slightly different view. Hold your hand up about 12 or 16 inches in front of your face. Notice what happens if you look at your hand first with only one eye and then just with the other eye. The image seems to jump slightly, and some objects are visible when you use one eye but not when you use the other eye. Other objects become visible only when you use the other eye.

   In the visual cortex, the two different views are fused in a process called *stereopsis*. The result is that objects appear to jump out sharply in three dimensions.

There are cameras available that can be used to take 3-D slides. The cameras are built so that two slightly different pictures are taken simultaneously. One picture is displaced to the left or right of the other picture. When the two pictures are processed, they are placed in a single cardboard frame, one picture slightly to the left or right of the other. When you look through a 3-D viewer, the left picture is located in front of the left eye and the right picture is in front of the right eye. The result is a picture that appears to have considerably more depth than pictures taken with conventional cameras. The 3-D camera and viewer supply the two different images we normally see when looking at a scene, and the visual cortex fuses the two images. Conventional cameras supply a single view, and conventional pictures tend to look somewhat flat as compared with the actual scene.

If our eyes were closer together than they actually are, the two images would be more similar. If the images were similar enough (if our eyes were very close together), stereoscopic vision would be impaired. A minimum discrepancy between the images is needed for stereopsis to work. But if our eyes were very far apart, the two images would be completely different. Imagine that you are a fish. Your eyes are located on different sides of your head, and the view through your left eye is completely different from the view through your right eye. The two images cannot be fused and stereopsis cannot occur. In fact, the only depth cues you have are the monocular cues. (Of course, you have the advantage of being able to see large areas on your left and right without having to swing your head from one side to the other, the way people do.) Perhaps animals whose eyes receive completely different views have developed a different method of interpreting visual information. Their brains may first sample the information coming from one eye, then the information from the other, back to the first, and so on. Our brains join together the information from both eyes to provide a single composite view.

The ability to perceive in depth is critically important for survival. Any animal that hunts moving prey must have good depth perception if it's going to eat. Just think about the requirements of birds that spot their prey while in flight and then swoop down after it, or of frogs that flick out their tongues after moving flies. In addition, the ability to perceive in depth is necessary for the avoidance of dangers; animals that crawl or walk must be able to recognize a drop-off before they plunge into it.

Because depth perception is important, we might ask at what age it develops. The answer is, at an extremely young age. Experiments have been performed using a piece of apparatus called the *visual cliff*: a thick piece of glass is placed several feet above the floor, and patterned paper is placed directly beneath half of the glass; The same paper is placed far below the other half of the glass (on the floor).

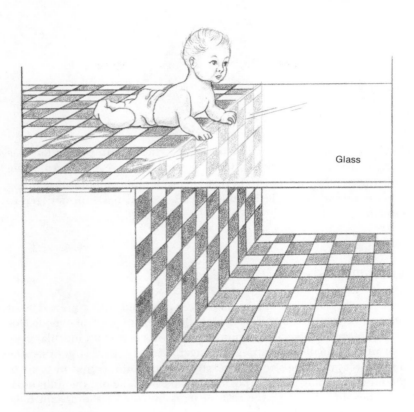

Glass

When very young animals (kitten, puppies, young goats, and human children, as soon as they can crawl) are placed on the glass, they inevitably scurry to the side where the patterned paper is just beneath the glass even though they can feel a solid surface beneath them no matter where they are on the glass. Evidently animals at a very young age can perceive depth visually, and they react to it in a very pronounced way.

Even though young animals can perceive depth, they must practice depth perception if they are to function normally when they get older. If kittens are placed on the visual cliff when their eyes first open, they move to the side with the patterned paper just beneath the glass. They clearly demonstrate that they come "prewired" to see in depth; they don't need any training sessions. However, if kittens are raised in complete darkness or in harnesses that prevent them from seeing the movements of their own body, they become quite abnormal. When given a chance to move about without a harness in a lighted room, they bump into things, move clumsily and, if placed on a table, they are likely to walk off the edge of the table. Their depth perception was normal at birth but, deprived of normal visual experiences while growing up, they demonstrate that a considerable amount of learning must go on early in life if the ability to interpret visual information is to remain normal.

Visual Illusions

Usually when we look at a scene, we are provided with a great deal of redundant information. If you look out over an area of woods, for example, you receive a large number of monocular and binocular cues that all indicate the same thing. The nearby trees appear larger than the distant trees (relative size); the nearby trees cut off the view of some of the more distant trees (interposition); you can make out the individual branches and leaves of the nearby trees but not of the distant ones (details); the more distant trees appear to be higher up than the nearby ones (height in the horizontal plane); parallel rows of trees appear to meet in the distance (geometric perspective); when you look at a nearby tree and then a distant one, different groups of extraocular muscles contract (convergence); the two eyes receive slightly different views of the woods that are merged by the brain (stereoscopic vision). Because of this rich array of cues, there is little confusion in interpreting the scene. However, if we arrange situations in which there are few cues or the cues contradict each other, things can get confusing.

   Suppose, for example, I have two pieces of cardboard and I arrange them as follows.

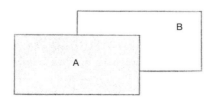

You are likely to say that A is in front of B because A appears to cut off the view of B (interposition). But suppose when I separate the two pieces of cardboard, you discover that they are actually shaped like this.

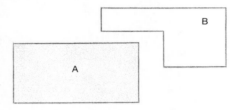

Now your interpretation of the original arrangement might be quite different.

Or, consider the following.

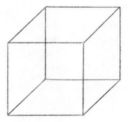

The drawing, called the *Necker cube,* is a *reversible figure:* the cube can be viewed as having its front face pointing downward and to the left, or it can be viewed as having its front face pointing upward and to the right. If you keep staring at the cube, you can see it shift from one position to the other (blinking often helps when you are first trying to get the cube to reverse). Most people initially see the front face pointing downward and to the left because the only depth cue that's available is height in the horizontal plane (when the front face is seen as pointing downward and to the left, the rear and more distant side appears higher up). The cube is reversible because there are so few depth cues that either position is possible. Suppose we start adding additional depth cues, such as interposition.

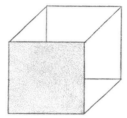

The cube is still reversible, but it is a bit more difficult to see the front face as pointing up and to the right. We can add relative size and geometric perspective.

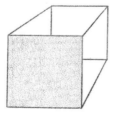

Now it is even more difficult to get the cube to reverse, although it is still possible.

The point is that, as we add additional, redundant cues, the situation becomes less ambiguous. We are always trying to interpret visual information. Most of the time, we don't have serious problems with the interpretation but, whenever the cues are changed or eliminated, the interpretation becomes tricky. (Think back over the moon illusion discussed in Chapter 4. Our judgment of the size of the full moon depends upon the presence or absence of depth cues.)

Usually people think of visual illusions as "tricks" that can be designed to "fool" the visual system. You should realize that visual illusions are not really special ways to "fool" the visual system. We always try to interpret visual information, and we always use the same rules for the interpretations. Normally when one object cuts off the view of another, the object is indeed in front. And we always interpret the information in that way unless strong cues signal that something else is going on. In a sense, interpreting the cardboard A as being in front of B is no more or less an illusion than interpreting the trees that cut off the view of the rest of the woods as being in front or closer to you. Visual illusions reveal the rules for interpretations. They do not reveal new rules and, in that sense, they are not "tricks" that "fool" the visual system.

Summary

Make sure you understand and can define all the italicized terms.

Visual perception is a vast topic. We've discussed just a few areas. First, we examined the nature of *dark adaptation* and *light adaptation* and found that the presence of both rods and cones in our eyes provides us with two different mechanisms for seeing under dim and bright conditions. We then discussed *difference thresholds*, describing *Weber's Law* and *Fechner's Law* (with a brief trip into the world of *logarithms*) as well as the *Stevens Power Law*. When we discussed the *absolute threshold*, we found that the ideal viewing conditions can be specified by taking into account the nature of rod vision, the *Bunsen–Roscoe Law*, and *Ricco's Law*.

The absolute-threshold experiment provided three findings: (a) only 5 to 14 rods must be activated in order for us to perceive light;   (b) each rod can be activated by absorbing just one quantum of light;   (c) by comparing the results of the experiment with the *Poisson probability distributions*, it was found that the variability in the results was due to the nature of light and not to the nature of people.

Finally, we discussed our ability to interpret complicated visual information. In particular, we described the *monocular cues* (*relative size, interposition*, etc.) and *binocular cues (convergence* and *stereoscopic vision)* to *depth perception.* Experiments have revealed that, although depth perception is present in very young animals, visual experiences are necessary for the maintenance and development of normal vision later in life. And we considered the nature of some *visual illusions,* concluding that they are examples of situations in which visual cues are minimal or contradictory.

Recommended Readings

There are two paperbacks well worth reading.

Gregory, R. L.   *Eye and Brain,* 2nd ed. World University Library, McGraw-Hill, 1973.

Mueller, C. G.   *Sensory Psychology.* Foundations of Modern Psychology Series, Prentice-Hall, 1965. (Chapters 1 and 2.)

There are several good advanced books that will give you additional information about visual perception. Three particularly good ones are the following.

Cornsweet, T. M.   *Visual Perception.* Academic Press, 1970.

Geldard, F. A.   *The Human Senses,* 2nd ed. Wiley, 1972. (Chapters 2–5.)

Gibson, J. J.   *The Perception of the Visual World.* Houghton Mifflin, 1950.

Specific articles of interest include the following.

Gibson, E. J., and R. D. Walk.   "The Visual Cliff," *Sci. Amer.,* April 1960 (Offprint #402).

Gregory, R. L.   "Visual Illusions," *Sci. Amer.,* Nov. 1968 (Offprint #517).

Hecht, S., S. Shlaer, and M. H. Pirenne.   "Energy, quanta and vision," *J. Gen. Physiol.,* 1942, 25: 819–840. (Also reprinted in *Stimulus and Sensation,* ed. W. S. Cain and L. E. Marks. Little, Brown & Co., 1971.)

Julesz, B.   "Texture and Visual Perception," *Sci. Amer.,* Feb. 1965 (Offprint #318).

9

The Ear and Sound

The ear is usually regarded as having three sections: the *outer ear*, the *middle ear*, and the *inner ear*.

The Outer Ear

The section called the outer ear consists of those structures that can be seen from outside the skull. The first and most obvious structure is the fleshy piece of tissue known as the *pinna*. In many animals (e.g., cats and horses), the pinna can be pivoted around so that sound waves are reflected from it toward the ear canal. In us, the pinna is relatively small, flat, and immobile—yet it still reflects some sound waves toward the ear canal.

The next structure is the ear canal, which extends from the pinna to the eardrum. The ear canal is technically known as the *external auditory meatus.* It carries sound waves inward. The eardrum, correctly called the *tympanic membrane* (if you realize that a kettledrum is often called a tympanum, you should have no trouble remembering the word "tympanic"), is a thin sheet of tissue that forms the last structure in the outer ear. When sound waves travel down the external auditory meatus, they bounce up against the tympanic membrane, and it begins to vibrate. *(ear canal)*

Along the walls of the external auditory meatus, especially toward the area where the tympanic membrane is found, there are glands that secrete a waxy substance. The waxy material coats the delicate tympanic membrane and the walls of the external auditory meatus, preventing the tissues from drying out.

The Middle Ear

Just inside the tympanic membrane, there is a cavity in the skull bone that houses the three smallest bones in the body. The first bone, called the *malleus,* rests against the tympanic membrane. The second bone, called the *incus,* rests against the first; and the third bone, called the *stapes* (pronounced "stay'-peas"), rests against the second. Whenever the tympanic membrane vibrates, the malleus begins to move. Its movements make the incus vibrate. The incus, in turn, sets the stapes into movement. The three bones, as a group, are called the *ossicular chain* ("ossicle" means "little bone," so "ossicular chain" means the "little bony chain"). The ossicular chain and the cavity that houses it are called the middle ear.

The Inner Ear

The stapes rests against a thin, flexible membrane in the side of a coiled structure that forms the inner ear. Inside the coiled structure are the auditory receptors—the cells that transform sound information into neural information. The coiled structure looks something like a very tiny snail shell and it gets its name, *cochlea* (pronounced "cock'-le-ah"), from a Latin word for snail. The cochlea is filled with fluids and, when the stapes moves in and out against the cochlea's flexible membrane, waves are created in the fluids. From the cochlea, a collection of axons called the *auditory nerve* carries the neural information to the brain. We can diagrammatically sketch the ear as follows.

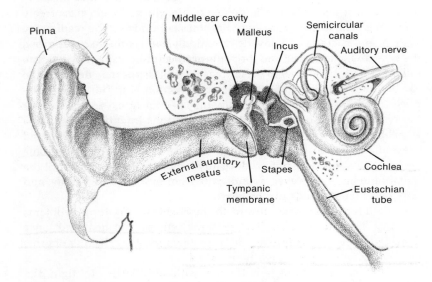

Notice that the middle-ear cavity connects to the *eustachian tube* which, in turn, connects to the throat. The primary purpose of the eustachian tube is to allow the air pressure on both sides of the tympanic membrane to be equalized. If you descend suddenly (in an airplane or elevator or when diving), the air pressure on the outside of the tympanic membrane becomes greater than the pressure within the middle ear cavity. As a result, the tympanic membrane bulges inward, and you experience a feeling of pressure or pain. When you swallow, some air from the throat cavity is forced, through the eustachian tube, into the middle-ear cavity. The pressure on the two sides of the tympanic membrane becomes equal, and the membrane returns to its normal position and shape. If you ascend quickly, the air pressure within the middle ear cavity will be greater than the pressure outside. As a result, the tympanic membrane bulges outward and, again, you feel pressure or pain. When you swallow, some of the air in the middle-ear cavity is released via the eustachian tube. This equalizes the pressure on both sides of the tympanic membrane and it returns to its normal position and shape. Whenever the tympanic membrane bulges in either direction, it becomes taut, and it cannot freely vibrate when sound waves bounce up against it. Because of this, sounds seem muffled and distant.

If you have a throat infection, the eustachian tube may become inflamed. If it becomes swollen enough, air will no longer pass freely through it. The middle-ear cavity becomes cut off from the respiratory system, and bacteria may invade the middle ear. As the bacteria grow, the tympanic membrane and the walls of the middle-ear cavity become inflamed. The blood flow to these areas increases; pus may develop; the ear becomes painful; and a middle-ear infection is in full swing. The pressure inside the middle-ear cavity may become great enough to tear the tympanic membrane (sometimes physicians intentionally make a small hole in the tympanic membrane to relieve the pressure and prevent a large tear from occurring). Because the tympanic membrane heals readily, this does not produce any long-term problems. Until the membrane heals, however, sounds will seem muffled and hollow, and only fairly loud sounds can be heard.

If the infection spreads inward to the cochlea, long-term problems are very likely to develop. The receptor cells do not heal and, once damaged, they are lost forever. Because new receptor cells do not grow in, hearing will be permanently impaired.

Usually ear infections are treated with antibiotics, to fight the infection, and with antihistamines and decongestants, to reduce the swelling of the tissues. Often ear infections are accompanied by dizziness. This occurs because the inner ear is directly linked to the vestibular system, the system that detects movements of the head. (This is the system that becomes very active when you're subjected to constant, jerky motions and that is involved in "motion sickness." We'll talk about the vestibular system in Chapter 13.) Whenever the middle and inner ears are strongly stimulated, whether because of an ear infection or by very loud sounds, the vestibular system will also be activated.

The Nature of Sound

In order to understand why the ear is built the way it is, it's necessary to understand the nature of sound. Imagine that we have a container of air and that we can see all the molecules in the air. The molecules are fairly evenly spread out through the container. But if we tap one side of the container, the molecules right near the container wall will be pushed forward. These molecules will bump into the molecules ahead of them. Those molecules will be pushed forward and they, in turn will bump into the next group of molecules. This will go on, like a chain reaction, through the container.

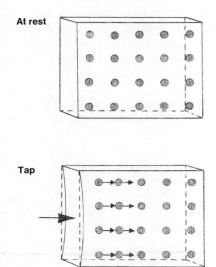

When a molecule moves forward and bumps into the next molecule, two things happen: (1) the first molecule bounces backward because of the collision, and (2) the second molecule moves forward until it too bumps into another molecule and is bounced backward. Each molecule actually moves only a very short distance.

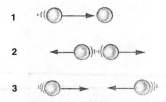

But the wave of molecule movement is carried all the way down the length of the container.

Suppose we repeatedly tap the container wall. Each tap produces a wave of molecule movement. If we put in the container a device that could count the number of molecules in one "slice" of the container, the device would alternately measure many molecules (as some crowded in, following a tap), very few molecules (as the ones that had crowded in moved backward and the others moved forward), and so on.

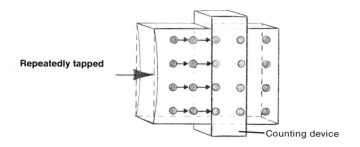

Each tap produces a "bunching up" and then "spreading out" of the molecules. The counting device would give us information that we can easily graph.

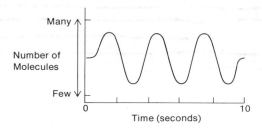

The graph is a representation of a *sound wave*. Sound waves are made up of a series of cycles of "bunching up" and "spreading out." When a sound wave reaches the tympanic membrane, the molecules bounce up against it. Each "bunching up" of the molecules pushes the tympanic membrane slightly inward, and each "spreading out" allows the tympanic membrane to push slightly outward.

If we tap the container at a faster rate, the molecules "bunch up" and "spread out" more often.

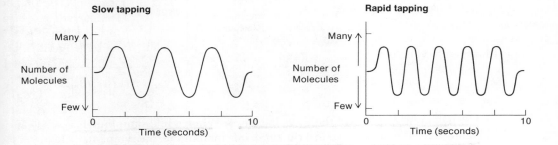

One way to describe what's happening is to say that the frequency of the cycles of sound wave has increased (that is, the number of "bunchings up" and "spreadings out" per second has gone up). The tympanic membrane will move in and out more often. What we hear is a change in pitch; the higher the frequency of the wave, the higher the frequency of movement of the tympanic membrane will be, and the higher the pitch of the sound will seem to us. We can hear sound waves whose frequencies range from about 20 to 20,000 *cycles per second* (abbreviated *cps*, often known as *Hertz*, pronounced "hurts", or *Hz*). The note of middle C has a frequency of 262 Hz. The notes that are higher in pitch (more soprano) have a higher frequency, and the notes that are lower in pitch (more bass) have a lower frequency. Notes whose frequencies are multiples of each other have a special relationship: we call them *octaves*. The frequency of middle C is 262 Hz, and the frequency of the next highest C is 524 Hz (twice 262), while the frequency of the next lowest C is 131 Hz (half of 262). Each of these notes is separated from middle C by one octave.

Let's go back to our container of air. Suppose we tap the container at a steady rate, but we tap it harder. What happens? The molecules "bunch

if tap harder

up" and "spread out" at the same rate but, the harder we tap, the more the molecules are jostled.

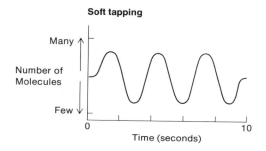

Soft tapping

Number of Molecules

Many ↑

Few ↓

0   10

Time (seconds)

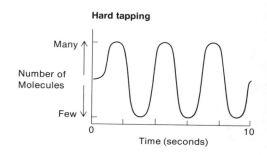

Hard tapping

Number of Molecules

Many ↑

Few ↓

0   10

Time (seconds)

The height or *amplitude* of the wave increases. When a high-amplitude sound wave bounces up against the tympanic membrane, the tympanic membrane moves more. (It doesn't move more often. It does move a greater distance). What we hear is a change in *loudness;* the greater the amplitude of a sound wave, the more the tympanic membrane will move, and the louder the sound will seem to us.

Now we can describe sound as follows.

Sound	Our Perceptions
1. Molecules alternately "bunch up" and "spread out" in cycles.	1. We hear sounds as a result of the molecules bouncing up against the tympanic membrane.
2. The *frequency* of the sound wave changes.	2. We hear sounds of different *pitch* as a result of the tympanic membrane moving in and out, more or less often.
3. The *amplitude* of the sound wave changes.	3. We hear sounds of different *loudness* as a result of the tympanic membrane moving over a greater or lesser distance.

In case you've been bothered by the fact that, when we described *light waves*, we referred to their *wavelength* and, when we describe *sound waves*, we refer to their frequency—don't let it confuse you. Wavelength and frequency are measures of the same thing. A wave with a short wavelength has a high frequency (if cycles are short, many of them can occur in one second); a wave with a long wavelength has a low frequency (if the cyles are long, only a few of them can occur in one second). The two measures are reciprocals of each other, and we could talk about the wavelength of sound waves, instead of their frequency. Middle C, with its frequency of 262 Hz, has a wavelength of 4.31 feet. (Sound waves have surprisingly long wavelengths! Remember that we measured the wavelength of light in nanometers. One nanometer is one ten-millionth of a centimeter, and one centimeter is less than half an inch). The note one octave above middle C has a frequency of 524 Hz and a wavelength of 2.16 feet. The note one octave below middle C has a frequency of 131 Hz and a wavelength of 8.62 feet. When describing sound, the frequency numbers are a bit easier to manipulate than the wavelength numbers.

Tones and Noise

If a sound wave is made up of just one frequency, the pattern of its cycles repeats itself again and again, as long as the sound remains on. This is called a *pure tone*. But most sound waves contain a mixture of several different frequencies. These are called *complex tones*.

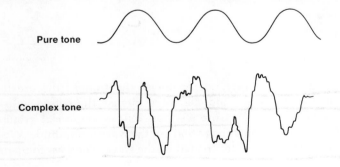

Pure tone

Complex tone

Complex tones are combinations of two or more pure tones. If we combine all the pure tones we can hear, we have an extremely complicated sound wave that appears to be irregular and that is called *white noise*. (Remember that the mixture of all the wavelengths of light we can see is called white light). White noise sounds like the hissing static you can pick up on your radio. It has no particular pitch and is best described as a "shush" sound.

The Measurement of Intensity

As we've said, sound consists of repeated cycles of the "bunching up" and "spreading out" of molecules. Instead of talking about the numbers of molecules that are found during a "bunching up" or "spreading out" phase, we could talk about the *pressure* created by the molecules as they crowd into and then leave an area. If we examine one cycle of a sound wave, we can see that the greatest pressure occurs during the crest, and the smallest pressure occurs during the trough.

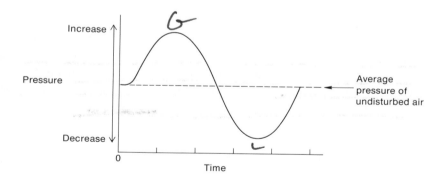

The higher the crest and the lower the trough, the greater the amplitude of the wave and the more intense the sound will seem. Suppose we want to measure just how loud a sound is. Certainly we would need to do something to find out the wave's amplitude. We do so by measuring the pressure created by the wave. Then we compare that average pressure to the known average pressure of a standard, reference sound:

$$\text{Intensity} \approx \frac{\text{Pressure}_?}{\text{Pressure}_R},$$

where Pressure$_?$ = the average pressure of the sound we want to measure;
      and
      Pressure$_R$ = the average pressure of the standard reference sound.

Notice that, in any sound wave, the size of the crest is equal (but opposite) to the size of the trough. If we measured the *average* pressure of any sound wave, we'd end up with a number that is identical to the average pressure of undisturbed air (the maximum pressure at the crest and the minimum pressure at the trough would cancel each other out). To get out of this dilemma, we resort to a math trick: we measure the average *squared* pressure of the wave. Consider the following example. Suppose the average pressure of the undisturbed air is 5 pounds per square inch. The first sound wave we create produces a pressure of 6 pounds per square inch during the crest and 4 pounds per square inch during the trough. The second sound wave we create is more intense: it produces 7 pounds per square inch during the crest and 3 pounds per square inch during the trough. Each wave produces an average pressure of 5 pounds per square inch:

$$\frac{6 + 4}{2} = 5, \quad \text{and} \quad \frac{7 + 3}{2} = 5.$$

However, the waves produce different average *squared* pressures:

$$\frac{6^2 + 4^2}{2} = \frac{36 + 16}{2} = 26, \quad \text{and} \quad \frac{7^2 + 3^2}{2} = \frac{49 + 9}{2} = 29.$$

The average squared pressure reflects the fact that the waves are, indeed, different.
Now we can change our equation:

$$\text{Intensity} \approx \frac{\text{Pressure}_?^2}{\text{Pressure}_R^2}.$$

As in many other sensory systems, it turns out to be useful to use a logarithmic scale when describing sounds. Thus, we can change the equation again:

$$\text{Intensity} \approx \log \frac{\text{Pressure}_?^2}{\text{Pressure}_R^2}.$$

(Think about logarithmic scales. Recall our earlier discussion of logarithms. What happens when we convert to a logarithmic scale?) The unit of measurement of sound intensity is called the *bel*:

$$\text{Number}_{bel} = \log \frac{\text{Pressure}_?^2}{\text{Pressure}_R^2}.$$

Often, we work with sounds that are less than one bel, and there is a unit of measurement that is smaller than a bel. The *decibel* (abbreviated, *db*) is one-tenth of a bel. Now we have

$$\text{Number}_{db} = 10 \log \frac{\text{Pressure}_?^2}{\text{Pressure}_R^2},$$

Multiply exponent by no. preceding logarithm

or

$$\text{Number}_{db} = 20 \log \frac{\text{Pressure}_?}{\text{Pressure}_R}.$$

(When using logarithms, you can remove an exponent by multiplying it by the figure that precedes the logarithm.)

Notice that the intensity of a sound is always stated in relative terms: the db scale always implies that we are making a comparison between the average squared pressure of the sound we want to measure and the average squared pressure of a reference sound.

Two different reference sounds are used. One is the *sound pressure level* (abbreviated *SPL*), which is defined as a wave having a pressure of 0.0002 dyne/cm². The other is the *sensation level* (abbreviated *SL*) which is the pressure of a sound that is at the threshold of human hearing. SPL and SL actually do not differ very much, but you will sometimes see a sound rated as 30 db SPL or 10 db SL, signifying which reference sound was used.

Because the average squared pressure is equal to the *power of a wave*, we can write the equation for the number of db in a third way:

$$\text{Number}_{db} = 10 \log \frac{\text{Power}_?}{\text{Power}_R}.$$

If one sound is ten times more powerful than the reference sound, we'd say that the sound's intensity is 10 db:

$$\text{Number}_{db} = 10 \log \frac{\text{Power}_?}{\text{Power}_R} = 10 \log 10 = 10 \times 1 = 10.$$

(The logarithm of 10 is 1.)

If one sound is 100 times more powerful than the reference sound, we'd say that the sound's intensity is 20 db:

$$\text{Number}_{db} = 10 \log \frac{\text{Power}_?}{\text{Power}_R} = 10 \log 100 = 10 \times 2 = 20.$$

(The logarithm of 100 is 2.)

If our to-be-measured sound has the same power as the reference sound, we'd say that the sound's intensity is 0 db:

$$\text{Number}_{db} = 10 \log \frac{\text{Power}_?}{\text{Power}_R} = 10 \log 1 = 10 \times 0 = 0.$$

(The logarithm of 1 is 0.)

Notice that a sound rated as 0 db is truly a sound: 0 db does not mean the absence of sound; it means a sound that is equal to the reference sound. In fact we can have sounds that are less than 0 db. These sounds have less power than the reference sound. For example, a sound that has one-tenth the power of the reference sound is rated as −10 db:

$$\text{Number}_{db} = 10 \log \frac{\text{Power}_?}{\text{Power}_R} = 10 \log 0.1 = 10 \times -1 = -10.$$

(The logarithm of 0.1 is −1.)

Use the following logarithmic table to solve the problems that follow the table.

Table of Logarithms

Number	Log	Number	Log
1.0	0.0000	4.5	0.6532
1.5	0.1761	5.0	0.6990
2.0	0.3010	5.5	0.7404
2.5	0.3979	6.0	0.7782
3.0	0.4771	6.5	0.8129
3.5	0.5441	7.0	0.8451
4.0	0.6021	7.5	0.8751

47.71

1. Figure out the number of decibels in a sound that is 3 times more powerful than the reference sound.

2. Figure out the number of decibels in a sound whose average squared pressure is $5\frac{1}{2}$ times the average squared pressure of the reference sound.

3. Using SPL, figure out the number of decibels in a sound that has a pressure of 0.0004 dyne/cm^2.

One reason for using a logarithmic scale is to take into account the fact that a particular difference in the powers of two loud sounds appears to us to be less than the same amount of difference in the powers of two soft sounds. Another way to think of this is to note that we perceive the ratio between the powers of sounds rather than the actual difference between their powers. (I hope this reminds you of our discussion of logarithms in Chapter 8.)

The following table will give you an idea of the db ratings of some common sounds.

Rustle of leaves in gentle breeze	10 db
Quiet car, 10 feet away	50 db
Ordinary conversation	60–70 db
Pneumatic drill, 10 feet away	90 db
Phonograph putting out 10 watts, 10 feet away	110 db

The Function of the Ossicular Chain

You now know that sounds are really pressure cycles. The variations in pressure make the tympanic membrane move in and out. The ossicular chain is attached to the tympanic membrane; whenever the membrane moves, first the malleus, then the incus, and finally the stapes will move. The stapes pushes and pulls a flexible membrane in the wall of the cochlea. This flexible membrane is called the oval window and, when it moves, waves are created in the fluids of the cochlea. The receptor cells become active as a result of the movements of the fluids, and they send information to the neurons that make up the auditory nerve.

But why should there be an ossicular chain between the tympanic membrane and the cochlea? The answer lies in the fact that movements of air molecules must be translated into movements of fluid molecules.

The fluids inside the cochlea are considerably denser than air; that is, there are many more molecules per unit volume of fluid than there are molecules per unit volume of air. Because of the higher concentration of molecules in the fluids, they offer more resistance (or "impedance") to movement than the relatively sparse air molecules do. Stated another way, we would have to apply greater force against the fluids than against the air if we wanted to create equal effects on them.

In essence, the ossicular chain provides the mechanism for supplying more force against the cochlear fluids than the force created by movements of air molecules in the external auditory meatus. As it does so, the ossicular chain effectively cancels out the difference between the resistance ("impedance") of fluids and of air. This function of the ossicular chain is called, logically enough, *impedance matching.*

The chain accomplishes impedance matching by transferring the movements of the relatively large tympanic membrane to movements of the very small oval window. The tympanic membrane is actually about 20 times larger than the oval window. Pressures against the entire tympanic membrane are funneled down, by the ossicular chain, to pressures against a membrane one-twentieth its size. In other words, the pressure per unit area of the oval window is some 20 times greater than the pressure per unit area of the tympanic membrane. This twenty-fold increase makes up for the higher impedance of the cochlear fluids.

Sometimes sound waves do not reach the cochlea via the ossicular chain. Instead, the bones of the skull vibrate, and the outer bony walls of the cochlea are set into motion. The vibrations of the cochlear walls make the fluids move. Sounds that reach the cochlea this way are called *bone-conducted sounds.* Bone-conducted sounds commonly occur whenever you speak because, as you move your tongue and lips and expel air, the bones of the skull vibrate. In fact, that's part of the reason why, when you hear your voice on tape, it sounds so strange; when you listen to the tape, you do not receive the bone-conducted sounds that you normally hear when speaking.

Bone-conducted sounds form the basis for distinguishing between two general kinds of deafness. If an individual cannot hear sounds that reach the cochlea via the tympanic membrane and ossicular chain, but can hear the bone-conducted sound produced by resting the base of a vibrating tuning fork against the skull, we know that the problem must be in the outer or middle ear. If the individual can't hear either airborne or bone-conducted sound, the cochlea and/or auditory nerve must be damaged. The first kind of deafness is called *conduction deafness*; the difficulty is located somewhere along the route by which airborne sounds are conducted to the cochlea. The second kind of deafness is called *nerve deafness*; the difficulty is in the cochlea or auditory nerve.

Summary

Think about the steps involved from the time a sound wave is produced until waves occur in the fluids of the cochlea. (Make sure you understand and can define all the italicized terms.)

Sound waves consist of slight to-and-fro movements of molecules, which result in alternating increases and decreases in *pressure*. The waves may differ in *frequency* or in *amplitude*. When they differ in frequency, we hear sounds of different pitches. Sound waves may be *pure tones, complex tones,* or *white noise,* depending on the number of different frequencies that are present. When waves differ in amplitude, we hear sounds of different *loudnesses.* The intensity of any particular sound wave can be specified in *decibels.*

Sound waves reach the *pinna* and travel down the *external auditory meatus* to the *tympanic membrane* (these three structures are collectively called the *outer ear*). When the tympanic membrane moves, the *ossicular chain* of the *middle ear* is set into vibration. The *malleus, incus,* and *stapes* perform *impedance matching.* When the stapes moves against the *oval window,* waves are created in the fluids of the *cochlea* (the cochlea comprises the *inner ear*).

If an otherwise deaf individual can hear *bone-conducted sounds,* the individual is said to have *conduction deafness.* If bone-conducted sounds cannot be heard, the individual has *nerve deafness.*

Recommended Readings

For an excellent discussion of the ear, try this article.

von Bekesy, G.   "The Ear," *Sci. Amer.*, Aug. 1957 (Offprint #44).

For more information about sound and hearing, there is a very fine, well-written paperback.

van Bergeijk, W. A., J. R. Pierce, and E. E. David.   *Waves and the Ear.* Anchor Books, 1960.

There is also a fine book with lots of illustrations and a very readable text.

Stevens, S. S., and F. Warshofsky.   *Sound and Hearing.* Time Inc., 1965.

10

The Cochlea

The cochlea is a very small, snail-shell-shaped structure embedded in the bone of the skull. It is difficult to remove the cochlea from the skull; it is hard to examine the interior of the cochlea; it is not easy to understand the cochlea's construction. Yet, if you don't understand how the cochlea functions, it is not possible to understand audition (hearing).

Please read the following description of the cochlea's structure slowly and carefully. Try to visual it as a three-dimensional structure. Remember that it twists around itself, forming a spiral.

The Anatomy of the Cochlea

The cochlea is made up of three long chambers. Picture three soda straws, arranged so that the first one lies above and to the right of the second one, and the third one lies directly below the second one.

If you looked at the ends of the straw, you would see the following.

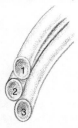

If we held the three in this arrangement with tape, they would form a kind of cable, which could be curled around itself.

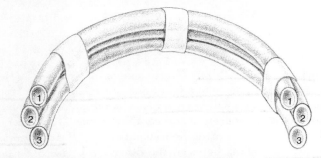

We could continue to curl the cable and pile each twist on top of the last twist, turban fashion. If we cut straight down the center of the turban, we'd see this.

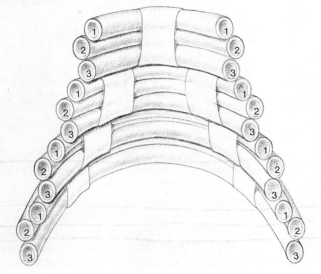

The cochlea's three "straws" are named as follows. (1) *Scala vestibuli.* (As a mnemonic, you might think of La *Scala* Opera House in Italy. Think of *scala* as a hall or chamber. Then think of the small front room found in many houses; it's called a "vestibule." And, then, scala vestibuli means "the front or first chamber.") (2) *Scala media* (the chamber located *midway* between the other two). (3) *Scala tympani* (remember the drum called a *tympanum*). The first coil in the cochlea appears, in cross-section, as follows.

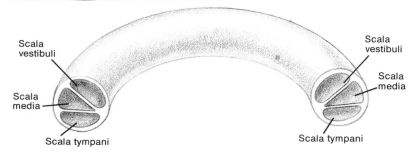

There are approximately three and a half coils in the human cochlea, and the complete structure has a height roughly the same as the width of the tip of your pinky fingernail. It really is small.

Each scala is divided from the next one by a very thin membrane. Scala vestibuli is separated from scala media by *Reissner's membrane;* scala media is separated from scala tympani by the *basilar membrane.*

Try to imagine that we could untwist the cochlea. Then we'll slice it, along its length, right down the middle. If we throw out the right half and look at the left half from the cut side, we'll see something like this.

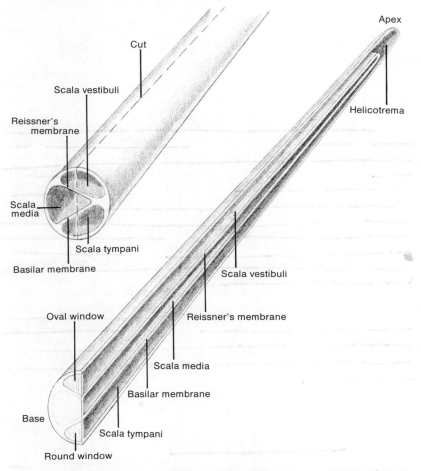

Notice that Reissner's membrane and the basilar membrane do not extend the length of the cochlea. At the apex, they join. The opening between them that's created at the apex is called the *helicotrema*.

The three cochlear chambers contain fluid. Because scala vestibuli and scala tympani communicate with each other at the helicotrema, it shouldn't surprise you to discover that they contain the same fluid, called the *perilymph*. Scala media contains a slightly different fluid called the *endolymph*. (If you have trouble remembering which fluid is found where, think of scala vestibuli and scala tympani as being on the *peri*meter of scala media, and they are the ones that have *peri*lymph.)

The walls of the cochlea are made of bone except at two places along the cochlea's base. There we have two flexible membranes. The membrane that covers the base of scala vestibuli is called the *oval window*. Recall that we said in the last chapter that the stapes pushes in and out against the oval window. As it does so, waves are set up in the perilymph of scala vestibula. The waves travel down the length of scala vestibuli. And, through the helicotrema, the waves continue into the perilymph of scala tympani. At its base, scala tympani also has a flexible membrane, called the *round window*. As the perilymph surges against it, the round window bulges out and in, providing a kind of damping mechanism for the waves.

Reissner's membrane and the basilar membrane are extremely thin tissues. Because of this, whenever waves occur in the perilymph, waves will also occur in the endolymph. Thus, scala media will also be affected when the stapes pushes in and out against the oval window. Because the receptor cells are located in scala media, we need just such an arrangement.

The Cochlear Duct

Because the receptor cells are in scala media, we need to look carefully at everything associated with this portion of the cochlea. In fact this portion—which includes Reissner's membrane, scala media and its endolymph, the receptor cells and their associated structures, and the basilar membrane—has been given its own label: it's called the *cochlear duct*.

The receptor cells and their associated structures are located along the entire length of the basilar membrane. The receptor cells have tips that look very much like extremely thin and short hairs. For this reason, the receptor cells are called the *hair cells*. They jut up out of *supporting cells* that rest on the portion of the basilar membrane nearest the inner, narrow side of scala media. Resting on top of the hair cells, there is a flap of tissue called the *tectorial membrane.* Let's take a close look at these structures and how they fit into the cochlea.

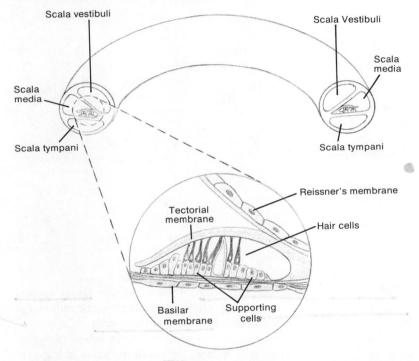

The collection of supporting cells, hair cells, and tectorial membrane is called the *organ of Corti.* Notice that there are two groups of hair cells. One group juts out of the supporting cells nearest the base of the tectorial membrane. These are termed the *inner hair cells,* and there are two rows of them. The *outer hair cells* are more numerous; there are 4 to 6 rows of them. All the hair cells bear very small, bristle-like endings called *cilia,* which touch the underside of the tectorial membrane. When the tectorial membrane moves relative to the cilia, the cilia are deformed by the movement. Somehow this activates the hair cells. And lying just underneath the bases of the hair cells, among the supporting cells, are dendrites of neurons. The somas of the neurons are located in the bony, central core of the cochlea, and their axons travel together toward the brain, forming the *auditory nerve*.

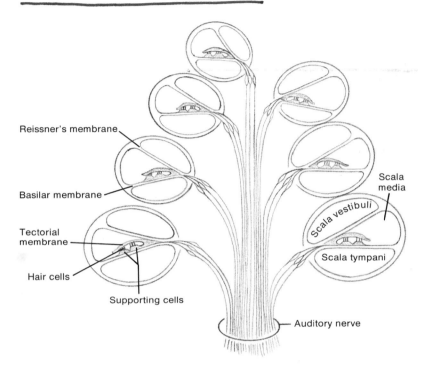

Reissner's membrane

Basilar membrane

Tectorial membrane

Hair cells

Supporting cells

Scala media

Scala vestibuli

Scala tympani

Auditory nerve

When the hair cells become active, they somehow create graded potentials in the dendrites. If the graded potentials are sufficiently large by the time they reach the axons, action potentials occur.

Although we are once again in that mystery world where receptors translate physical energy into neural information, some things are known about the processes involved. First of all, it's clear that the critical step is to get the tectorial membrane to rub across the cilia. What's important is the bending of the cilia from side to side. This is called the *shearing force*, and it occurs because the tectorial membrane and the basilar membrane (on which the hair cells rest) move at different rates and in slightly different directions when waves are set up in the endolymph. Part of the reason for the differences in their movements has to do with the fact that the tectorial membrane is anchored at only one edge, while the basilar membrane is anchored along both edges. The net result is that the tectorial membrane tends to slide (back and forth) across the basilar membrane, bending the cilia.

The second thing that's known is that shearing forces causing bending in opposite directions tend to produce opposite effects. If the cilia are bent one way, the dendrites become depolarized (an excitatory response); if the cilia are bent in the opposite direction, the dendrites become hyperpolarized (an inhibitory response).

Finally, it is suspected that the activation of hair cells is somehow related to changes in the distribution of ions in the endolymph immediately surrounding the cilia. The precise way in which the shearing of the cilia creates ionic changes is not known.

Intensity Changes and the Cochlea

When the amplitude of a sound wave is increased, the sound seems to us to get louder. You already know that, as the wave's amplitude is increased, the tympanic membrane will move over a greater distance. As a result, the malleus, incus, and stapes also will move over a greater distance.

Picture the stapes as a piston that moves in and out, against the oval window. When the stapes moves over a greater distance, it pushes the oval window further in and pulls it further out. This creates larger waves in the perilymph and, indirectly, in the endolymph. As a consequence, the tectorial membrane and the cilia will have larger and larger relative motions. The shearing force will be increased. The degree of activity in the hair cells is proportional to the amount of shearing force. The dendrites produce responses that vary with the degree of activity in the hair cells. Therefore, the dendrites will produce larger graded potentials when the shearing force is increased. When the dendrites produce large depolarizations, the axons will be more likely to produce more action potentials. When the dendrites produce large hyperpolarizations, the axons will be less likely to produce action potentials. As a result, a sound wave of large amplitude will produce, alternately, many and very few spikes. A sound wave of small amplitude will produce, alternately, small increases and decreases in the firing rates of the axons. We interpret the change from small increases and decreases in the firing rates to large increases and decreases as an increase in the sound's loudness.

It is conceivable that we could make a sound wave's amplitude so large that the stapes would drive right through the oval window. That would create obvious problems. There is a protective mechanism that usually prevents the stapes from moving far enough to damage the oval window. When the amplitude of a sound wave becomes sufficiently large, two very small muscles in the middle ear reflexly contract. One muscle, called the *tensor tympani*, connects the malleus to the wall of the middle-ear cavity. The second muscle, the *stapedius muscle*, connects the stapes to the wall of the middle-ear cavity.

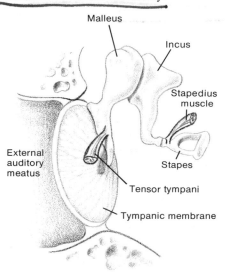

When these muscles contract, two things happen. First, the malleus is pulled slightly to one side, and it doesn't impart as much of its movement to the incus as it normally would. Because the incus moves less than it otherwise would, it doesn't impart as much movement to the stapes. Second, the stapes is no longer free to move in and out, like a piston, against the oval window. Instead it rocks from side to side against the oval window. The net result is that the oval window is not pushed or pulled as much; the oval window is not torn by the stapes, and the waves created in the cochlea are not as large as they would otherwise be. The sound will seem less intense than it actually is.

The reflex contraction of these *middle-ear muscles* sometimes occurs even when a very loud sound is not present. When you yawn, for example, the tensor tympani and stapedius muscle briefly contract.

And you may have noticed that, during a yawn, sounds seem less intense and somewhat muffled.

This protective reflex suffers from two problems. First of all, you should realize that the muscles will not contract until just after a very loud sound begins. The muscles contract when efferent neurons that synapse on them produce action potentials. These efferent neurons receive their information from neurons of the auditory nerve. When a very intense sound occurs, the neurons of the auditory nerve activate the efferent neurons which, in turn, activate the muscles. Notice that a very intense sound must occur and have its effect on the cochlea before the muscles will contract. During the period of sound reception before the muscles contract (the so-called *latency* of the protective reflex), the oval window is subjected to a great deal of pushing and pulling. Fortunately, the latency is rather brief (on the order of milliseconds), and the oval window is not subjected to intense movements of the stapes for long.

Even a very brief period of intense movement might prove disastrous were it not for the fact that the tympanic membrane, the ossicular chain, and the oval window all have inertia, and it takes more energy to get them moving initially than it does to keep them moving. If you've ever tried to push a stalled car, you know that it takes a great deal more energy to move the car from its stopped position than it does to keep the car going once it's already moving. The principles are the same, whether we're dealing with stalled cars or the apparatus that carries sound information to the cochlea. Much of the energy of the initial cycles of a sound wave is spent getting the apparatus going. It is not until after the apparatus has started moving that most of the energy is translated directly into effective movements of the stapes against the oval window. During the "start-up" phase, enough energy is spent in movements of the stapes against the oval window to create rather large waves in the cochlea. The auditory neurons become activated, and some of these activate the efferent neurons that synapse on the middle-ear muscles. Usually, at about the time the apparatus is beginning to move easily, the middle-ear muscles have contracted. Needless to say, the more intense the sound is and the more suddenly it comes on, the greater the probability will be that some damage will occur during the latency period.

If you listen very carefully to a moderately loud and sustained sound that comes on suddenly, you may be able to detect a slight change in the sound's loudness. Initially, the sound seems just a bit louder than it does subsequently. What you're hearing is a reduction in the effectiveness of the sound waves created by the contraction of the middle-ear muscles.

The second problem associated with the middle-ear muscles is the fact that, like all muscles, they cannot maintain contractions indefinitely. The muscles fatigue and, the longer the intense sound remains on, the less the muscles will be able to protect the cochlea. As the muscles tire, more and more of the sound energy is translated directly into piston-like movements of the stapes against the oval window. If the sound is intense enough and if it remains on long enough, the stapes may indeed tear the oval window.

A problem far more common and insidious than a rupture of the oval window is associated with loud sounds: the loss of hair cells. We do not keep developing new hair cells throughout our lifetime. We are born with one set of them and, if hair cells are destroyed, replacements for them do not grow. Obviously, if all the hair cells are destroyed, the neurons of the auditory nerve will not be activated as a result of sound waves; there will be nothing to translate the physical energy of sound into neural information, and the individual will be deaf. If only some of the hair cells are destroyed, the individual will have impaired hearing.

The Loss of Hair Cells

As the tectorial membrane and the hair cells move in relationship to each other, the shearing forces can become very substantial. If the hairs are sufficiently bent, they may, in fact, break off. This can occur during the latency period of the protective reflex if the sound is sufficiently intense and sudden. However, it is far more likely to occur during prolonged exposures to intense sounds when the middle-ear muscles begin to fatigue. In fact, there is a trading ratio between the intensity of sound and the duration of the exposure to it that will cause damage. Extremely loud sounds will result in the loss of hair cells after a very brief exposure; somewhat less intense sounds will result in hair-cell losses after a somewhat longer exposure.

The deafness that results from hair-cell loss is a form of nerve deafness (as opposed to conduction deafness) and is usually called *noise-induced deafness.* It cannot be corrected. Hearing aids, which are really miniature amplifiers, can increase the amplitude of the sound waves that arrive at the tympanic membrane. However, if there are no hair cells or fewer than the full complement of hair cells, increasing the amplitude of sound waves will not improve hearing substantially. Hearing aids are most effective when used in conjunction with conduction deafness. Because they increase the amplitude of sound waves, they force the tympanic membrane and ossicular chain to move more than they otherwise would. This means that the defective conduction apparatus will respond with movements that more closely approximate the movements of a normal tympanic membrane and ossicular chain.

We are only recently beginning to appreciate the degree to which hair-cell losses occur because of exposures to loud sounds. The cumulative effects of all the sounds we hear, day in and day out, take their toll. By the age of about 20 (for unknown reasons, males are affected at a younger age than females), our hearing is already impaired. And, as we get older, the impairment gets steadily worse. The initial hearing loss is restricted to very high-pitched sounds. Most adults cannot hear the very high-frequency sounds created by timing devices in traffic lights, but young children often complain about the high-pitched sound when they sit in a car waiting, with their insensitive (literally insensitive) parents, for a red light to change. The hearing loss gradually extends to lower-pitched sounds as we grow older. The age of onset, the degree of hearing loss, and the rate at which it increases are related to the amount of loud sound we're exposed to. That fact has created substantial interest in the amount of environmental sound we're exposed to and in controlling the level of *noise pollution.* ("Noise" in this context does not mean only those sound waves that contain a mixture of many frequencies. Rather, it simply means unnecessary and unwanted sound.)

There are dramatic examples of hearing losses created by very loud sounds. Infantrymen who are repeatedly exposed to the sounds created by large weapons usually show marked hearing losses. People who often work with riveters or jackhammers commonly suffer from serious noise-induced hearing losses. Were it not for the large "ear muffs" worn by airport runway personnel, they too would rapidly show noise-induced deafness. Most of us are not repeatedly exposed to sounds of this intensity (a rifle blast creates a sound on the order of 150 db; riveters and jackhammers produce sounds that reach 120 db for the user; a nearby jet engine can produce 155 db). However, many of us are repeatedly exposed to somewhat less intense sounds. People who live or work near airports may be exposed to as much as 120 db each time a jet takes off or lands. Subways and trains may produce 100 db as they go past us. Heavy automobile traffic may produce 80 db; a noisy typewriter may produce 75 db. Remember that the amount of hearing loss is related to both the intensity of the sound and the duration of the exposure to it: four hours of work at a lathe that produces 95 db is just as damaging as 15 minutes near the starting line of a drag strip, where sounds of 140 db may be produced. (I hope this trading ratio between intensity and length of exposure reminds you of the Bunsen–Roscoe Law in vision.)

Some legislation now protects us against prolonged exposures to noise pollution. The Walsh–Healey Public Contracts Act (May 1970) specifies permissible noise exposures for factories, offices, and apartment buildings. Individuals may not be exposed to sounds of at least 90 db for more than 8 hours per day. Exposures to sounds of at least 100 db may not exceed 2 hours per day. Exposures to sounds in excess of 115 db may not exceed 15 minutes a day. The legislation is a step in the right direction, but it probably will not affect the noise-pollution levels to which people willingly expose themselves.

One of the most common situations in which people freely subject themselves to dangerously loud sounds is when they listen to amplified music. A speaker putting out 10 watts produces sounds of 110 db at a distance of 10 feet. In concerts, amplified music may reach 120 db at some locations in the audience (the Walsh–Healey Act specifies that exposures to 110 db should not exceed 30 minutes per day, and that exposures to 120 db should not exceed 15 minutes in a day). There is substantial concern that current listening habits, especially those prevalent among young people, are creating earlier and far more profound hearing losses than have ever occurred before. Hearing tests conducted among college-age people have repeatedly revealed widespread, premature noise-induced hearing losses. It is not an exaggeration to say that many 20-year-olds of today have the hearing of 40- or 50-year-olds. Keep in mind that the hearing loss is permanent; it cannot be corrected.

The prevention of the problem is relatively simple: don't expose yourself to unduly loud sounds. It's difficult to know how loud a sound has to be before it becomes "unduly loud." But there is a rough index you can use. If you're exposed to a dangerously loud sound, you'll notice that a hum or ringing in your ears seems to go on after the sound has gone off. Once the sound is loud enough to produce this effect, it is loud enough to destroy your hair cells. (The hum or ringing is the result of extreme activation of the structures of the ear. The structures have been stimulated so much that it takes quite a bit of time for all the movement to die down after the sound stops.) If you're listening to a speaker, turn the volume down. If you're at a concert, back away from the speakers. [Sound-intensity levels follow the inverse square law: as you increase the distance between you and the sound source, the power (or pressure^2) drops by a factor that is $1/$(distance in feet)^2. If you stand 2 feet from the speaker, the power is $\frac{1}{4}$ of what it is just 1 foot from the speaker. If you stand 5 feet from the speaker, the power is $\frac{1}{25}$ of what it is just 1 foot from the speaker.] When you back away from the speakers in an enclosed setting rather than outdoors, you need to make sure that you don't end up in an area where the sound waves bouncing off the ceilings, walls, and floor all meet and reinforce each other. Find a spot where the sound seems much softer.

There is another source of hair-cell loss you should be aware of: certain medications, if given in sufficiently large dosages, destroy hair cells. The most common of these medications are kanamycin, neomycin, streptomycin, and quinine. (Please note that not all mycins have this side-effect. Aureomycin, for example, does not appear to attack the hair cells.) Kanamycin, neomycin, and streptomycin are antibiotics used to combat infections. If one of these is prescribed for you, ask if a different antibiotic could be used instead. Quinine is used in the treatment of malaria, and there is no proven, adequate substitute. Why these particular medications should destroy hair cells is unknown.

Frequency Changes and the Cochlea

When the frequency of a sound wave is changed, the sound seems to us to change in pitch. You already know that, as the wave's frequency is changed, the number of to-and-fro movements of the tympanic membrane will change. As a result, the number of to-and-fro movements of the malleus, incus, and stapes will also change. The stapes will move in and out against the oval window more rapidly when the sound waves have a high frequency, and more slowly when the sound waves have a low frequency. The reactions within the cochlea turn out to be rather complicated. Historically, there have been two kinds of theories about the reactions within the cochlea: *frequency theories* and *place theories*. Let's briefly discuss one example of each kind of theory. Keep in mind that these particular examples were proposed long before very much was known about the structure of the cochlear duct.

Frequency Theories

All frequency theories propose that the entire basilar membrane moves at the same frequency as the stapes. According to them, if we turn on a sound of low frequency, the stapes would move in and out against the oval window relatively few times each second; as we increase the sound's frequency, the stapes would move in and out at a faster rate. Frequency theories hypothesize that the basilar membrane moves up and down in time with the movements of the stapes.

The most well-known frequency theory is *Rutherford's Telephone Theory*. Ernest Rutherford proposed that the basilar membrane's behavior is similar to the behavior of the diaphragms in telephones. When you speak into a telephone, the speaker diaphragm vibrates at different frequencies, depending upon the frequencies of sound waves in your voice. The diaphragm is thin and light enough to be moved back and forth by the movements of air molecules right near it. In effect, each movement of the diaphragm modifies an electrical circuit, permitting different amounts of current to pass through the circuit. The listening diaphragm moves as a result of changes in the amount of electricity passing through its circuit. As it jumps back and forth, it pushes air molecules in its path. The molecules move forward, collide with other molecules, and return to their original position to be pushed forward again the next time the diaphragm moves. The net result is that sound waves are produced and they travel to your ear.

Notice that the diaphragms don't analyze or code anything. They simply move at the same frequency as the driving stimulus (sound for the speaker diaphragm; electrical impulses for the listening diaphragm). Rutherford proposed that the basilar membrane works the same way: it too moves at the same frequency as its driving stimulus (the movement of the stapes). According to Rutherford, a sound of 25 Hz moves the basilar membrane up and down 25 times per second. A sound of 250 Hz moves it up and down 250 times per second.

Place Theories

All place theories propose that the basilar membrane does not respond as a single, unitary structure. They propose that different portions of the basilar membrane react to sounds of different frequencies. These theories postulate that sounds of different frequencies each activate a particular place along the length of the basilar membrane.

The most well-known of the older place theories is *Helmholtz's Resonance Theory*. Hermann von Helmholtz began by considering the shape of the basilar membrane. He noticed that it was narrow at the base of the cochlea and broad at the cochlea's apex.

The best way to understand the basilar membrane's shape is to imagine, once again, that we can unroll the cochlea. We'll place it with scala tympani down on the table and then we'll slice horizontally along the cochlea, as if we were cutting a long roll to make a submarine sandwich. When we remove the top half, we can look down onto the basilar membrane.

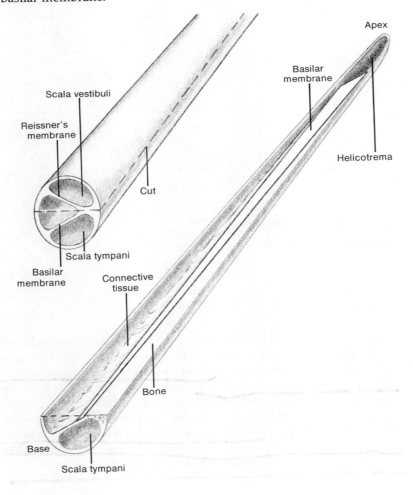

Helmholtz looked at that and thought of musical instruments that are made of a series of stretched strings of various lengths.

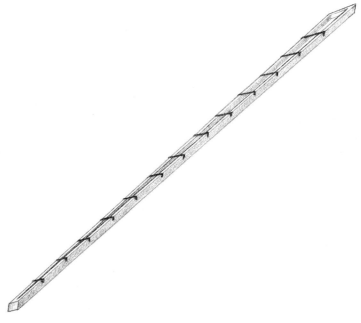

When a short string is plucked, a high-pitched sound will be produced by the string's vibration. When longer strings are plucked, lower-pitched sounds are produced. The rate at which any particular string vibrates is called its *natural frequency*. But it isn't necessary to pluck the strings in order to get them to vibrate. If a vibrating tuning fork is brought near the strings without touching them, some of the strings will be induced to vibrate. Those strings whose natural frequencies are the same as (or are multiples of) the tuning fork's frequency will vibrate. Inducing the strings to vibrate in this way is called *resonance*.

Helmholtz reasoned that the basilar membrane might operate in the same way, as if it were made of a series of stretched strings. High-frequency sounds would cause vibrations in the narrow end of the basilar membrane. Sounds of lower and lower frequency would produce vibrations in the middle or wide portions of the basilar membrane.

Notice that for Helmholtz to be correct, the basilar membrane must be under considerable transverse tension. (If the strings of the instrument are slack, they won't resonate. They must be taut. Helmholtz suggested that this is also true of the basilar membrane.) Many years after Helmholtz proposed his theory, a researcher named Georg von Békèsy (pronounced "beck'-a-she") directly tested Helmholtz's theory by making a small horizontal slit in the middle of the basilar membrane. If the membrane were under transverse tension, it should have ripped open. As it turned out, the basilar membrane did not rip open, and von Békèsy concluded that the basilar membrane is normally quite slack. Helmholtz's Resonance Theory was wrong. But the general notion of place theories was not wrong.

The Traveling-Wave Theory

Von Békèsy managed to drill a small hole in the wall of the cochlear duct, sprinkle some very fine shavings of aluminum on the basilar membrane, cover the hole with glass, and then watch what happened when the stapes moved at different frequencies. (The aluminum shavings were needed because the basilar membrane itself is so thin as to be virtually transparent.) What he discovered is that the place theories are essentially correct: different portions of the basilar membrane react to sounds of different frequencies. When the stapes moves at high frequencies, the narrow end of the basilar membrane moves up and down the most. As the frequency of stapes movement is lowered, the location of the maximum movement of the basilar membrane shifts toward the wider end at the apex of the cochlea.

The movement of any particular location along the basilar membrane is created by very complicated waves in the fluids, which are set up by movements of the stapes and reflections of waves off the walls of the cochlea. As waves reflect off the walls, they reinforce or cancel out both each other and the additional waves being generated by the movements of the stapes. The outcome is that some portions of the basilar membrane are subjected to strong waves, while other portions remain relatively still. We can schematically represent this as follows.

High-frequency sound

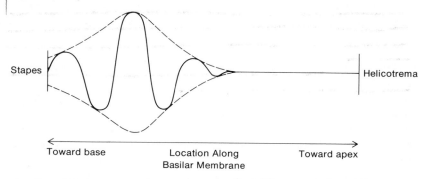

Stapes   Helicotrema

Toward base   Location Along   Toward apex
                     Basilar Membrane

Medium-frequency sound

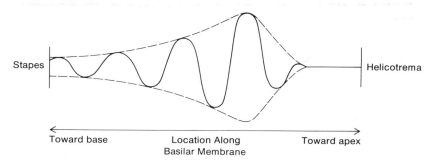

Stapes   Helicotrema

Toward base   Location Along   Toward apex
                     Basilar Membrane

Low-frequency sound

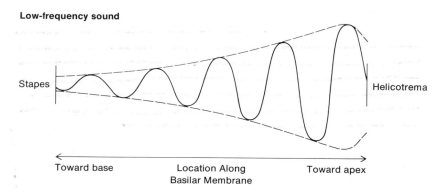

Stapes   Helicotrema

Toward base   Location Along   Toward apex
                     Basilar Membrane

When we draw in the dashed "envelopes," it becomes clear that different portions of the basilar membrane are maximally affected by different sound frequencies. The more a region of the basilar membrane moves, the more the tectorial membrane bends the hair cells of that region. And the more the hair cells are bent, the more their associated neurons will change their firing rates. Thus, sound frequency is signaled by the identity of the group of neurons that produces the greatest changes in firing rates. (This is a good place to pause and reconsider our discussion of the importance of the *pattern of activity* created by a stimulus. Do you recall that in Chapter 7 we noted that our visual perceptions depend upon making comparisons among neurons? Here, we are indicating that our auditory perceptions also depend upon comparisons of the relative activity of different neurons.)

This approach to understanding the cochlea is called *von Békèsy's Traveling-Wave Theory*, and it correctly describes the movements of the basilar membrane in response to sounds above 500 Hz (remember that we can hear sounds ranging from 20 to 20,000 Hz). Sounds that have frequencies less than 500 Hz create up-and-down movements equally throughout the entire length of the basilar membrane; as a result, hair cells throughout the cochlea are equally affected by sounds below 500 Hz. Therefore, the principle behind frequency theories is correct when it comes to low-frequency sounds, and the principle behind place theories is correct when it comes to moderate- and high-frequency sounds.

You already know that, as a sound's amplitude is increased, the movements of the basilar membrane increase. If a high-frequency tone (perhaps 19,000 Hz) is made louder and louder, the narrow end of the basilar membrane continues to move more than any other portion. But all the movements of the basilar membrane will be larger. If an individual is exposed to a very loud sound with a frequency of 10,000 Hz, the hair cells in the middle region of the basilar membrane are the ones that are bent the most; they are therefore the ones most likely to be damaged. This would produce noise-induced deafness to sounds of or about 10,000 Hz. If the individual is exposed to a very loud sound composed of several frequencies, the hair cells located in those regions of the basilar membrane that move most in response to the particular frequencies will be damaged. The individual would have hearing losses corresponding to each of the particular frequencies.

Why, as we get older, do we first lose our ability to hear high frequencies? The answer is to be found in the "envelopes" of basilar movement. All sounds create at least some movement of the portion of the basilar membrane near the base of the cochlea. Even low-frequency sounds create some movement there. The hair cells in that region are bent whenever we hear any sound. They are usually the first to go simply because they are used so much. The next-most-used region is the middle of the basilar membrane and, eventually, these hair cells also go, resulting in impaired hearing of progressively lower frequencies.

Summary

Make sure you understand and can define all the italicized terms.

First try to picture the overall structure of the cochlea. Think about the *oval window, scala vestibuli, Reissner's membrane, scala media,* the *basilar membrane, scala tympani,* and the *round window.* Think about the *perilymph* and the *endolymph.* Think about the way in which scala vestibuli and scala tympani communicate at the *helicotrema.*

Now focus on the *cochlear duct.* Picture the *organ of Corti* with its *supporting cells, inner* and *outer hair cells,* and the *tectorial membrane.* What must happen in order to produce changes in the firing rates of axons in the *auditory nerve?*

Think about what happens when the amplitude of a sound wave is increased. Describe what happens when the *middle-ear muscles* contract, and describe the two problems associated with this protective reflex.

Stop and consider your own environment. How much *noise pollution* are you exposed to? What are the chances that you are developing *noise-induced deafness?*

Now think about the *place theories* and *frequency theories* that have been proposed as decriptions of what happens inside the cochlea when sounds of different frequencies are heard. Make sure you can describe *von Békèsy's Traveling-Wave Theory.*

Recommended Readings

There is a difficult, advanced book you may wish to scan. It contains the remarkable work of a remarkable investigator.

von Békèsy, G.   *Experiments in Hearing.* McGraw-Hill, 1960.

For more information about noise pollution:

Report to the President and Congress on Noise, Senate Document No. 92-63. U.S. Government Printing Office, 1972.

11

The Auditory System

As you recall, in the visual system there is only one synaptic area (the lateral geniculate nuclei) between the optic nerve and the visual cortex. By contrast, in the auditory system there are four sets of synaptic areas (nuclei) between the auditory nerve and the neurons of the auditory cortex. At each of the synaptic areas, information may be compared, modified, analyzed, deleted, etc.

The Nuclei

The first-order neurons of the auditory system collect information from the hair cells of the organ of Corti. These axons travel as a bundle called the *auditory nerve* to the brainstem. Many of the axons synapse in brainstem synaptic areas called the *cochlear nuclei*. There are four cochlear nuclei, two on each side of the brainstem. One of each pair is termed the *dorsal cochlear nucleus*. It lies just behind the *ventral cochlear nucleus* ("dorsal" means toward the back side; "ventral" means toward the front or belly side). Axons of the left auditory nerve synapse primarily in the left dorsal and ventral cochlear nuclei, although some synapse in the cochlear nuclei on the right side. Similarly, the right auditory nerve sends most of its information to the right cochlear nuclei, but some is sent to the left cochlear nuclei.

Some of the axons of the auditory nerve do not synapse in any of the cochlear nuclei. Instead, they synapse in nearby regions called the *superior olivary nuclei*. There are two such nuclei, one on the left and one on the right. Once again, most of the axons synapsing in the left nucleus come from the left auditory nerve, but there is some "crossing over." There are even some interneurons that just carry information between the two superior olivary nuclei.

The second-order neurons carry information from the cochlear nuclei and/or superior olivary nuclei up into the brain. They synapse in the *inferior colliculi*. (Remember the superior colliculi? They are nuclei involved in controlling the extraocular muscles. In neuroanatomy, the terms "superior" and "inferior" have nothing to do with being "better" or "worse." They are terms used to signify location: "superior" means above, and "inferior" means below.)

The third-order neurons carry information from the inferior colliculi to the *medial geniculate nuclei,* which are the portions of the thalamus devoted to audition. Finally, the fourth-order neurons carry the information to the *auditory cortex*.

Notice that the auditory system is *bilateral:* information from each ear ends up being sent to both sides of the brain. At virtually every synaptic area, there is more and more mixing of the information that originated in the two ears; by the time the information reaches the cortex, there is an almost equal amount of information from each ear arriving on each side of the cortex.

The Auditory Cortex

You already know that the auditory cortex is located in the temporal lobe. As was the case with the visual cortex, the auditory cortex contains subdivisions. The first subdivision is called *AI* ("A" for auditory; pronounced "A-one"). It's located along and below the Sylvian fissure. Below AI, there is another subdivision, called *AII* (pronounced "A-two"). Lying alongside AI and AII is the subdivision known as *Ep* (pronounced "ee-pe").

If we place a microelectrode into any of these subdivisions, we find that each neuron responds most to a small number of tones. For example, neurons located in AI closest to the Sylvian fissure respond most to high-frequency tones; neurons located in AI furthest from the Sylvian fissure respond most to low-frequency tones. In between these two areas of AI, there are neurons that respond most to tones of moderately high or moderate or moderately low frequency. The neurons are laid out systematically, so the neurons that respond most to a tone of 1,100 Hz, for example, are located between neurons that respond most to 1,000 Hz and those that respond most to 1,200 Hz, etc.

In AII, there is a similar arrangement: the neurons are systematically laid out according to the frequency that has the greatest effect on them. However, in AII, the sequence is reversed. Neurons that respond most to low-frequency tones are located toward the front of AII; those that respond most to high-frequency tones are toward the back.

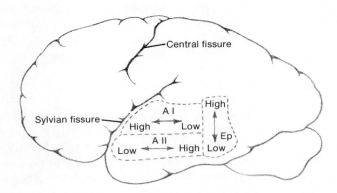

Each systematic arrangement of this kind is called a *tonotopic map*, and each subdivision of the auditory cortex contains its own tonotopic map. (This should remind you of the systematic arrangement, the so-called retinotopic mapping, we met in the visual system.) In Ep, the high-frequency tones are represented at the top and the low-frequency tones are represented at the bottom. Some researchers feel there may be as many as eight different tonotopic maps on each side of the cortex (including one called AIII that is located in the area just in front of the Sylvian fissure, not in the temporal lobe). Because there appear to be so many tonotopic maps, a large portion of the cortex seems to be involved in audition. It is rather difficult to figure out what each subdivision, with its own tonotopic map, does because destroying any one subdivision does not produce any obvious hearing problem. It is very likely that

each subdivision performs a complicated analysis of auditory information, but that the loss of a particular subdivision doesn't produce a
marked effect because a great deal of the analysis continues to occur in
the undamaged subdivisions. Somewhat surprising, however, is the
fact that, if most or all of the subdivisions are destroyed in a laboratory
animal such as a cat, the animal still has the ability to discriminate
between tones of different frequencies or intensities and the ability to
tell what direction a sound is coming from. The destruction of the
auditory cortex does profoundly disturb some aspects of hearing.
Before we describe the results of damaging the auditory cortex, let's
examine what can be discovered by placing electrodes at different
locations in the auditory system.

Recordings from the Cochlea

Because the cochlea is made up of three canals, we can begin by finding
out whether there are any electrical differences among them. We can
compare scala vestibuli and scala tympani, or we can compare either
one of these with scala media. When there is no sound present, each
canal differs electrically from the other two. Because the cochlea is "at
rest" when no sound is present, these electrical differences are called the
cochlear resting potentials.

If one electrode is placed in scala vestibuli and the other is placed in
scala tympani, we record a rather small resting potential: scala vestibuli
is about 2 to 4 mV more positive than scala tympani. Because scala
vestibuli and scala tympani both contain perilymph, this small cochlear
resting potential is called the *perilymphatic potential.*

If one electrode is placed in scala media and the other is placed in
either of the other canals, we record a large resting potential: scala
media is some 80 mV more positive than either scala vestibuli or scala
tympani. This large cochlear resting potential is called the *endolymphatic
potential.*

Both kinds of cochlear resting potentials appear to be created by the
presence and particular location of the cochlea's rich blood supply. A
group of blood vessels runs along the outer wall of scala media,

throughout the length of the cochlea. The blood vessels form a noticeable band or stripe, and they are called *stria vascularis*.

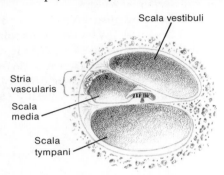

Small capillaries carry blood into the depths of the canals supplying the required oxygen and carrying off wastes. But the mass of larger vessels is found along scala media's outer wall, somewhat closer to scala vestibuli than to scala tympani. (Do you recall our discussion of the location of blood vessels in the eye? We concluded that there is an important reason for having them located in the choroid, behind the outer segments of rods and cones; there they can service the rods and cones without interfering with the light coming into the eye. There is an equally important reason for the location of stria vascularis. These blood vessels are quite large. They are able to service the cochlea via small capillaries. If stria vascularis were located within the cochlea, rather than along its outer wall, the pulsing of blood through the vessels would produce substantial disturbances in the cochlear fluids; as a result, we would hear a continuous roar. In effect, we would have a difficult time hearing anything other than the sounds created by movements of our blood.)

In general, any area in the body that contains a rich blood supply is electrically more positive than the surrounding tissues, and the cochlea is no exception. The resting potentials are, in fact, an excellent example of this principle. Because scala vestibuli is slightly closer to the blood supply than is scala tympani, scala vestibuli is slightly more positive. Because scala media is considerably closer to stria vascularis than either of the other canals, it is considerably more positive.

Suppose we place one electrode anywhere in the vicinity of the cochlea and we place our other electrode in a neutral location (in a neck muscle or in a toe; any place where we are fairly sure there will be no neural response to sound). If we then turn on a sound, we can measure the overall electrical response of the cochlea. This overall response of the cochlea is called the *cochlear microphonic*.

The name is very descriptive because the response is almost an exact replica of the sound that is played. If we play a particular melody into the ear, we can compare the sound waves of the melody with the overall responses of the cochlea. Perhaps the easiest way to do this is to use the information from the electrodes to drive a loudspeaker. The sounds that come out of the loudspeaker sound virtually identical to the sounds we play into the ear.

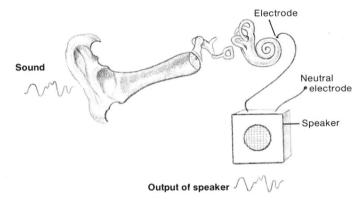

If we hum "Home Sweet Home" into the ear, "Home Sweet Home" comes out of the loudspeaker. In other words, we can say that the cochlear microphonic faithfully reproduces the input. In a sense, the cochlea behaves like a microphone, responding in a way that insures that the output is a faithful reproduction of the input. The cochlear microphonic is probably best viewed as the result of the shearing of hair cells throughout the cochlea. This view is supported by the fact that, if a high-frequency tone is used as the input, the cochlear microphonic is largest when the electrode is placed near the base of the cochlea; if the input is of low frequency, the cochlear microphonic is largest when the electrode is placed near the apex of the cochlea.

There are two aspects of the cochlear microphonic that require some further discussion. The first has to do with a shift from the ear's resting potential. Before the sound begins, the cochlea has an overall resting potential (due to the stria vascularis) that is slightly more positive than many other tissues. When the sound begins, the cochlea becomes less positive.

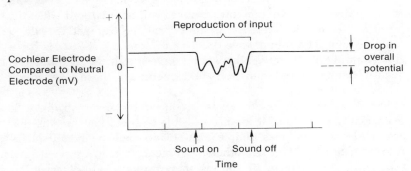

The drop in the overall potential is called the *summating potential*. It represents a general use of energy by the hair cells.

The second aspect of the cochlear microphonic is a bit more complicated. We've indicated that the cochlea's response to a sound is almost an exact replica of the sound. Notice the word "almost." There are some small but important differences between the input and the output. The differences occur because the ear introduces distortions of its own whenever a sound is played into it. In fact, any acoustical system introduces distortions. Tape recorders, stereos, telephones, microphones, and musical instruments create distortions. Inexpensive tape recorders tend to sound flat and "tinny" because they produce only a limited number of frequencies. Some of the richness of the original sound is lost. Furthermore, the tape recorder may add some frequencies that weren't present in the original sound, or it may overemphasize or underemphasize some of the frequencies of the original sound. In part, what is happening is that the tape recorder contains components that vibrate most easily at certain frequencies (their natural frequencies). Whenever a component is disturbed, it will tend to vibrate at one of these frequencies, even if the original sound does not contain these frequencies.

The introduction of distortions is not always something undesirable. Consider musical instruments. If I play middle C on a piano, a violin, and a trumpet, you can probably tell which instrument is producing each middle C, even if you can't see the instruments. Because each instrument produces middle C, each produces a sound that has a frequency of 262 Hz. But each instrument also produces additional frequencies. It's the additional frequencies that allow you to distinguish among the instruments. A middle C on the piano is a mixture of tones, the most prominent of which has a frequency of 262 Hz. The mixture of tones is created by the vibrations of various parts of the instrument. The density of the wood, the shape of various portions of the piano, the tightness of the joints, the construction of the keyboard, and so on—all will help determine what mixture of tones will be produced when the piano key is struck. Similarly, middle C on the trumpet is really a complex tone. The sound wave that has a frequency of 262 Hz has a greater amplitude than the other sound waves produced by the shape, quality, and design of the instrument. Nonetheless, those other sound waves do occur.

The collection of sound waves produced by any instrument is aesthetically important. If it were possible to build instruments that produced only pure tones, middle C on a piano would be indistinguishable from middle C on any other instrument. In fact, we would not experience the richness of sounds that results when different instruments all play the same note; the sound would seem to get louder and louder if we played a piano, then added a violin, then a trumpet, etc. But if each produced only pure tones, the sound would not seem to get richer or fuller.

In reality, no acoustical instrument produces pure tones. Tuning forks do not introduce as many distortions as pianos, but any object that vibrates introduces some distortion. Tuning forks introduce distortions primarily when they first begin to vibrate and then, again, when they stop vibrating. Suppose we have a tuning fork that is built so that its natural frequency is 500 Hz. We know that, if we disturb the tuning fork (by striking it against a table top, for example), it will vibrate at 500 Hz. However, parts of the tuning fork may initially vibrate at other frequencies. Typically these other frequencies are very small in amplitude, and most of them soon die out. As the tuning fork gradually stops vibrating, it does not go from 500 Hz directly to zero vibrations. Rather, it vibrates at other, lower frequencies. If you listen carefully to a tuning fork as it stops vibrating, you can hear the sound getting softer (the amplitude of vibration is getting smaller) and the pitch changing (the frequency of vibration is changing).

Any acoustical system produces a set of frequencies when it begins to vibrate and as it stops vibrating. The ear is an acoustical system, and it too produces these distortions. As we've seen, most acoustical systems (including the ear) also produce distortions during a sound because of the frequencies at which various components most easily vibrate. The distortions created by musical instruments produce the characteristic quality (often called the *timbre*, pronounced "tam'-burr") that identifies the kind of instrument. The distortions created by the ear produce what are called the *aural harmonics*.

If a very careful comparison is made between the sound played into the ear and the cochlear microphonics that are produced, it becomes clear that the two are not identical. The differences are the aural harmonics created by the components of the ear.

You should notice that, because all acoustical systems introduce distortions, none of them can produce a pure tone. In fact, a pure tone is something that exists only in theory. The tones we hear are complex tones. Some are more complex than others (that is, some contain a wider variety of frequencies than others), but not one is truly a pure tone. Even if we could somehow find a way to produce a pure tone, we could never hear a pure tone because the ear always introduces distortions.

Recordings from the Auditory Nerve

If we place a fairly large electrode near the auditory nerve, we can record the overall activity that occurs in all the axons in response to a sound. This kind of recording does not permit us to see the individual action potentials that occur; it only allows us to see the gross (that is, average or overall) activity. Because the auditory nerve is often called the VIIIth cranial nerve, this kind of recording allows us to see what's called the *gross VIIIth nerve response.*

Usually, the sound that's used as a stimulus is a click. If the click is quite soft, hair cells throughout the cochlea will be bent slightly, and axons in the auditory nerve may each produce just one action potential. If the click is louder, the hair cells will be bent more and the auditory nerve axons may each produce two or more action potentials. The gross VIIIth nerve response will reflect the sound intensity as follows.

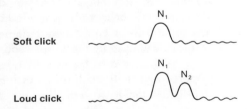

Each "hump" represents the production of action potentials by the auditory-nerve axons. In response to a soft click, we'll have some axons respond, and we'll have a single "hump" called the N_1 *response.* If the click is louder, we'll have two humps, called the N_1 *response* and the N_2 *response.* The N_1 response is larger than it was with a soft click because more axons will produce at least one action potential. The N_2 response represents the second action potential produced by at least some of the axons.

We could go on and on, making the click louder or longer. But if we want to know more about the activities of the individual axons, we'll need to use a microelectrode so that we can penetrate the auditory nerve and record individual action potentials.

When a microelectrode is placed in the auditory nerve, the first thing that's noticed is that the axons have a *maintained discharge:* they produce action potentials at a relatively steady rate when no sound is present. (Do you recall that we first met the concept of a maintained discharge during our discussion of the visual system in Chapter 6?) When an appropriate sound is presented to the ear, an axon may either increase its firing rate or decrease its firing rate. This is reminiscent of the situation we discovered in the optic nerve.

With this in mind, we can refine our ideas about the gross VIIIth nerve response. The N_1 and N_2 responses actually represent changes from the maintained discharge levels in many axons. Strictly speaking, they don't represent the production of one or two action potentials; rather they represent overall changes in the firing rates of many axons.

When we use microelectrodes to study the responses of individual axons, it becomes obvious that different axons respond to different sounds. Suppose we place our microelectrode near one axon. The axon has a maintained discharge and we're going to systematically vary the sounds we play into the ear, trying to identify those sounds that alter the axon's firing rate. We might begin with a tone of 1,000 Hz (that is, we'll use a "relatively" pure tone) at -10 db. If the axon does not alter its firing rate, we can increase the intensity to -5 db, then to 0 db, and so on, until we find that a change in the firing rate occurs. Then we can begin again at -10 db with a tone of 2,000 Hz and repeat the same procedure. As we continue to test with different frequencies, we'll find that the axon will respond to some tones when they are soft and to others when they are loud, and that the axon will not respond at all to some no matter how loud we make them. We can summarize all this in a graph.

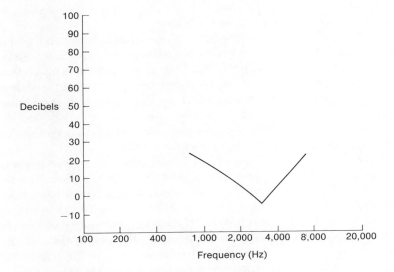

What's indicated on the graph is the lowest intensity to which the axon responds when the tone is varied from 800 to 8,000 Hz. When the tone is 3,000 Hz, the sound need not be very intense in order to produce a change in the axon's firing rate. When the tone is 2,000 or 4,000 Hz, it must be made more intense in order to produce a change in the axon's firing rate. If the tone is 7,500 or 8,000 Hz, the axon's firing rate remains at the maintained discharge level no matter how intense the tone is.

What we have graphed is the axon's *response area:* all the tones located within the V will produce a change in the axon's firing rate. None of the sounds outside the V will alter the axon's firing rate. Each axon in the auditory nerve has its own response area; that is, each axon will respond only to a certain group of tones. And within the response area, there will be one frequency to which the axon is especially sensitive. That frequency is called the axon's *characteristic frequency.* The axon we graphed has a characteristic frequency of 3,000 Hz. Others may have characteristic frequencies of 1,000 Hz or 8,000 Hz or 12,000 Hz. But each axon will, in a sense, be "tuned to" just one frequency, although it will respond over a range of frequencies when the intensities are increased.

Imagine that we make recordings from three different axons, and we discover that their characteristic frequencies are 1,500 Hz, 5,000 Hz, and 13,000 Hz. Can you guess which hair cells in the cochlea are responsible for activating these three axons?

Recall von Békèsy's findings: he discovered that, as long as the sound is above about 500 Hz, the principle of the place theories is correct. Tones of different frequencies have their primary effects on different locations in the cochlea. High-frequency sounds result in traveling waves that have their greatest effect on that portion of the basilar membrane near the base of the cochlea. Low-frequency tones produce traveling waves that have their greatest effect on that portion of the basilar membrane nearest the apex of the cochlea.

Now, from what portions of the basilar membrane are our three axons collecting their information? The axon with a characteristic frequency of 1,500 Hz must be part of a neuron whose dendrites synapse with hair cells near the apex of the cochlea. The axon with a characteristic frequency of 13,000 Hz must be getting its information from a portion of the basilar membrane near the base of the cochlea. And the axon with a characteristic frequency of 5,000 Hz collects its information from a middle region of the basilar membrane.

Let's concentrate on this last axon. If it collects its information from just a few hair cells in the middle region of the basilar membrane, why should it respond to tones that are substantially above or below its characteristic frequency when these tones are made louder? Why should the axon have a response area at all? Why doesn't it just respond to 5,000 Hz tones only?

The answer has to do with the fact that the basilar membrane does not operate as if it were made up of separated subsections. If one portion of the basilar membrane moves, the rest of the basilar membrane also moves. If you press a pencil point against your skin, the area just underneath the point is deformed the most but neightboring regions are also deformed. As you press harder against the skin, the immediately neighboring regions are deformed more, and more distant regions begin to be deformed. Your skin, like the basilar membrane, does not react as if it were made up of disconnected subsections.

The axon with a characteristic frequency of 5,000 Hz is part of a neuron whose dendrites synapse with hair cells in the middle region of the basilar membrane. If a tone of 5,000 Hz is played, those hair cells are bent more than hair cells at other locations. If a tone of 3,000 Hz is played, the same hair cells will be bent, but only slightly. (A tone of 3,000 Hz will have its major effect on a portion of the basilar membrane located slightly closer to the cochlea's apex.) If the 3,000 Hz tone is made louder, the same hair cells will be bent more (just as pressing harder on the skin produces a greater deformation in a neighboring region). If the 3,000 Hz tone is made loud enough, the same hair cells will be bent enough to produce a large postsynaptic potential that will travel down the dendrite to the soma and axon hillock. If the graded potential is still sufficiently large, the activity of the axon will be affected. Notice that, the greater the difference between an axon's characteristic frequency and the other tone, the more intense that tone must be in order to affect the axon. That is sensible because a tone that is very different from the characteristic frequency will have its major effect on a more distant portion of the basilar membrane. If the tone is different enough, the axon may not respond to it, regardless of how intense the tone is. The tone is producing its major effect at such a distance from the relevant hair cells that even intense stimulation of that distant site will result in very little bending of those hair cells. (If you press a pencil against the back of your hand, even very intense pressure will not deform the skin beyond a certain distance.)

In the auditory nerve, axons may have their characteristic frequencies anywhere between about 500 Hz and 20,000 Hz. We can hear sounds that are as low as 20 Hz, but there are no axons with characteristic frequencies below 500 Hz. In order to understand why, think back again about von Békèsy's findings. He discovered that, when tones below 500 Hz were played, the basilar membrane moved (as a unit) up and down at the same frequency as the sound. If the entire basilar membrane moves, hair cells throughout the cochlea will be equally affected. No one particular location along the basilar membrane will be involved and consequently, no one set of hair cells will be bent. Instead, all the neurons that collect information from all the hair cells will be affected and, if the sound is made sufficiently loud, all the axons of the auditory nerve will respond. If the sound is 25 Hz, the axons will tend to react 25 times per second. If the sound is 100 Hz, an individual axon may not respond to each cycle but it may respond to every second cycle, producing 50 changes per second in its maintained discharge. Another axon may respond to the first, third, and fifth cycle, and so on. In this way, the axons "platoon" themselves so that no one axon must respond at an impossibly high rate, but each cycle of the sound wave produces a response in some of the axons. This "platooning" behavior has been termed the *Volley Principle.* We can represent this behavior as follows.

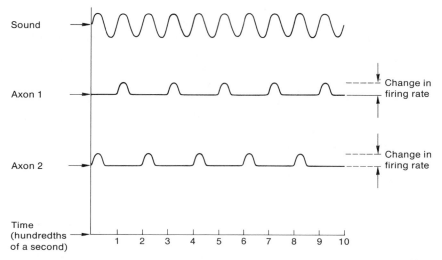

If an axon responds to a particular sound of low intensity, it will typically respond more and more as the sound's intensity is increased. We can now indicate that, in the auditory nerve, the frequency of a sound is signaled either by the group of axons that responds (for sounds above 500 Hz) or by the rate at which axons respond (for sounds below 500 Hz), and that the intensity of a sound is signaled by the amount of the response of the axons.

Recordings from Synaptic Areas

Neurons of the cochlear nuclei, superior olivary nuclei, inferior colliculi, medial geniculate nuclei, and auditory cortex also have response areas and characteristic frequencies. There are three general differences between the activity of these neurons and the activity of the auditory-nerve axons. First, the axons of the auditory nerve respond only to sounds that arrive at one ear; because the auditory system is a bilateral system, neurons at all the other locations may respond to sounds that arrive at either ear. We can refer to the auditory nerve axons as being *monaural* ("one-eared") and the other neurons as being *binaural* ("two-eared").

Second, the response areas tend to get more narrow as we record first from the auditory nerve, then from the cochlear nuclei, then from the superior olivary nuclei, then from the inferior colliculi, and finally from the medial geniculate nuclei. The neurons of each successive synaptic area are less and less inclined to respond to a broad range of sounds, even when the sounds are made quite loud. As an example, we can graph the response areas of one auditory-nerve axon and one medial geniculate neuron.

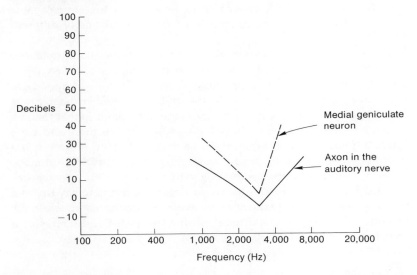

We can describe this by saying that the neurons become more selective as we march upward through the auditory system from the auditory nerve to the medial geniculate nuclei. Evidently there is an interplay of excitation and inhibition that produces the narrowing of the response areas. This interplay is, in many ways, similar to the on and off areas that are juxtaposed in so many receptive fields in the visual system.

However, neurons in the various subsections of the auditory cortex tend to have rather broad response areas. In fact, their response areas may be broader than those of the auditory-nerve axons. In some ways, this parallels what occurs in the visual system: the ganglion cells have a few requirements concerning which lights they will react to. Some of the neurons of the lateral geniculate nuclei are more specific; they require lights of certain wavelengths. In the visual cortex, the simple, complex, and lower-order hypercomplex cells are even more specific. They demand that the light be of a particular width or angle of orientation or length. Each kind of cell responds to a narrower range of stimuli. But the higher-order hypercomplex cells are somewhat less choosy. They don't require the light to be of a particular orientation.

In the auditory system, with its many synaptic areas, increasingly specific requirements (i.e., a smaller range of frequencies) occur from one synaptic area to the next. The cells that finally receive the information at the cortex are somewhat less specific. In both the visual and auditory systems, it appears that the analysis of information is progressively refined up until the final groups of cells. These final cells seem to collect broader kinds of information and are therefore capable of an overview of the information or broad comparisons of different kinds of information.

The third difference between the auditory-nerve axons and the remainder of the auditory system is that the neurons of the synaptic areas increasingly set an upper limit to the intensities of sounds to which they'll react. If an axon in the auditory nerve responds to a low-intensity 2,000 Hz tone, it will continue to respond to that tone no matter how loud it becomes. In fact, the axon responds more and more (up to a limit, of course) when the tone is made louder. However, if a neuron in the cochlear nuclei, for example, responds to a low-intensity 2,000 Hz tone, it will stop responding to that tone once the tone reaches a particular intensity level. One way to describe this is to say that the response areas of the auditory nerve axons are open-ended, while the response areas of neurons throughout the rest of the auditory system tend to have a closed "top" on them.

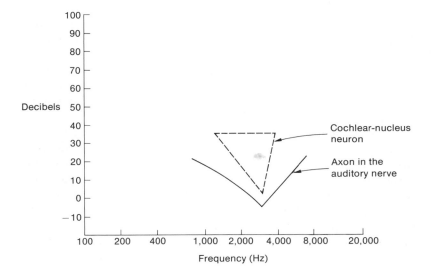

Thus, the neurons are not only more selective about the range of frequencies to which they'll respond; they are also more selective about the range of intensities.

We said earlier that, if the auditory cortex of a cat is removed, the ability to discriminate between tones of different frequencies or intensities is not seriously impaired. It should be clear to you now that a great deal of analysis concerning the frequency and intensity of a sound occurs in the synaptic areas between the auditory nerve and auditory cortex. Removing the auditory cortex does not affect the functioning of these synaptic areas, and both frequency and intensity discriminations can still be made.

We also said that removing the auditory cortex does not impair the ability to tell what direction a sound is coming from. This ability to perform what's called *sound localization* requires some explanation.

Sound Localization

Turn on a radio or stereo, or sit in a room where people are talking. Close your eyes and try to figure out how you can tell where the sounds you hear are originating.

The most obvious clue you have is the *relative intensity* of the sounds arriving at each ear. If the sound source is off to your left or right, the ear closest to the sound source receives a sound of greater intensity. The more distant ear is in an acoustical shadow created by your head. If the sound source is directly in front, overhead, or behind you, both ears receive the same intensity. In fact, if you keep your head still, it's very difficult to discriminate among sound sources in these three positions. You need to move your head so that one ear is partially blocked before you can figure out whether the sound is coming from directly in front, overhead, or behind.

There are two other clues we use in sound localization. They also involve differences in the sound as it arrives at the two ears. The first difference is the *time of arrival* of the sound. If you are sitting in a quiet room and a sound source to your left is turned on, initially your left ear receives the sound before your right ear. The second difference is the *phase* of the sound. As the sound continues, while the left tympanic membrane is being pushed in by the bunched up air molecules, the right tympanic membrane may be returning to its resting position as the molecules near it spread out. In other words, the sound waves at the two ears may not have their cycles in register with each other. The waves are said to be out of phase; when the sound source is off to one side or the other, the head gets in the way and, as sound waves travel around it, they do not "keep time" with the sound waves arriving at the ear closest to the sound source.

Many of the neurons of the superior olivary nuclei seem to perform just the kind of analysis that would permit us to discriminate among sounds coming from different directions. These neurons receive binaural information, and many of them are sensitive to the differences in sounds arriving at the two ears. Some superior olivary neurons respond most if the sound arrives first at one ear and then, after a brief delay, at the other ear. Some respond most when the left ear "leads"—others, when the right ear "leads."

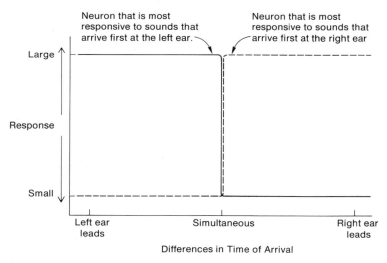

These neurons provide precisely the kind of information that's required to perform sound localization. And they not only respond to particular time-of-arrival arrangements, they also respond to particular relative-intensity arrangements. (In fact, we could talk about a trading ratio between time of arrival and intensity.) Suppose we consider a neuron that responds most if the sound arrives at the left ear first. We might examine that neuron's behavior when we turn the sound on simultaneously in the two ears, but we make the intensity different at the two ears.

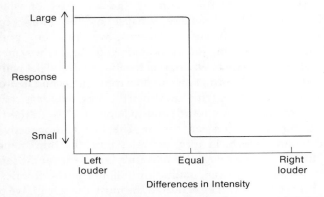

Differences in Intensity

Notice that the neuron responds more when the sound is louder at the left ear. In natural situations, when a sound source is off to the left, the sound arrives first at the left ear and the sound is also louder in the left ear. As a result, the neuron responds a great deal. When the sound source is off to the right, neither requirement of this neuron is met (the sound will arrive first at the right ear and it will be louder in the right ear), and this neuron does not respond. Because there are many neurons, each with its own time-of-arrival and relative-intensity requirements, different neurons will respond when the sound source is in different positions.

One interesting model has been proposed to explain how these neurons manage to have time-of-arrival requirements. The model is called a *cross-correlator*. Imagine that we have two series of neurons, one collecting its information from the left ear and one from the right, and a set of "collecting" neurons that systematically gathers information from the two series. We can schematically represent the situation as follows.

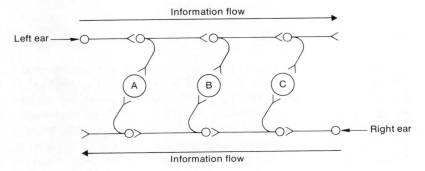

Each series contains four neurons, the last three of which have branched axons. The branches synapse on the three "collector" neurons, marked A, B, and C. Suppose we "turn on" both series simultaneously by having sounds occur in both ears at the same time. In the left-ear series, activity will start in the first neuron. That will activate the second neuron. Information will flow from the second neuron to the third neuron and to "collector" A. When the third neuron is activated, it sends information to the fourth and to "collector" B. In the right-ear series, a similar progression occurs. The first neuron activates the second neuron which, in turn, activates both the third neuron and "collector" C, etc. If we begin by activating both series at the same time, then "collector" B receives simultaneous input from both series. Of the three "collectors," B will be activated the most. But what if we begin by activating the left-ear series first and later the right-ear series? Information in the left-ear series will be "ahead" of the right-ear series. By the time information has traveled to the last neuron in the left-ear series, it might have traveled only to the second neuron in the right-ear series. In that case, "collector" C would be the one that received simultaneous activation from both series, and it would be activated more than A or B. Imagine now that the "collectors" represent superior olivary neurons; A would be a neuron that responds most when the sound arrives first at the right ear, and C would be a neuron that responds most when the sound arrives first at the left ear. B would be a neuron that responds most to sounds arriving simultaneously at both ears.

Remember that this is a *model* of how the superior olivary neurons *might* operate. It's not meant to be an accurate description of how they work, but it does provide an excellent way to begin thinking about the problem.

The Olivocochlear Bundles

The auditory system contains a mechanism that exaggerates the differences between sounds arriving at the two ears. The mechanism involves neural pathways that run from each superior olivary nucleus to the *opposite* ear. The pathways are called the *olivocochlear bundles* ("olivo-" meaning from the superior olivary nuclei; "-cochlear" meaning to the cochlea; "bundles" for collections of axons), or *OCB* for short. We can represent the OCB arising from the left superior olivary nucleus in a schematic diagram of the auditory system. Notice in the diagram that only the pathways from the left ear have been drawn in.

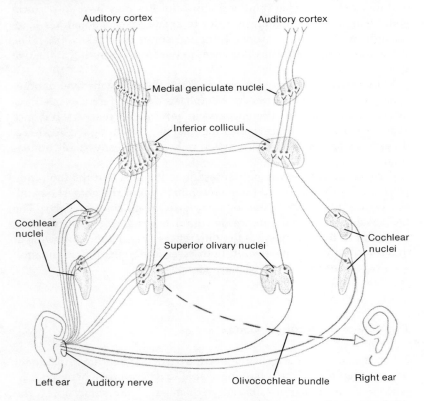

Notice that the information flows *from* the superior olivary nuclei *to* the cochleas, and that the arrangement is *contralateral*. In addition, each OCB has an *inhibitory* effect on the information arising from the opposite cochlea. The OCB axons synapse onto the neurons of the opposite auditory nerve and inhibit them.

What does this do? To begin, remember that, although each superior olivary nucleus receives binaural information, it gets more information from the ear on the same side than from the ear on the opposite side. If a sound arrives at the left ear, the left superior olivary nucleus becomes more active than the right superior olivary nucleus. The left OCB becomes active and it inhibits the right auditory nerve. If sound now arrives at the right ear, the right auditory nerve will not respond as much as it would otherwise. What may actually be just a small difference in the intensity of sound at the left and right ears will seem to be a larger difference, and what may actually be a small time-of-arrival difference may seem to be a larger difference. (Because the right auditory nerve is being inhibited, the dendrites may have to perform some temporal summation in order to create graded potentials large enough to activate the axons. Temporal summation takes *time*.) The OCB thus exaggerates the differences in the sounds arriving at the two ears.

I hope that it's occurred to you that the OCB provides yet another example of our nervous system's emphasis upon differences in stimulation. In this case, the differences occur between the two ears. But once again, we have evidence indicating that we are designed to detect differences or changes in stimulation rather than steady-state stimulation.

Perhaps what's even more interesting is the idea that the inhibition provided by the OCB and the lateral inhibition of the horseshoe-crab eye we discussed at the end of Chapter 6 create similar effects. The OCB exaggerates the differences in stimulation arriving at the two ears; lateral inhibition exaggerates the differences in stimulation arriving at different portions of the eye. In both cases, differences in stimulation are singled out for very special attention.

The Role of the Auditory Cortex

When the auditory cortex is removed, a particular hearing impairment occurs. The individual is no longer able to discriminate between *tonal patterns*; if we play two different sequences of the same notes, the individual is unable to distinguish between the sequences. Suppose we pick middle C (262 Hz) and C one octave above (524 Hz). We could play these in the following sequences: 262 Hz—524 Hz—262 Hz, or 524 Hz—262 Hz—524 Hz. Individuals with normal hearing describe these as two different "melodies"; individuals whose auditory cortex has been extensively damaged cannot tell them apart. Because removal of the auditory cortex doesn't seriously disrupt the ability to discriminate between sounds of different frequencies (the person can distinguish between 262 Hz and 524 Hz), the problem seems to be related to remembering the order in which the sounds occurred. Researchers have suggested that the auditory cortex has as its chief function the storage of auditory information or, put simply, that the auditory cortex is the location of auditory memory.

Without auditory memory, it becomes extremely difficult to appreciate music or to make anything meaningful out of the sounds we call speech. If you cannot remember the sequence of individual sounds and syllables, speech becomes a jumble of disconnected sounds.

Summary

By way of a review, make a schematic diagram of the auditory system. Be sure to include the *cochleas, auditory nerves, cochlear nuclei, superior olivary nuclei, inferior colliculi, medial geniculate nuclei* (remember that they're part of the thalamus), and the *AI, AII,* and *Ep* subdivisions of the *auditory cortex.* Remember to indicate that the auditory system is increasingly *bilateral* as you go from the cochlear nuclei to the auditory cortex.

Now think about the kinds of responses you can record from each location (make sure you understand and can define all the italicized terms).

1. Cochlea: *perilymphatic potential, endolymphatic potential,* and the *cochlear microphonic* (don't forget the *summating potential* and *aural harmonics*).

2. Auditory nerve: the *gross VIIIth nerve response* (made up of the N_1 *response*, N_2 *response*, etc.), and the *response areas* and *characteristic frequencies* of individual axons.

3. Synaptic areas: think about the three ways in which the response areas here differ from those of the auditory-nerve axons (*binaural* vs *monaural*, narrow vs broad, closed "top" vs open-ended.)

4. Auditory cortex: think about the *tonotopic map* of each subdivision, and about the response areas of neurons in the auditory cortex.

Finally, consider the following questions.

1. Why aren't there axons with characteristic frequencies below 500 Hz?

2. How are sounds of different intensities signaled?

3. How are sounds of different frequencies signaled?

4. How does *sound localization* take place?

5. What is meant by *tonal-pattern discrimination?*

Recommended Readings

You may wish to try the following somewhat difficult articles in *Sensory Communication,* ed. W. A. Rosenblith, MIT Press, 1961.

Katsuki, Y.   "Neural Mechanism of Auditory Sensation in Cats," pp. 561–584.

Neff, W. D.   "Neural Mechanisms of Auditory Discrimination," pp. 259–278.

Woolsey, C. N.   "Organization of Cortical Auditory System," pp. 235–258.

Also take a look at the following book and articles.

Griffin, D. R.   *Listening in the Dark.* Yale University Press, 1958.

Roeder, K. D.   "Moths and Ultrasound," *Sci. Amer.,* April 1965 (Offprint #1009).

Rosenzweig, M. R.   "Auditory Localization," *Sci. Amer.,* Oct. 1961 (Offprint #501).

12

Auditory Perception

The study of auditory perception poses two problems we haven't encountered before. First, any study of auditory perception must take into account the fact that sound waves interact with each other and with objects in rather complicated ways. Suppose we place a loudspeaker in a large, open field. You already know that the intensity of sound will vary inversely with the square of the distance from the speakers. If we place two speakers in the field, we have to keep this inverse square law in mind, but we also have to recognize that the sound waves produced by the two speakers will sometimes reinforce and sometimes cancel out each other.

Imagine that the speakers face each other. If they both produce the same sound waves at the same time, the waves will reinforce each other where they meet. If the waves produced by the speakers are out of phase, the waves will cancel out each other.

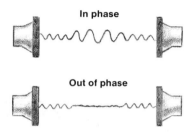

In either situation, the sound's intensity changes drastically if you stand at various locations between the speakers. If you wanted to test your auditory thresholds, you would have to measure the sound's intensity at the spot where you were standing. Just measuring the intensity in front of each speaker would be insufficient.

If the speakers were in a room rather than an open field, the situation would become extremely complicated. Not only would the sound waves interact directly with each other, but they would also interact with sound waves reflected from the walls, floor, and ceiling. Any objects in the room would also reflect some sound waves. The result would be a very complicated pattern of reinforcements and cancellations. Depending upon the shape and size of the room, the locations of the speakers, the materials used for the room's surfaces (rough materials such as drapes or carpeting or acoustical tiles tend to trap sound waves; smooth materials tend to reflect sound waves), and the nature of the sounds created by the loudspeakers, the patterns can vary considerably. Any one pattern will create some "dead spots" in the room and some places where the sounds are extremely intense.

Suppose you wanted to test an individual's hearing. If you allowed the individual to wander around the room (so-called *free-field* testing), you would have considerable difficulty figuring out exactly how much sound the person received at any given moment. In free-field situations, the intensity can increase or decrease several-fold when the person moves just a few feet to one side or the other.

Free-field situations are so complicated that the designing and building of concert halls are as much art forms as they are science. It is not a simple matter to create a setting in which there are few dead spots and there is minimal distortion. Often acoustical reflectors and baffles have to be experimented with after the hall is built; upholstery and draperies may be changed; seats may be moved.

In the study of auditory perception, the use of free-field situations is almost always avoided because of the difficulties created by the interactions of sound waves. Earphones are used, so that sound can be delivered directly to the ears. When earphones are used, the intensity of sound arriving at the ears can be precisely determined and controlled.

The second problem encountered in the study of auditory perception has to do with the fact that we produce sound. Our breathing, heartbeats, the rush of blood through arteries and veins, and the movements of our body—all produce sound. Thus it's impossible to place an individual in a truly sound-free situation. External sounds can be minimized or eliminated by using acoustical insulation, but internal sounds cannot be eliminated. This is quite different from the situation we encountered when describing the study of visual perception; our bodies don't produce light, so it is relatively easy to place an individual in a light-free environment. All we can do is recognize the problem and keep in mind the fact that our own production of sound occurs in any setting.

Auditory Thresholds

We've said earlier that human beings can hear sounds that range in frequency from 20 to 20,000 Hz. However, we are not equally sensitive to all these frequencies. If we measure the thresholds of young people who are not suffering from any hearing disorders, we find that the thresholds to sounds in the range from 1,000 Hz to 2,000 Hz are lower than the thresholds to other frequencies, and that the thresholds increase gradually in the lower and upper frequency ranges.

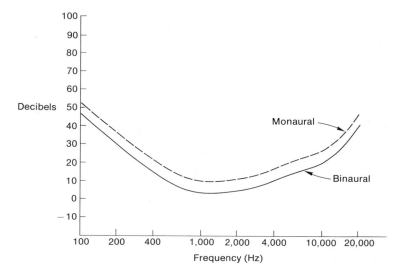

Notice that, when the sounds are presented to only one ear (the *monaural* curve), all the thresholds are higher than when the sounds are presented to both ears (the *binaural* curve).

With advancing age, the thresholds for high-frequency sounds increase.

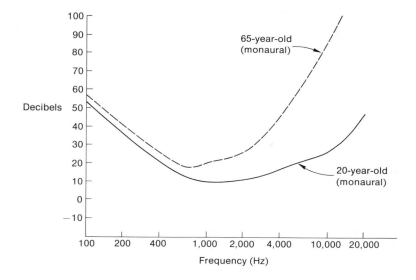

As we've previously indicated, this high-frequency hearing loss occurs as a result of damage to the hair cells near the base of the cochlea.

If hair cells throughout the cochlea are damaged by disease or by exposure to loud noises (containing many frequencies) or by the use of those drugs that attack the hair cells, all the thresholds increase. If, however, an individual is exposed to very loud sounds of particular pitches, the thresholds are elevated only for those frequencies. Such a narrow range of elevated thresholds is often called a *tonal gap*.

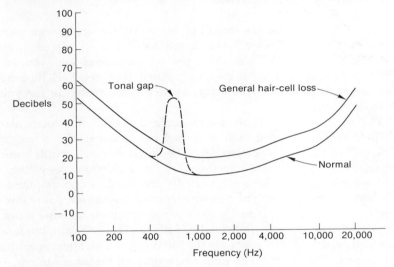

Rather than measuring an individual's thresholds to sounds of different frequencies, we could measure an individual's ability to discriminate between two sounds that differ in either intensity of frequency. In either case, we would be measuring the individual's difference thresholds. As you already know, *Weber's Law* applies to audition as well as to vision: two tones will have to differ by a particular ratio in order to be discriminable.

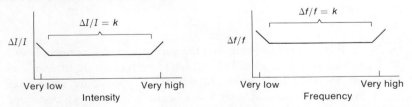

The curve on the left indicates that, over the broad middle range of intensities, two sounds must differ in intensity by a particular ratio if they are to be perceived as being different. The curve on the right indicates that, for two sounds to be perceived as having different pitches, their frequencies must differ by a particular ratio. In both cases, Weber's Law accurately describes our difference thresholds over the broad middle range of sounds we can hear. At the extremes, Weber's Law is not correct.

The Theory of Signal Detection

Let's closely examine the situation in which we could test your thresholds to sounds of different amplitudes. You are placed in an acoustically insulated room. You put on earphones and you are instructed to pay attention to a warning light in the room. Each time the warning light comes on, you are asked to report whether or not you heard any sound.

The experimenter begins by selecting a sound of a particular frequency. The warning light is turned on, and then the sound is delivered through the earphones. The experimenter records your report: either "yes, I heard something," or "no, I didn't hear anything." The same frequency sound is repeatedly presented, and its amplitude is systematically varied. The experimenter may begin with a very low-amplitude sound and gradually increase the amplitude; at other times, the sound may be made quite loud initially, and then the amplitude is gradually reduced. We might get the following results after repeating the sequence 10 times. (The numbers signifying the sound intensity level are arbitrary.)

Sound Intensity Level	Percentage "Yes"	Percentage "No"
1 (low)	0	100
2	20	80
3	40	60
4	60	40
5	80	20
6 (high)	100	0

Notice that the results indicate that the softest sound was never heard (0% "yes") and the loudest sound was heard each of the 10 times it was turned on (100% "yes"). Intermediate sounds were only sometimes heard. For example, sound level 2 was heard on 2 of the 10 occasions when it was turned on (20% "yes"). On the other 8 occasions when this same sound was presented, it was not heard. This should remind you of

a similar situation we encountered when talking about visual thresholds: the responses of the individual vary when we repeatedly present a
stimulus. When we explored the problem before, we found that the
reason the responses vary is that lights vary. They do not always
produce the same number of quanta. In audition, the problem has been
tackled in a slightly different way. The approach that is used is called
The Theory of Signal Detection, or *TSD* for short.

Let's begin by considering the responses to sound level 3. Out of a
total of 10 presentations, that sound was heard 4 times but it was not
heard 6 times. For the moment, let's think about the situation: there you
are, sitting in a quiet room with earphones on, watching a warning light,
listening for a very soft sound. Maybe you sometimes reported hearing
the sound simply because you knew there was "supposed to be" a
sound. If you knew that a sound was supposed to come on each time the
warning light came on, you might tend to say that you heard it even if
you didn't.

One way we could test this idea would be to have some "catch" trials:
the experimenter could occasionally turn on the warning light without
turning on any sound at all. Suppose we have the experimenter present
10 "real" trials during which sound level 3 comes on and, intermingled
among them, 10 "catch" trials during which no sound comes on. Then
we could keep track of the percentage of your "yesses" and "noes" on
each kind of trial

	Percentage "Yes"	Percentage "No"
"Real" trials	40	60
"Catch" trials	20	80

We can call those instances when you said "yes" and there really was
a sound present, *hits.* If you said "no" and there really was a sound
present, we'll call it a *miss.* If you said "yes" but no sound was present,
we have a *false alarm.* And if you said "no" and no sound was present,
we have a *correct response.*

	"Yes"	"No"
"Real" trial	Hit	Miss
"Catch" trial	False Alarm	Correct Response

How are we going to interpret the false alarms? Are they an
indication that you were just "guessing"?

Let's go a step further. Suppose we test an individual five different
times. Each time we will have 100 trials (the warning light will come on

100 times), but one time we'll have 90 "real" trials and 10 "catch" trials, the next time we'll have 70 "real" trials and 30 "catch" trials, and so on. In every case, the "real" trials will all involve turning on the same intensity of sound. We'll tell the individual how many "catch" trials to expect. Then we'll keep track of the percentages of hits and false alarms.

Number of Catch Trials	Percentage (Hit)	Percentage (False Alarm)
10	90	50
30	85	40
50	75	30
70	60	20
90	30	5

When there were 10 "catch" trials out of the total of 100 trials, the individual said "yes" on 50% of the "catch" trials (5 times) and on 90% of the "real" trials (81 times). When there were 70 "catch" trials out of the total of 100 trials, the individual said "yes" on 20% of the "catch" trials (14 times) and on 60% of the "real" trials (18 times). Notice that both the hits and the false alarms vary, depending on the number of "catch" trials that are introduced. And keep in mind that, no matter how many "catch" trials we have, the "real" trials are always exactly the same sound at the same intensity. Something strange is going on: sometimes the individual reports hearing the sound 90% of the time it's presented, and sometimes the individual reports hearing exactly the same sound only 60% of the time it is presented. Maybe we just won't be able to decide whether or not the individual "really" hears the sound at all!

Before we come to that conclusion, let's explore this some more. Notice that, the more "catch" trials there are, the less often the individual says "yes." ("Yes" scores either a hit or a false alarm. Because both hits and false alarms decrease when there are more "catch" trials, the individual must be saying "no" more often and scoring more misses and correct responses.) Maybe when there are lots of "catch" trials, the individual builds up a tendency to say "no."

Let's try making a graph of our results, plotting the percentage of hits against the percentage of false alarms.

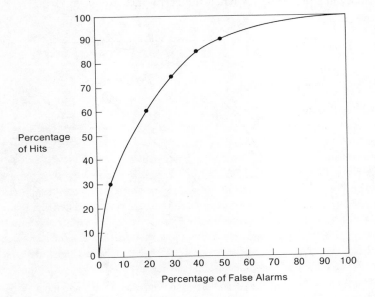

This graph is called the *receiver-operating characteristic* or, for short, the *ROC*. What would the ROC look like if, unknown to us, our individual had never put the earphones on? The only thing the individual would know is about how many "catch" trials to expect. He or she could not ever hear the sound because the earphones weren't on, and all the individual could do is guess "yes" or "no" each time the warning light came on. If the individual knows that there will be very few "catch" trials, he or she is likely to guess "yes" most of the time. That means that both the hits and false alarms will be high. If the individual knows that there will be a great many "catch" trials, he or she is likely to guess "no" most of the time, and both the hits and false alarms will go down.

The ROC would be a straight line, running from lower left to upper right. This is called the *guessing line*, and we can compare it to our individual's performance when the earphones are worn.

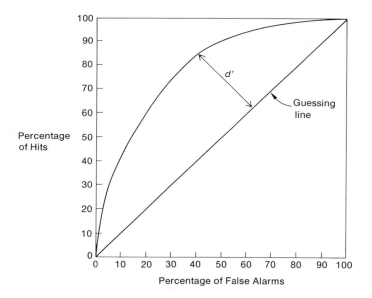

The maximum distance between the two curves is called d' (pronounced "dee-prime"), and it is a measure of how much better than guessing our individual's performance was.

Suppose we re-run the five sequences of trials just as before, but this time we use a louder sound during the "real" trials. The louder the sound is, the more easily our individual will be able to discriminate between the "real" trials and the "catch" trials. Perhaps now when there are 10 "catch" trials out of the total of 100 trials, the individual scores only 20% false alarms but gets 95% hits, and when there are 70 "catch" trials, he or she scores 10% false alarms but gets 80% hits. If we added the curve for these sequences to the ROC, we'd get.

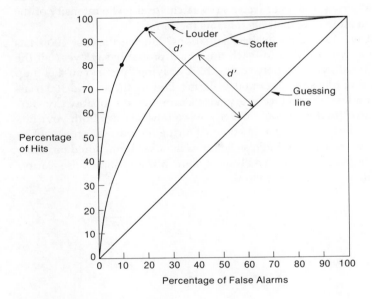

The curve is more bowed and we can summarize the difference by saying that d' is larger; the individual's performance is better than it was before. Now we can make two statements. First, if we use a more intense sound, the individual's overall performance will be better (that's not surprising). Second, whatever sound intensity we use, the individual's performance will change depending upon the numbers of "catch" trials and "real" trials the person expects. The second point is perhaps surprising, especially when you consider that we began all this by trying to discuss thresholds. Now we've come to a point where the individual's "thresholds" seem to vary depending upon something that has nothing to do with the sound itself.

We can examine this second point in another way. Suppose we test our individual all over again. This time we'll always give the individual 100 trials, 25 of which will always be "catch" trials. On the "real" trials, the sound will always be the same; we'll keep it quite soft. Before the first 100 trials, we tell our individual that he or she will win 5¢ for each hit that is scored. Then we run the 100 trials. Before the next 100 trials, we tell our individual that he or she will now lose 5¢ for every false alarm. Again, we run the 100 trials. Finally, before the last 100 trials, we tell our individual that he or she will win 5¢ for every hit but lose 5¢ for every false alarm. Notice that the only thing that changes from one set of trials to the next is the payoff. Each set contains 100 trials, 75 of which are "real" trials and 25 of which are "catch" trials. The intensity of the sound on all the "real" trials remains the same.

What would you do in these situations? During the first 100 trials when you win a nickel for each hit, you'd probably say "yes" all the time (after all, you can only score a hit by saying "yes"). You'd end up with a lot of hits and a lot of false alarms. During the second 100 trials when you lose a nickel for every false alarm, you'd probably say "no" all the time (that way you'd never score a false alarm). Both your hits and false alarms would go way down. During the third 100 trials, when you win 5¢ for each hit but lose 5¢ for each false alarm, you'd probably be as careful as possible. You'll score some hits and some false alarms. The ROC would look as follows.

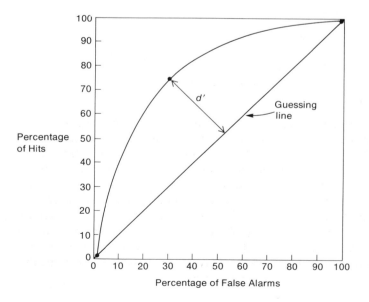

What would happen if we re-ran this payoff game, but we used a more intense sound on all the "real" trials? Again, when you were faced with the situations in which you either won a nickel for every hit or lost a nickel for every false alarm, you'd say "yes" or "no" all the time. When you were faced with the situation in which hits earned nickels and false alarms cost nickels, you'd once again be very careful. Because the "real" trials are now more intense, you'd probably end up doing better in the win–lose situation than you did before. Let's add these results to the ROC.

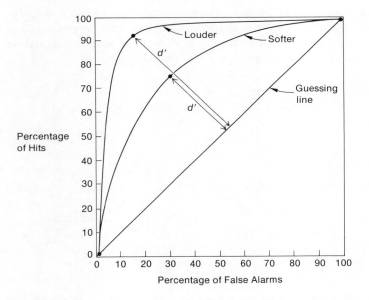

Just as we noticed before, your overall performance is certainly affected by the intensity of sound that's used on the "real" trials. But in addition, your performance is affected by something that has nothing to do with the sound itself; your performance depends, in part, on the payoff you'll receive.

What we are now saying is that your ability to hear a sound can be influenced by the situation in which you are tested. But we started all this by trying to understand auditory thresholds, and now we're talking about something very different from thresholds.

In fact, TSD suggests that the concept of a threshold is inappropriate. The theory suggests that we can measure how much better than guessing an individual will do (d') in various circumstances, but that the circumstances in large part determine the individual's performance.

Those who support TSD argue that there really is no such thing as "the threshold." They propose that we should forget about that concept and concentrate instead on an individual's performance in a particular situation.

All of that seems reasonable enough, but how can we reconcile it with the conclusions we reached when discussing the experiment on the absolute visual threshold? Should we just forget about the concept of a threshold when we're dealing with audition, but use the concept of a threshold when dealing with vision? Let's see if there's a way to reconcile the work in audition and vision.

Remember that I said that we produce sound: breathing, heartbeats, the rush of blood, and the movements of our body are noisy. The amount of sound we produce varies from moment to moment, and we can represent our sound production as follows.

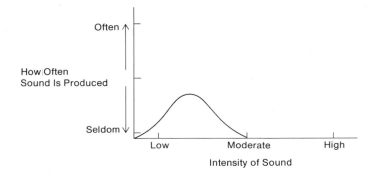

This graph indicates that, on the average, we produce a relatively low level of sound. Once in a while, we produce considerably less or more.

If a sound of a particular intensity is delivered to our ears through earphones, the amount of disturbance it creates in the cochlea varies. Sometimes the middle-ear muscles will be semicontracted (this happens when we yawn, swallow, or clench our jaws), and the stapes will not move in and out against the oval window as much as it otherwise would. Sometimes there will be a slight gap between the earphones and the pinna and, as a result, not all the sound intensity will be delivered to the eardrum. Then again, sometimes everything will be working perfectly, and the sound will create a larger disturbance in the cochlea than the sound usually does. Notice that the sound intensity, as it comes out of the earphones, is kept constant. It is the intensity of the effect of the sound on the cochlea that varies.

Suppose the sound coming out of the earphones is moderately soft. We can represent the intensity of the sound's effect on the same graph we used before.

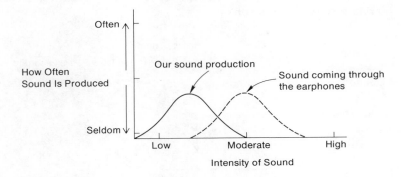

If the sound coming out of the earphones is fairly soft, the two distributions will overlap quite a bit as indicated in the graph. If the earphone sound is very loud, its distribution will be shifted to the right, and the two distributions will overlap very little.

Imagine that the sound is fairly soft. You are sitting, with earphones on, trying to decide whether a sound came through the earphones when the warning light came on. If no sound came through the earphones, you would hear only the sounds produced by your body. If a sound did come through the earphones, you'd hear the effects of that sound plus the sounds created by the body. Suppose you heard something that seemed quite loud. You'd probably decide that a sound must have come through the earphones, because your body rarely produces a loud sound. If you heard something very soft, you'd probably decide that no sound had come through the earphones, and that what you'd heard was sound produced by your body. But what if you heard something that was moderately loud? Such a sound would correspond to the region of overlap between the distributions, and you might have some trouble deciding whether or not something came through the earphones. The sound could have been produced by your body alone, or it could have been the combination of sound produced by your body and sound coming through the earphones. You'd have to decide, somewhat arbitrarily, just how loud the sound would have to be before concluding that something had come through the earphones. The loudness level you choose is called your *criterion cutoff*. If you had to make sure you never missed a sound that came through the earphones but it didn't matter how many false alarms you made, you'd set the criterion cutoff quite low. If you had to make sure that you never scored a false alarm but it didn't matter how many misses you made, you'd set the criterion cutoff rather high. If both hits and false alarms were important, you'd set the criterion cutoff in the middle. We can represent these three criterion cutoffs on the graph.

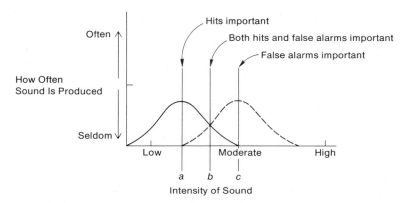

Suppose you had picked the lowest cutoff. You'd say "yes, I heard a sound" whenever the intensity was above that cutoff. You'd score lots of hits, but you'd also score lots of false alarms. If you had picked the highest cutoff, you'd score few hits, but you'd also score few false alarms.

We can represent the situation in which a more intense sound was used on the "real" trials as follows.

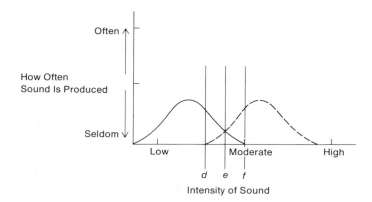

Notice that the degree of overlap between the two distributions has changed. The criterion cutoffs also shift. Now if you apply the middle criterion cutoff, you will score more hits and fewer false alarms than you scored when you used the middle criterion cutoff but the "real" trials involved a less intense sound.

What we've described is really the basis for the ROC curves. Each criterion cutoff is represented in the ROC as one point on a curve. The two different sound intensities are represented as two different curves.

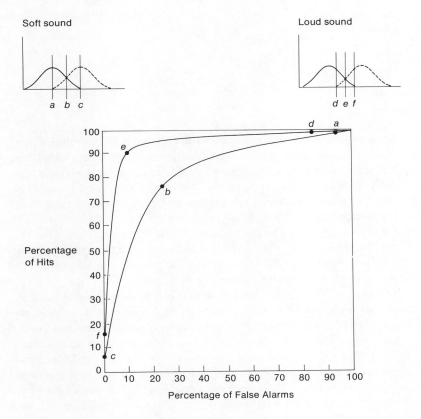

In the circumstances we described earlier, when the payoffs for hits and false alarms do not change but the percentages of "real" trials and "catch" trials do, something very similar is going on. In that case, individuals establish criterion cutoffs based on their expectations of the proportions of "real" and "catch" trials that will occur.

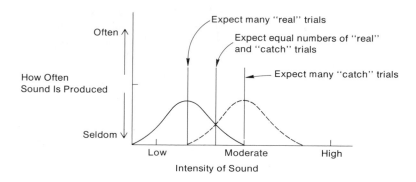

Let's now return to the experiment dealing with the absolute visual threshold. Remember that Hecht, Shlaer, and Pirenne concluded that people require a certain number of quanta in order to see a light. For some people, 5 quanta are required. For others, it may be 6 or 7. The number of quanta required can be thought of as a criterion cutoff. In other words, the results of the experiments by Hecht, Shlaer, and Pireene can be viewed as *one* point on *one* ROC curve. If we reran the experiment with "catch" trials and either we varied the proportions of "real" and "catch" trials or we varied the payoffs for hits and false alarms, we could generate a complete ROC curve.

In the case of audition, we know that our bodies make noise and, when we try to detect a sound coming in from the "outside" world, we have to make a decision about whether what we hear is just our bodily noise or something else. In the case of vision, our bodies do not make light. However, the axons in the visual system do produce nerve impulses even when no physical light is present. This ongoing activity produces a situation that is perfectly analogous to the one in audition. When we try to detect a light coming in from the "outside" world, we have to make a decision about whether what is going on in the visual system is just the maintained discharges of axons or something else.

Let's summarize what TSD is saying. The level of activity in a sensory system varies from moment to moment because of variations in both the system itself and the effects of any "outside" physical stimulus on that system. Even under the most rigorously controlled conditions, the variations will exist. Faced with the uncertain and confusing results of ever-changing activity, people will adopt rules for making decisions. The rules will be determined by factors that are not part of the sensory system itself, but are linked to such considerations as expectations and consequences.

But what happened to the idea of an absolute threshold? What happened to the apparently reasonable notions that a particular minimum amount of light is required for seeing and that a particular minimum amount of sound is required for hearing? We may still want to talk about the threshold of a receptor cell or neuron, but the decision-making properties of organisms confronted by uncertainty cannot be denied. We can determine an individual's sensitivity in a particular setting, but we cannot find a fixed, unchanging, absolute threshold.

Ohm's Acoustic Law

Rather than discussing what occurs when relatively pure tones of varying intensities or frequencies are heard, we can focus our attention on what occurs when combinations of tones are heard. Suppose, for example, I strike three piano keys at once. What would you hear? How does that compare with what happens if you look at a light composed of three different wavelengths?

The difference is somewhat remarkable when you think about it. The auditory system analyzes a complex sound in such a way that we hear the individual components. The visual system analyzes a light in such a way that we see a blend but not the individual components. If I strike three piano keys, you can hear the three notes. If you look at a mixture of red, green, and blue light, you see something white and you have no perception of the original colors.

In order to understand the kind of analysis that takes place in the auditory system, let's reconsider the nature of sound. If we could create a truly pure tone, we would have a situation in which each cycle of the sound wave was identical to every other cycle of that wave. Such a regularly repeating wave is called a *sine wave*. We've already indicated that it's not possible to produce or hear a pure tone. The best we can do is have a relatively pure tone. One way to think about a relatively pure tone is to imagine that it is the combination of a few truly pure tones. For example, if we add together two pure tones that differ in frequency, amplitude, and phase, we'll get the following.

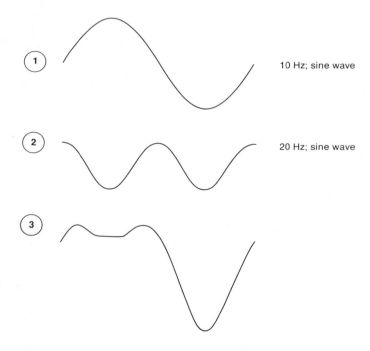

(1)   10 Hz; sine wave

(2)   20 Hz; sine wave

(3)

The first two waves are sine waves. Notice that these waves are made up of regularly repeating cycles. The third wave is not a sine wave. It is, however, the sum of the two sine waves. The first two waves have just been added together algebraically. Let's see how this works.

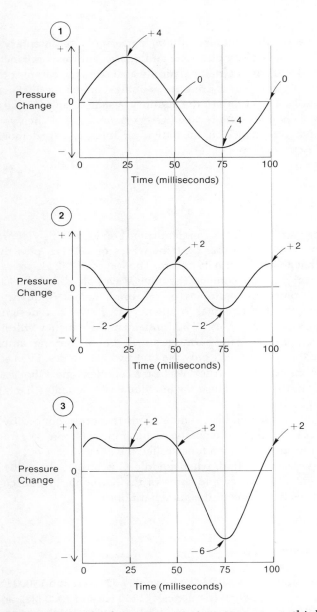

Thus, although our third wave is not a sine wave, we can think of it as the sum of a series of sine waves. And any wave, no matter how complicated, can be thought of in this way. When you take a wave and represent it as the sum of a series of sine waves, you are performing what's called *Fourier* (pronounced "foor'-yay") *Analysis.*

In a sense, the auditory system performs a rudimentary Fourier analysis: it takes a complex tone and figures out the components. The auditory system is not mathematically analyzing the complex tone into a series of sine waves, but it is doing something that's roughly comparable. The ability of the auditory system to analyze the components of a complex tone is called *Ohm's Acoustic Law*. When you hear a chord and you can pick out the individual notes, you are demonstrating Ohm's Acoustic Law.

The Individual Note

Suppose I strike middle C on the piano. You know this will produce a complex sound wave that contains waves of 262 Hz, plus the other waves that give the piano its timbre. The waves of 262 Hz are called the *fundamental frequency;* some of the other waves are called the *harmonics.* The harmonics are multiples of the fundamental frequency. If we designate the fundamental frequency as f, we can designate the harmonics as $2f$, $3f$, $4f$, etc. The fundamental frequency will have the largest amplitude. The harmonics will be of varying amplitudes. Imagine that we can hear only the first two harmonics. Even so, when the note of middle C is struck, we hear a complex tone. Ohm's Acoustic Law tells us that we will hear the individual components (that is f, $2f$, $3f$) instead of a blend.

In addition, we will hear some sounds that are produced by the ear itself. Recall our discussion of the cochlear microphonic. We found that the ear introduces its own tones called the *aural harmonics.*

Now we can say that, when middle C is struck, we will hear the fundamental frequency and some of the harmonics produced by the piano, as well as some of the aural harmonics.

Combination Tones

Suppose I simultaneously strike two notes, 1200 Hz and 1500 Hz. There will be two fundamental frequencies (1200 Hz and 1500 Hz), and there will be two sets of harmonics (multiples of 1200 Hz and 1500 Hz). In addition, there will be the aural harmonics.

And there will be even more. There will be *combination tones* which, as their name implies, are the results of the interactions of the original tones. The combination tones are not physically present in the sounds.

They are, however, present in our perception of the sounds. There are two kinds of combination tones: *summation tones* and *difference tones.*

The summation tone sounds like a tone that has the frequency of the sum of the original tones. In our example, the original tones were 1200 Hz and 1500 Hz. Their summation tone has a pitch identical to a tone of 2700 Hz.

The difference tone sounds like a tone that has the frequency of the difference between the original tones. In our example, the difference tone has a pitch identical to a tone of 300 Hz.

The harmonics of the original tones will also interact to produce summation tones and difference tones. Now we can say that, if two tones are played, we hear the fundamental frequencies, their harmonics, the aural harmonics, and the combination tones created by the fundamental frequencies, as well as their harmonics.

Where do the combination tones arise? Do they occur in the ear or in the brain? One way to answer the question is first to arrange things so that both tones (the 1200 Hz and 1500 Hz) are sent to one ear (a *monaural* arrangement), and then to arrange things so that one tone goes to one ear while the other tone goes to the other ear (a *binaural* arrangement). When we use the first arrangement, we can hear the combination tones but, when we use the second arrangement, there are no combination tones.

In both arrangements, the brain receives information about both tones. If the combination tones occur because of the way the brain interprets auditory information, we should expect to hear combination tones in both arrangements. But if combination tones occur because of the way the ear works, we should expect to hear combination tones only in the monaural arrangement. The outcome is that combination tones occur only in the monaural arrangement; therefore, they occur in the ear. They probably arise in the cochlea, where the traveling waves interact with each other and activate hair cells at particular locations along the basilar membrane.

Beats

If you listen to two tones that are very similar in frequency, you don't hear the usual combination tones. Instead you hear *beats.* The beats sound like a waxing and waning of loudness. As an example, suppose we simultaneously play tones of 1000 Hz and 1010 Hz. We would hear the fundamental frequencies, the harmonics, the aural harmonics, and an additional, beating tone. The beating tone seems to have a pitch comparable to the frequency midway between the fundamental frequencies, and it seems to beat at a rate that is equal to the difference between the fundamental frequencies. In our example, the beating tone would have a pitch comparable to a tone of 1005 Hz, and its loudness would seem to wax and wane at a rate of 10 times per second.

Beats are used in tuning instruments. Suppose we're trying to tune a violin's middle C to a piano's middle C. We'd tighten or loosen the appropriate violin string so that the two instruments produced approximately the same note. To make the tuning precise, we'd play the violin and piano at the same time. Suppose the violin actually produces 260 Hz and the piano produces 262 Hz. It is difficult to hear the difference in these notes if they're played individually. However, if they're played together, we will hear a third tone of intermediate pitch whose loudness seems to increase and decrease twice per second. When the instruments are precisely tuned, there will be no tone whose loudness seems to wax and wane.

Where do the beats arise? Once again, we can use a monaural arrangement (both tones delivered to one ear) and a binaural arrangement (one tone delivered to each ear). In both cases, we hear beats if the two tones are quite similar in frequency. In the binaural arrangement, the loudness of the beating tone doesn't appear to wax and wane. Instead the beating tone seems to move back and forth inside the head, from left to right (for this reason, *binaural beats* are often called *rotating tones*). The rate at which it moves back and forth depends upon the difference between the frequencies of the original tones.

Despite this perceptual difference between monaural and binaural beats, we can say that beats occur whether or not both tones go to one ear. We can conclude that beats occur because of the way the brain interprets auditory information.

Masking

It's beginning to seem that we should hear a huge number of sounds when only two notes are played. Yet we know that we don't hear all the harmonics or all the combination tones. Why not?

Some of the harmonics may be "too soft" to hear. But what does this really mean? Consider the following: in a quiet room, you may be able to hear the quiet hum of a fan or air-conditioner or heater. If the room becomes noisy, you may not be able to hear the hum any longer, even though it is still present. We could say that the louder sounds hide or *mask* the hum.

Any sound can mask another sound if it is intense enough. Sounds that are similar in frequency to the masker are masked most easily. In order to mask sounds that are very different in frequency, the masker must be made more intense.

Where does masking arise? Masking occurs in both monaural and binaural arrangements. But in the binaural arrangement, the masker must be made considerably more intense than in the monaural arrangement. In fact, it is sometimes argued that binaural masking only occurs when the masker is made so loud that it is carried as bone-conducted sound to the other ear. In a sense, this is no longer a binaural arrangement because both sounds actually arrive at one ear.

Although there is disagreement over binaural masking, researchers agree that masking does not occur because the masker somehow prevents the other sound from reaching the ear or having its effect on the cochlea. Even when a sound is masked, information about it can be found in the cochlear microphonic. Evidently masking represents a failure of the auditory system to extract all the information that's available from the cochlea.

Summary

Be sure you understand and can define all the italicized terms.

Studies of auditory thresholds have shown that our *binaural thresholds* are lower than our *monaural thresholds,* that *Weber's Law* accurately describes our ability to discriminate among sounds of different intensities or frequencies over the middle ranges, and that thresholds vary considerably. The variability of auditory thresholds was discussed under the framework of *TSD.*

In TSD, the *hits* and *false alarms* are graphed on *ROC* curves. The results reveal that the ability of individuals to detect a sound depends critically upon the situation in which the individuals are tested. The concept of a *criterion cutoff* underlying our sensitivity (as measured by d') is substituted for the traditional concept of an absolute threshold.

Our perceptions of sounds were described with reference to *Ohm's Acoustic Law, fundamental frequencies* and the *harmonics, aural harmonics, combination tones, beats,* and *masking. Monaural* and *binaural arrangements* were described as methods of determining whether some of the effects occur in the ear or in the brain.

Recommended Readings

Here are three books that contain excellent chapters dealing with audition.

Alpern, M., M. Lawrence, and D. Wolsk.   *Sensory Processes.* Brooks/Cole, 1967. (Chapter 3.)

Geldard. F. A.   *The Human Senses,* 2nd ed. Wiley, 1972. (Chapters 6–8.)

Mueller, C. G.   *Sensory Psychology.* Foundations of Modern Psychology Series, Prentice-Hall, 1965. (Chapters 3 and 4.)

In addition, you may wish to read the following book, which more fully discusses many aspects of audition.

Yost, W. A., and D. W. Nielsen.   *Fundamentals of Hearing.* Holt, Rinehart & Winston, 1977.

13

The Skin Senses

Think for a moment about all the sensations you can perceive through your skin. The sensation most people think of first is touch. Vibration and tickle can be thought of as particular kinds of touch. But in addition to touch and its variations, there are also temperature (the perceptions of warmth and cold) and pain sensations.

It would be nice if we could examine the receptors contained in the skin, discover that there are several different types of receptors, and then demonstrate that each type of receptor is sensitive to just one form of stimulation. If we could accomplish this, we would be justified in identifying one type of receptor as the touch receptor, another as the cold receptor, and so on. Early investigators tended to assign receptors in just this way. However, more recent work has complicated the picture. Before we get involved in the complications, let's take a look at the structure of skin.

The Structure of Skin

Skin is actually rather interesting stuff. The outermost layer of skin, called the *epidermis*, is made up primarily of dead cells. The thickness of epidermis varies considerably from one body region to another: on your face, the epidermis is quite thin, while on the soles of your feet this outer dead layer is usually very thick, especially over those areas that are weight-bearing.

Underneath the epidermis, there is a rather thick layer of living cells. This layer, called the *dermis*, constantly produces new cells that are progressively moved to the surface, replacing epidermal cells (which continuously slough off). The dermis has a rich supply of blood vessels, sweat glands, sebaceous (oil-producing) glands, hair roots, and receptors.

The epidermis and the dermis, taken together, make up skin. Underlying the skin, there is a layer of connective tissue containing, among other things, fat.

Imagine that we could cut out a small cube of skin and the underlying connective tissue. Looked at from the side, it would have the following appearance.

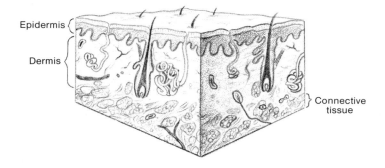

As you look at this sketch and think about the skin, you should keep in mind that skin is a resilient, flexible structure that is made even more resilient by the underlying pad of connective tissue. The receptors are found within the dermis, surrounded by tissues that absorb some of the impact of stimulation applied to the skin's surface. It shouldn't surprise you to realize that, when pressure is applied to the epidermis, only a fraction of that pressure ever reaches the receptors. Similarly, when heat or cold is applied to the epidermis, the receptors are partially insulated from the temperature change by the surrounding tissues.

(Furthermore, the blood vessels in the dermis bring a constant supply of body-temperature blood to the area. This unending, constant-temperature supply also tends to minimize the effects of hot and cold stimuli.)

The Receptors

Receptors in the dermis come in a bewildering variety of shapes and forms. They are all essentially the dendritic endings of neurons that collect information from the skin and carry it to the spinal cord. (We should stop here for a moment and clarify the term "dendritic ending." Information is carried from the receptor, along a neuronal filament, toward a cell body located near the spinal cord. Because the neuronal filament conducts information toward a cell body, it seems appropriate to call that filament a dendrite. The neuronal filament that arises from the cell body and carries information into the spinal cord is the axon. However, in some instances, both filaments are capable of producing nerve impulses. In other words, the filament we are calling a dendrite fits only part of the usual description of dendrites: it conducts information toward a soma, but it produces spikes rather than graded potentials. These atypical dendrites are found, here and there, throughout the nervous system, particularly in neurons that collect information from the skin, muscles, tendons, and joints. We'll continue to call them dendrites so that the direction of information flow will be clear.) However, most of these dendritic endings bear some kind of elaborate structure that is nonneural. Over the years, anatomists examined the structures and christened them with such delightful names as the Krause end bulb, the Ruffini cylinder, and the Meissner corpuscle (as you may have guessed, anatomists tend to name their discoveries after themselves or other anatomists). It then remained for physiologists to discover the function of each type of receptor.

The basic procedure was straightforward enough: select one region of the skin, explore it with a variety of stimuli, and then try to correlate the sensations you feel with the receptors found in that area. You might, for example, warm a blunted needle to a given temperature and then touch the needle to different spots on the back of your hand. When you locate a spot that seems especially sensitive to the warmed needle, you could cut out that portion of skin and examine it under a microscope. The same procedure could be used with a cooled, blunted needle or with a body-temperature needle that was either blunted (to locate touch spots) or sharpened (to locate pain spots). In each case, you would search the appropriate piece of skin under the microscope, looking for the receptors. The expectation was that a spot especially sensitive to one kind of stimulation would contain one kind of receptor. However, the results were confusing. Some researchers seemed to agree that Krause end bulbs are always found in spots especially sensitive to cold, that Ruffini cylinders are always found in spots especially sensitive to warmth, and that Meissner corpuscles are associated with touch spots. But, all too often, a variety of receptors would be found in all the spots, or a Ruffini cylinder might appear where a Krause end bulb or Meissner corpuscle ought to be. More and more researchers made little holes in their skins, but the self-sacrifice didn't make things any clearer. One of the reasons why researchers persisted in this painful exercise was their belief that each kind of receptor should be capable of signaling just one kind of stimulation. Their conviction was founded on a well-accepted tenet of physiology, which was first formulated during the nineteenth century, and which had since guided a considerable amount of research. That tenet is called the *Law of Specific Nerve Energies.*

The Law of Specific Nerve Energies

The Law of Specific Nerve Energies is really quite simple. It states that, no matter how a nerve is stimulated, it will produce the same sensation. If, for example, we stimulate the optic nerve by shining a light in the eye, of course we experience a visual sensation. If the optic nerve is stimulated by pressure on the eyeball, we also experience a visual sensation. In fact, if we stimulate the optic nerve by warming it or cooling it or squeezing it, we experience a visual sensation. The important point is that our experience is determined by the area of the brain to which a nerve sends its information. The optic nerve sends information to areas of the brain responsible for interpreting visual information. The optic nerve does not "know" what stimulated it. It can only signal the fact that stimulation took place. Similarly, the areas of the brain involved in vision do not "know" what stimulated the optic nerve. They can only register the fact that the optic nerve was stimulated, and then they can interpret the stimulation in the one language available to them: the language of a visual event.

The law summarizes an important concept and , broadly speaking, it is correct. All stimulations of the optic nerve produce visual sensations; all stimulations of the auditory nerve produce auditory sensations; all stimulations of nerves collecting information from the skin produce skin sensations.

Researchers interpreted the Law of Specific Nerve Energies to mean that all stimulations of a nerve would produce sensations that are identical. Some of them went even further: they interpreted the law to mean that a particular *receptor* could produce one and only one kind of sensation. This interpretation of the law accounts for the zeal with which researchers excised pieces of their skin in the expectation of finding a one-to-one relationship between receptors and sensations.

It became increasingly clear that the receptors in the skin do not behave according to a strict interpretation of the Law of Specific Nerve Energies. Perhaps the best evidence in favor of abandoning the strict interpretation came from a study of the cornea. The cornea contains only one kind of receptor, the so-called *free nerve ending*. (The free nerve ending is simply a dendritic ending that bears no elaborate structure. Such naked dendritic endings are found throughout the dermis, along with the elaborate receptors.) In studies of the skin, some researchers had assigned the sensation of pain to free nerve endings. But, if a cold stimulus is applied to the cornea, we have the sensation of cold. If a warm stimulus is applied to the cornea, we experience warmth. We can also experience touch and pain if the appropriate stimuli are applied to the cornea. Now we have a situation in which four different sensations can be experienced, but only one type of receptor is present. Clearly, the Law of Specific Nerve Energies does not describe this situation. We can continue to accept the law in general terms, but we cannot use it to understand all receptors. Some receptors, such as the Pacinian corpuscle (which you'll meet in a little while), do respond to only certain kinds of stimulation, but others (such as the free nerve ending) are capable of responding to and signaling different kinds of information.

Pathways of the Skin Senses

Information from the skin receptors all over the body, below the level of the neck, is carried to the brain via the spinal cord. The actual pathways are a bit complicated; we need to take this somewhat slowly.

To begin, there are two distinctly different systems involved in getting information from the receptors to the brain: the *lemniscal system,* and the *extralemniscal system.* Both systems end up bringing information to the same general region of the cortex of the brain, but they follow very different pathways to the cortex. No one is sure why there should be two separate systems. Some researchers have suggested that the two systems carry different kinds of information. They suggest that the lemniscal system is primarily involved in carrying touch information, while the extralemniscal system deals primarily with pain and temperature information.

Others argue that the important difference between the two systems is the speed with which they conduct information. They note that the lemniscal system contains relatively few synapses. (In the lemniscal system, the first-order neurons bring the information all the way from the receptors to the lower portion of the brain, and the third-order neurons bring the information to the cortex. In the extralemniscal system, the first-order neurons bring the information only from the receptors to the spinal cord, and it may be a sixth- or seventh-order neuron that brings the information to the cortex.) Because synapses introduce delays, the lemniscal system conducts information more rapidly. Still others mention that the lemniscal system seems to have arisen relatively recently in the course of evolution, while the extralemniscal system seems to be evolutionarily very old.

We have a puzzle here and, truly, no one has fully sorted out the whys and howcomes. What we can be certain of is the fact that we are describing an arrangment unlike the ones we've encountered before.

The Lemniscal System

The first-order neurons in the lemniscal system can be extremely long. Their dendrites are part of the skin receptors; their axons do not synapse until they reach the lower portion of the brain. Imagine a skin receptor in your big toe. That receptor is basically a dendritic ending. The dendrite extends all the way from the receptor, up your leg, to the lower portion of the spinal cord. The cell body of the neuron is located alongside the spinal cord. The axon enters the dorsal portion of the spinal cord and runs up the entire length of the spinal cord to the brainstem. The whole collection of axons running up the spinal cord together is called the *dorsal tract.* There are actually two collections: the dorsal tract on the left side of the spinal cord, which carries information from the left side of the body, and the right dorsal tract, which carries information from the right side of the body. The dorsal tracts are fairly small at the base of the spinal cord; they become larger and larger toward the top of the spinal cord as additional axons join the tracts.

We can take a look at a sketch of a cross-section of the spinal cord, about midway between the base and top of the spinal cord. In the sketch, two neurons are indicated, one arising from the left side of the body and one from the right.

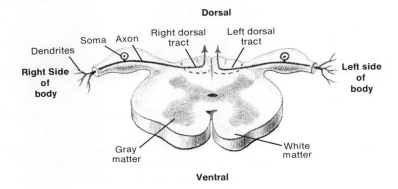

Imagine that the axons turn in the dorsal tracts and head upward, coming slightly out from the page. That is the direction in which they head on their way to the brain. Now imagine that the entire areas marked right and left dorsal tracts are bundles of axons heading up and out from the page. (By the way, are those dorsal tracts gray or white? Why?)

Those axons heading up and out from the page will finally synapse in a set of *nuclei* located in a lower portion of the brainstem called the *medulla.* Each of the dorsal tracts (right and left) has its own nuclei. The axons that arise from the nuclei in the medulla (that is, the axons of the second-order neurons) form two distinct bundles called the *medial lemnisci* (singular, lemnis*cus*). The nuclei of the right dorsal tract give rise to the right medial lemniscus, and the nuclei of the left dorsal tract give rise to the left medial lemniscus. (As you've probably guessed, the entire lemniscal system gets its name from the term, medial lemniscus. The word "lemniscus" comes from a Latin word for "ribbon," and indeed each medial lemniscus does look like a broad white ribbon coursing through the lower portion of the brain.)

The two lemnisci cross each other on their way from the dorsal tract nuclei to the thalamus. Thus, at the thalamus, the information that started out on the right side of the body is on the left side of the brain, and the information from the left side of the body is on the right side of the brain. The axons of the medial lemnisci synapse in an area of the thalamus devoted to the skin senses, called the *ventrobasal complex*. The axons that arise from the ventrobasal complex (that is, the axons of the third-order neurons) course upward to the area of the cortex just behind the central fissure. The neurons coming from the left ventrobasal complex go to the left side of the cortex; those coming from the right ventrobasal cortex go to the right side of the cortex. The area of the cortex just behind the central fissure is usually called *somatosensory cortex I*. Thus the left side of the body is represented on the right somatosensory cortex I, and the right side of the body is represented on the left somatosensory cortex I.

Let's now summarize the lemniscal system route.

First-order neurons: dendrites in skin;
                         axons ascend in the spinal cord, forming
                             the *dorsal tracts*.

Second-order neurons: dendrites collect information at the *dorsal
                             tract nuclei* located in the medulla;
                         axons form two broad ribbons, the *medial
                             lemnisci*, which *cross* each other on their
                             way to the thalamus.

Third-order neurons: dendrites collect information at the *ven-
                             trobasal complex* of the thalamus;
                         axons carry the information to *somatosen-
                             sory cortex I*.

The Extralemniscal System

The other system is, appropriately enough, called the extralemniscal system (the prefix "extra" means "other than," so this is a system "other than" the lemniscal system). It is also often called the *spinothalamic system*.

This system begins the same way as the lemniscal system: the first-order neurons have their dendritic endings in the dermis, and their axons enter the dorsal part of the spinal cord. However, these axons are short. They synapse just after they enter the spinal cord. The second-order neurons collect the information, carry it across the spinal cord to the opposite side, and then carry it up to the brain. The axons of these second-order neurons travel up the sides of the spinal cord in large bundles called the *spinothalamic tracts*.

Let's take another look at a sketch of a cross-section of the spinal cord. In this case, we'll include only one first-order neuron arising from the right side of the body.

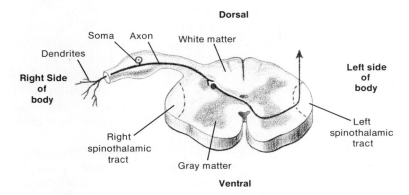

Again, you should try to imagine the spinothalamic tracts as bundles of axons heading upward and slightly out from the page.

It is important to keep in mind one of the profound differences between the lemniscal and extralemniscal systems: in the lemniscal system, information that starts out on the right side of the body travels up the right side of the spinal cord, while in the extralemniscal system information that starts out on the right side of the body travels up the left side of the spinal cord. Earlier in this chapter, I mentioned that some researchers believe that the lemniscal system carries touch information and that the extralemniscal system carries pain and temperature information. With this idea in mind, predict what would happen to an individual's skin senses if only the right side of the spinal cord were cut (imagine making the incision by sliding a blade parallel to the sketch above but only on the right side of the spinal cord). Do not read ahead until you've made your prediction!

All the axons arising along the right side of the spinal cord will be cut, and information from these axons will never reach the brain. The two bundles of axons of interest to us are the right dorsal tract and the right spinothalamic tract. The right dorsal tract is part of the lemniscal system. If it carries touch information from the right side of the body, this information would never reach the brain, and the individual would therefore be unable to sense touch on the right side of the body below the level of the cut. The right spinothalamic tract is part of the extralemniscal system. If it carries pain and temperature information from the left side of the body, the individual would be unable to detect pain or temperature on the left side of the body below the level of the cut. Notice that neither side of the body would be completely numb. Each side of the body would be insensitive to certain kinds of stimulation.

When an individual actually suffers the kind of damage we've described, that individual does indeed lose some sensitivity on both sides of the body. However, the actual loss of sensitivity is never quite as orderly as we've indicated. Usually some loss of touch, temperature, *and* pain sensitivity occurs on *both* sides of the body—even though the touch loss is greater on one side, and the pain and temperature loss is greater on the other side. What this means is that we can't neatly divide the lemniscal and extralemniscal systems simply on the basis of the kinds of sensations they carry.

But back to the extralemniscal system: the fate of the axons arising in the spinothalamic tracts is varied. Some of the axons go to the ventrobasal complex—the same thalamic area that receives information from the lemniscal system. More of the axons go to a different region of the thalamus, called the *posterior nuclear group.* Many of the axons go to the *reticular formation* in the brainstem. Still others may go to the cerebellum, via the *spinocerebellar system.* Eventually, either directly or indirectly, much of the information finally reaches the cortex. Although some of the information may reach somatosensory cortex I, most of the extralemniscal information ends up in a neighboring region of the cortex called *somatosensory cortex II.*

Let's now summarize the extralemniscal system route.

First-order neurons: dendrites in skin;
                        axons synapse as soon as they enter the
                            spinal cord.

Second-order neurons: dendrites collect information from first-
                            order neurons;
                        axons *immediately cross* to the opposite side
                            of the spinal cord and ascend as the
                            spinothalamic tracts.

Third-order neurons: may be part of the *ventrobasal complex* of the
                            thalamus;
                        may be part of the *posterior nuclear group* of
                            the thalamus;
                        may be part of the *reticular formation;*
                        may be in the *cerebellum.*

Fourth-order through
seventh-order neurons: there may be a whole series of neurons
                            that eventually bring the information to
                            somatosensory cortex II.

Skin Information from the Head

Receptors are found throughout the dermis of the head. Information from these receptors does not enter the spinal cord. Instead, information is carried directly to the *medulla* by cranial ("head") nerves. It is primarily the *trigeminal nerve,* the *facial nerve,* and the *vagus nerve* that innervate the head and upper-neck regions. However, the *glossopharyngeal nerve* ("glosso-" meaning tongue, "-pharyngeal" meaning pharynx) may contribute information from the mouth and throat. The axons of these cranial nerves synapse in nuclei in the medulla. From the medulla, information is sent to the thalamus (primarily to the ventrobasal complex), and from there to the cortex (primarily to somatosensory cortex I).

The Thalamic Relay Areas

As you now know, both the lemniscal and the extralemniscal systems have particular regions of the thalamus associated with them. The ventrobasal complex and the posterior nuclear group are dramatically different from each other. The differences between them should allow you to assess some of the differences between the lemniscal and extralemniscal systems.

Let's begin with the ventrobasal complex. The overwhelming majority of the neurons in it are associated with the lemniscal system. Perhaps the most outstanding feature of the ventrobasal complex is the orderly way in which the surface of the body is represented. Neurons that can be activated by stimulating the skin of the hand are grouped together in one location within the complex. Neurons that can be activated by stimulating the skin of the forearm are located nearby. Neurons that can be activated by stimulating the skin of the upper arm are found in another, neighboring location. And so on. The body surface is represented in such a way that relationships among body areas are preserved: the area representing the knee is found between areas representing the lower and upper leg. This kind of systematic mapping should not be new to you: we found something similar in the retinotopic maps within the visual system and the tonotopic maps within the auditory system. In the ventrobasal complex, we are dealing with the same principle. We can refer to it, logically enough, as *somatotopic mapping* ("somato-" meaning body).

The orderly arrangement doesn't stop there. Within each location in the ventrobasal complex, neurons are arranged so that those especially responsive to one kind of stimulation are grouped together. As an example, within the area of the ventrobasal complex representing the knee, all the neurons that are especially responsive to deep pressure on the skin of the knee are grouped together, and those that are responsive to changes in the position of the knee are grouped together. (We will take up the topic of our ability to detect the position of our limbs and the angles of our joints in the next chapter.) Thus within one component (the ventrobasal complex) of one structure of your brain (the thalamus), one-half of your entire body surface is systematically mapped out; and within each region of that map there is a further subdivision corresponding to the kind of stimulation applied to the skin. (The other ventrobasal complex in the other side of the thalamus takes care of the other half of your body.) If you are just a bit overwhelmed by this, you may want to reread the last few sentences. You should probably be more than just a bit overwhelmed by the intricacies of your nervous system!

Each neuron in the ventrobasal complex has a *receptive field*. Again, this concept should be rather familiar to you. Each neuron will be activated only when the appropriate area of skin is stimulated. Obviously a neuron that has collected information from the knee region will not react to stimulation of the skin overlying the ankle. More specifically, however, the neuron will react only to stimulation of one small region of the knee. Each neuron in the ventrobasal complex region representing the knee will have its own receptive field that differs slightly in location from all others, although two or more neurons may have overlapping receptive fields.

The sizes of receptive fields vary considerably and predictably. The most sensitive areas of the body (such as the hands and lips) have a very large concentration of receptors. Less sensitive areas (such as the back) have a much smaller concentration of receptors. Similarly, sensitive areas of the body are represented by great numbers of neurons in the nervous system, while less sensitive areas are represented by fewer neurons. When large numbers of neurons represent an area, the size of their individual receptive fields tends to be small. When few neurons represent an area, their individual receptive fields tend to be large. Thus the receptive field of a neuron involved in sensations from a finger may be only a few millimeters in extent. The receptive field of a neuron involved in sensations from the back may be several centimeters in extent.

Let's contrast all this with the situation in the posterior nuclear group. That region of the thalamus receives predominantly extralemniscal information. The differences are unmistakable. First, there is no systematic mapping out of the body surface in the posterior nuclear group. (A neuron that reacts to stimulation of the shoulder may be found right next to one that reacts to stimulation of the foot.) Second, there is no grouping of neurons based on the kind of stimulation to which they respond. In fact, many neurons respond to a wide variety of stimulation: a particular neuron may respond to light touch, deep pressure, cold, warmth, etc., applied to its receptive field. That brings up the third difference: the receptive fields tend to be extremely large. In fact, a neuron may respond to a wide variety of stimulations applied virtually anywhere along the body surface. Now *that's* a large receptive field!

The ventrobasal complex is astounding because of its precision and order. The posterior nuclear group is astounding because it is so higgledypiggledy (i.e., jumbled). No one knows how or why we came to have such an arrangement. There are some theories but, rather than discussing them (all of them are interesting but none is compelling), I think you should try to develop some theories of your own.

Somatosensory Cortex

You should be able to make some excellent guesses about somatosensory cortex I and II, based on what you now know about the ventrobasal complex and the posterior nuclear group. Just keep in mind that somatosensory cortex I receives most of its information from the ventrobasal complex, and somatosensory cortex II receives much of its information from the posterior nuclear group.

Somatosensory cortex I, located just behind the central fissure, is mapped out in an orderly way. The following sketches first identify the general location of somatosensory cortex I on the left side of the brain, and then give you a cross-sectional view of the left side of the brain through that area.

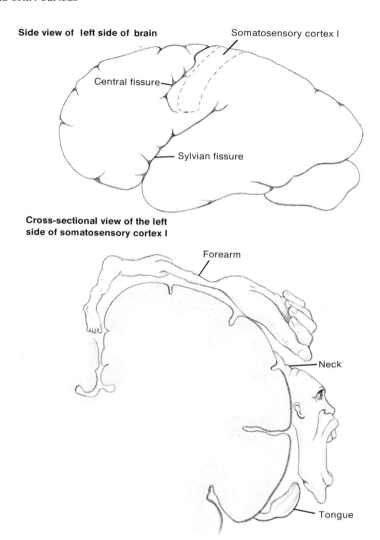

Side view of left side of brain

Somatosensory cortex I

Central fissure

Sylvian fissure

**Cross-sectional view of the left
side of somatosensory cortex I**

Forearm

Neck

Tongue

The weird "body" draped over the cross-sectional view shows you the way in which this area is mapped out. Notice that the map doesn't correspond very well to the shape or arrangement of your body. Although the foot, lower leg, and upper leg seem to be in the correct arrangement, the hand seems to be strangely positioned with reference to the head. Furthermore, the hand is enormous. So is the face. What the figure represents is the total area of somatosensory cortex I devoted to each body region. Those areas of the body that contain a great many receptors and are extremely sensitive are represented by large numbers of neurons in the cortex.

Don't be disturbed by the somewhat strange juxtapositions of body parts. The cortex does not need to have a representation of the body that is identical to the actual physical arrangement of the body. That correspondence is something that is learned—just as we found earlier that the true locations of up, down, left, and right are determined by experience, rather than by reference to actual directions on the retina or within the visual system. Once again, we must make note of the fact that the complex process by which this learning takes place is not well understood.

Somatosensory cortex I does, then, have a somatotopic map (even if its arrangement appears somewhat odd). There is the additional arrangement we discovered in the ventrobasal complex: neurons within each location on the cortex are further arranged so that those especially sensitive to one kind of stimulation are grouped together. The grouping in this case takes exactly the same form as the grouping we encountered in the visual cortex. The grouping is in the form of *columnar organization*: as an example, all the neurons that respond to light touch of the elbow are arranged in a column extending from the surface of the cortex inward to the depths of the cortex. Those neurons that respond to deep pressure of the elbow are located in a neighboring column, again running from the surface of the cortex inward, at right angles to the surface. Finally, the neurons all have receptive fields that are fairly small, although the neurons for the hand and face have the smallest receptive fields.

The receptive fields have been studied extensively. One of their most intriguing properties is the fact that they usually have outer inhibitory portions. In some ways, this is similar to what we found in the visual system with the center—surround receptive fields, and to the narrowing of the response areas in the auditory system. If the appropriate stimulus is applied to the outer edges of the receptive field, the neuron will decrease its firing rate. This arrangement probably adds to our ability to locate a stimulus on the skin. Touch a pencil point to your hand, without looking at your hand. You are probably able to determine, with considerable precision, the exact spot being touched. Recognize that when you touch your hand in this way, you are activating several receptors and many neurons. Because each neuron has a receptive field several millimeters in extent, the possible location of the pencil point could be anywhere within a fairly large area. But because you are simultaneously hitting the inhibitory areas of some receptive fields and the excitatory areas of others, you can narrow that fairly large potential area considerably, and you can locate the point being touched with more precision.

Let's move now to somatosensory cortex II.

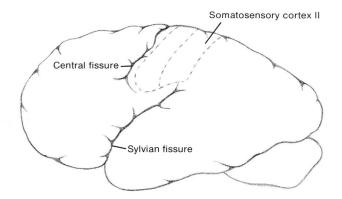

Although there is some mapping out of the body surface on somatosensory cortex II, it is not at all precise. Neurons representing a particular body area may be found roughly in the same general location but, beyond that, there is no somatotopic map. Neurons are not arranged in terms of the kind of stimulation to which they're sensitive. In fact, most neurons in somatosensory cortex II are sensitive to a variety of stimuli. The receptive fields are very large, and they do not contain discrete excitatory and inhibitory areas.

Somatosensory cortices I and II obtain their information from different sources and they are, in many ways, independent of each other. If, for example, somatosensory cortex II is removed, the neurons in somatosensory cortex I continue to function normally, and vice versa.

Now that we've examined the skin receptors and the pathways of the skin senses, we can take a closer look at the various kinds of sensations we can perceive through the skin.

Touch

Our sensitivity to touch stimuli varies considerably over the body surface. As you already know, our hands contain enormous numbers of receptors, and large portions of the somatosensory systems are devoted to neurons that process information coming from those receptors. Our legs, on the other hand, contain relatively few receptors, and proportionately smaller portions of the somatosensory systems are devoted to them. We can make systematic studies of various body regions; such studies can supply more exact information about this *regional variation* in sensitivity. We can, for example, determine how much weight must be applied against the skin in different regions before the individual will report feeling something. Suppose we blindfold you, and then rest different weights against the skin. You need only tell us "yes, I feel something" or "no, I don't feel anything." In this way we can discover the *threshold* for touch at a variety of locations. By now, such a threshold experiment should seem very familiar to you. As always, this kind of experiment is an attempt to discover the minimum amount of a stimulus required for the detection of that stimulus. As an example of the kind of results typically found in a threshold experiment on touch, take a look at the following.

Skin Region	Threshold in grams per mm^2
Tip of finger	3
Forearm	8
Leg	16
Sole of foot	250

If you carefully read the discussion of thresholds in audition and vision, you might be a bit concerned by now. Recall that, in those discussions, we decided that the results of any threshold experiment are influenced by the conditions of the experiment and by the uncontrollable variations in stimulation. In fact, we abandoned the idea that there is such a thing as "the" threshold. Those discussions still hold true, and it is certainly the case that the results of a threshold experiment in touch depend on these factors. For example, if we manipulated the consequences of "right" and "wrong" responses in a threshold experiment on touch, I'm sure we could substantially change the threshold figures. However, what is important here are not the exact threshold figures, but rather the *relative* threshold figures. As long as we take steps to insure that the conditions do not change throughout the experiment, we can make a legitimate comparison of the threshold on the fingertip versus the threshold on the forearm or leg or the sole of the foot. Thus, although we cannot conclude that a weight of less than 3 grams per mm^2 will never be detected at the fingertip, we can say with assurance that the fingertip is more sensitive than the forearm, that the forearm is more sensitive than the leg, etc.

Notice that the threshold figures are expressed in terms of grams per square millimeter. What this implies is that the appropriate stimulus to consider in any experiment on touch is the amount of weight applied against a *unit area* of the skin. This concept may be clearer if you consider the following question: will a penny placed on the skin seem to weigh more, less, or the same as a penny crushed to one-third its normal size placed on the skin? The true weight of the penny will not change, of course. But we are concerned with our perception of the weight. Because our perception depends upon the weight per unit area, the crushed penny will seem heavier to us. (Try this experiment. Cut two identical squares of aluminum foil, each about 3 inches on a side. Crumple one into a tight ball. Now place the flat square and the crumpled ball alternately on the back of your hand. Note the different weight sensations.)

Similarly, our perception of touch is dependent upon the amount of weight applied to the skin per *unit time.* If we lowered a penny onto the skin very, very slowly, that penny would seem to be lighter than one that was simply placed directly on the skin.

The fact that our perceptions depend upon the weight that is applied per unit area per unit time should not surprise you. We encountered the same thing in vision when we considered the trading ratios, and in audition when we considered the relationship between the intensity of sound and the length of exposure to the sound in producing noise-induced deafness. In the cases of vision and audition and in the present situation, we are simply recognizing the fact that our receptors and our nervous system are designed to integrate changes that occur within specified periods of time and within specified area limits. Perhaps the key word here is "changes." As you certainly know by now, we are not very good at detecting steady-state conditions. If a stimulus remains constant, we gradually adapt to it. Just as adaptation is a prominent feature of our visual and auditory perceptions, *adaptation* readily occurs in our perceptions of stimuli on the skin.

Adaptation in the skin senses is such a commonplace event that we rarely think about it: think for a moment about what happens when you wear a watch or a hat. When you put the article on, there is an initial period during which you're aware of sensations coming from your wrist or head. The longer the article remains in place, the less noticeable the sensations become. Usually you reach a point where the sensations cease. If your watchband or hatband is tight, it will take longer to reach the point when sensations cease. In formal language, we can describe this by saying that the rate of adaptation depends upon the intensity of stimulation. When you remove the watch or hat, you once again become aware of sensations arising from the wrist or head. Again, the sensations gradually subside.

Perhaps the best way to view all this is to think of adaptation as a process by which the nervous system resets its *baseline level*. Before you put on your watch, the neurons associated with the skin receptors maintain an ongoing level of activity (that is, the axons have a *maintained discharge*). The ongoing activity serves as a baseline against which any changes will be judged. When you put your watch on, the activity level is altered substantially but as this new activity level persists, the receptors and nervous system "accept" it as the new baseline against which changes will be judged. Then when you remove your watch, sensations arise because the ongoing activity will suddenly shift from the now-established baseline.

At the beginning of this chapter, we indicated that it is important to keep in mind the flexible, resilient nature of the skin. The receptors are cushioned by the surrounding tissues, and whatever force is applied to the surface of the skin will be "damped out" by the tissues. Therefore, a relatively mild stimulus to the skin's surface may be insufficient to activate the receptors. Furthermore, the skin's resilience tends to enhance adaptation in a purely mechanical way: when a constant stimulus is applied to the skin's surface, the tissues (because of their elasticity) tend to spring back to their original shapes and positions. As they do so, they reduce the forces reaching the receptors. This has the effect of reducing the effective intensity of the stimulation and thereby enhancing adaptation.

The Pacinian Corpuscle

One particular receptor in the skin has been studied in great detail. It is the *Pacinian* (pronounced "puh-sin'-ee-un") *corpuscle*. Unlike other skin receptors, the Pacinian corpuscle seems to be responsive to only one kind of stimulation, that of touch. The structure of this receptor is quite simple: it is a dendritic ending surrounded by layers of connective tissue. In longitudinal section, the receptor has the following appearance.

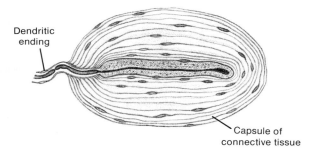

It is possible to place a recording electrode in or near the dendritic ending and to examine the responses of the receptor. When this is done, the first thing that becomes apparent is that the receptor responds neither to temperature changes of the skin, nor to such "painful" stimuli as a small incision in the overlying skin. It is, however, extremely responsive to pressure applied to the skin (the pressure can take the form of pushing or pulling on the skin). The receptor produces a graded depolarization, which increases in size as the stimulus intensity is increased.

One reason why the Pacinian corpuscle is of interest is that it provides an excellent system for studying adaptation. When pressure is applied to the skin or directly to the Pacinian's capsule of connective tissue and the pressure is then kept constant, the receptor responds with a graded potential that gradually wanes. When the pressure is removed, a graded potential is again produced and it too gradually wanes.

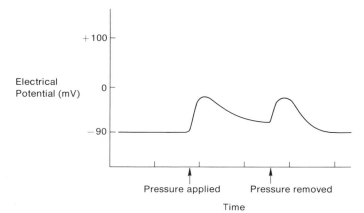

We might ask whether the waning of the graded potentials occurs because of a neural process or because of the springiness of the capsule. And we can answer the question by carefully stripping away the capsule and then repeating our experiment. What happens is that the receptor, even without its springy capsule, displays adaptation: the graded potential produced by either the application or the removal of the stimulus gradually wanes. However, the graded potential does not wane quite as much as it does when the capsule is in place. Thus, we can conclude that the basic mechanism of adaptation is neural, and that the springy capsule provides a mechanical means of enhancing adaptation.

Temperature

When people first begin thinking about our ability to detect stimuli of different temperatures, they often assume that this ability is based on a single "temperature sense." However, we now have a great deal of evidence indicating that we actually have two separate systems: a "warm sense" and a "cold sense." The most straightforward method of demonstrating our dual system is to make systematic explorations of a skin region with warmed and cooled stimuli. Suppose, for example, we mark out the back of the hand into very small squares. We can then touch a warmed probe to each square and identify those that seem especially sensitive to the stimulus. We can call those especially sensitive squares, the "warm spots." If we repeat the procedure with a cooled probe, we can also identify "cold spots." Although some squares are sensitive to both warmed and cooled probes, many of the squares are sensitive only to the warmed probe or only to the cooled probe (and some squares are quite insensitive to both probes). In other words, the "warm spots" and "cold spots" usually do not coincide. That bit of evidence certainly suggests that our ability to detect temperatures is not a unitary sense. We should point out that one sidelight of this kind of experiment is the discovery that, no matter what region of the body is explored, there are always more "cold spots" than there are "warm spots."

As you might expect, some regions of the body contain a larger complement of "warm" and "cold spots" than other regions. The hands (especially the fingers) and the face (especially the region around the lips) are areas particularly rich in these temperature "spots."

We indicated earlier that the skin, the underlying connective tissue, and the blood vessels found in the dermis all tend to reduce temperature changes before they affect the receptors. As an example of just how effective this "insulation" can be, consider the following: if we warm a probe that is 1.5 mm in diameter to a temperature 10°C warmer than skin temperature and place it on the skin's surface for 6 seconds, the maximum temperature increase that can be found just 1 mm below the skin's surface is only 1°C. If we use the same probe but cool it to 15°C below skin temperature and leave it in place for 6 seconds, the maximum decrease found just 1 mm below the surface is less than $\frac{1}{2}$°C. You should keep this insulation effect in mind whenever you consider our ability to detect temperature changes.

We can certainly demonstrate adaptation to temperature changes: think about what happens if you place one hand in a bucket of warm water. Initially you perceive the warmth but, if you let your hand remain in the water, gradually the water feels more and more neutral. If you then remove your hand from that bucket and place it in a bucket containing water of body temperature, you experience an initial sensation of coolness, followed by a gradual return to neutrality. This process is very much like the one we described for touch: the receptors and the nervous system establish a baseline level against which they compare any changes. In the present case, the baseline level is usually called *physiological zero*. Each skin area that is exposed to a given temperature will establish its own physiological zero, independent of other skin areas. With this in mind, think about what would happen if you placed your right hand in warm water and your left hand in cool water. After both hands had adapted, what would you experience if you simultaneously placed both hands in water of body temperature? (Try it!)

When we have a shift in physiological zero, our ability to detect temperature changes also shifts. In order to understand this point, think back about our discussions of the difference threshold. The question that is asked in any experiment on difference thresholds is, how different do two stimuli have to be before the individual notices that they are different? When our physiological zero is set at normal skin temperature (32°C), a stimulus must be at least 0.15°C warmer or cooler than 32°C for us to notice a difference. However, when our physiological zero is set at 40°C, we require a stimulus to be at least 0.5°C warmer or cooler than 40°C for us to notice a difference. Thus, when we adapt to a temperature, more than our physiological zero is changed; our sensitivity to temperature differences also changes.

Paradoxical Cold

It is possible to record from the axons entering the spinal cord and to locate those that produce nerve impulses when warmed or cooled probes are placed on the appropriate regions of the skin. These axons fall into two categories: those that react to warmed probes, and those that react to cooled probes. These have been logically named the *warm fibers* and the *cold fibers*. Both kinds of fibers display adaptation: they react to an appropriate stimulus with an initial burst of impulses that gradually subsides to a lower level, which persists as long as the stimulus is present.

Warm fibers, as you might expect, respond most to temperatures above the normal skin temperature. Cold fibers, on the other hand, react to temperatures below normal skin temperature. Take a close look at the following graph, which illustrates the responsiveness of these fibers.

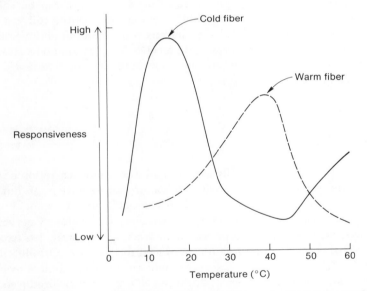

Notice that the warm fibers are not very responsive to temperatures above about 45°C. Notice that, although the cold fibers are very responsive to temperatures below 32°C, they are also responsive to temperatures above 45°C. That is strange indeed. No one knows why cold fibers should respond to high temperatures, but the fact that they do explains a strange phenomenon most of us have experienced: when the first few drops of a hot shower hit you, you often have the sensation of cold. What happens is that at least some of those first drops hit "cold spots" (remember that there are more cold spots than warm spots, so the odds are that more cold spots than warm spots will be hit; in addition, the cold fibers react faster than the warm fibers). The cold fibers collecting information from the "cold spots" respond vigorously, and our brain ends up interpreting that as "cold." As more drops of water hit you, more warm spots will also be hit, and the somewhat slower warm fibers will begin responding. At that point, both cold fibers and warm fibers are reacting, although the cold fibers are responding more vigorously. Our brain interprets the combination of moderate responding in the warm fibers and vigorous responding in the cold fibers as "hot." The initial perception of "cold" is usually called *paradoxical cold.*

Notice that the sensation "hot" does not arise because of a superstimulation of the warm fibers. In the language of the nervous system, "hot" means a particular *pattern of activity* that involves both sets of fibers. In fact, it is possible to produce the sensation "hot" even when no truly hot stimulus is presented. Two metal tubes can be coiled around each other and, if you hold the resulting double coil in your hand while one tube is filled with slightly warmed water and the other is filled with cooled water, you will perceive "hot." It should be clear to you that the sensation occurs because both sets of fibers will be activated by the double coil.

Pain

People usually think of pain as the result of extreme activation of the nervous system. After our discussion of the sensation of hot, it probably will not surprise you to discover that "pain" does not appear to be the result of superactivation. Extremely high rates of nervous-system activity can be produced by directing pulsating jets of air against the skin, but pain is not produced in that case. On the other hand, a fairly deep cut in the skin produces considerably less overall nervous-system activity yet, as I'm sure you know, pain is produced. In the language of the nervous system, "pain" is not synonymous with high levels of activity.

Perhaps the most interesting and exciting theory that attempts to explain the way in which the nervous system signals "pain" is the one developed by Ronald Melzack and Patrick Wall. The *Melzack–Wall Theory* begins with several well-founded and well-accepted concepts about the nervous system.

In the peripheral nervous system, axons can be classed into two distinct groups: those that are large in diameter, are heavily myelinated, and have relatively low thresholds (the so-called *L fibers*, "L" for large diameter); and those that are rather skinny, have little myelin, and have relatively high thresholds (the so-called *S fibers*, "S" for small diameter).

Afferent L fibers and S fibers bring information into the dorsal side of the spinal cord. Inside the spinal cord, there are several distinct layers of cells at this dorsal entry point. One of the layers encountered by the L fibers and S fibers as they enter the spinal cord is called the *substantia gelatinosa*. For the sake of simplicity, we can refer to this area as *SG*. Deeper within the spinal cord, there is a layer or region of cells that are called the *T cells* ("T" for transmission). These cells transmit information to other neurons within the spinal cord.

The L fibers, S fibers, SG, and T cells form the basic components of the Melzack—Wall Theory. According to the theory, the relationships among these components hold the key to understanding pain.

The theory stipulates that both the L fibers and the S fibers synapse onto both SG and the T cells. Some of the synapses are excitatory, while others are inhibitory. In particular, the synapses of the L fibers are all excitatory. The synapses of the S fibers onto the T cells are also excitatory, but the synapses of the S fibers onto SG are inhibitory. Finally, SG has an inhibitory effect on information reaching the T cells.

Let's put all this into a sketch that symbolically represents the components and the nature of their relationships. In the sketch, + and − refer to excitatory and inhibitory synapses, respectively.

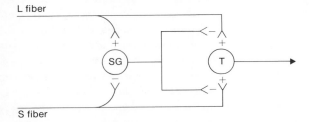

It takes a little while to get used to the sketch and the ideas it represents, so let's take this step by step. Imagine that we've activated only the L fiber. As the nerve impulse sweeps down the L fiber, it will activate SG. SG, in turn, will inhibit the axonal ending of the L fiber just before its synapse with the T cells. As a result, the T cells will not receive very much, if any, excitation.

Now imagine that we've activated only the S fiber. Nerve impulses in the S fiber will inhibit SG. When SG is inhibited, it is unable to exert its inhibitory effect on the axonal endings synapsing onto the T cells. The S fiber excites the T cells, and there will be some activation of the T cells.

Before you go any further, go back through the last two paragraphs *slowly*.

What will happen if both the L fiber and the S fiber are active? SG will receive both excitation (from the L fiber) and inhibition (from the S fiber). The net effect will be that SG will be less active than if only the L fiber were active, but it will be more active than if only the S fiber were active. As a result the axonal endings of the L and S fibers will be somewhat inhibited as they synapse onto the T cells. The net effect will be that the T cells will receive more excitation than if only the L fiber were active, but less excitation than if only the S fiber were active.

What is important to keep in mind is that Melzack and Wall argue that our perception of pain depends, in large part, on the amount of activity in the T cells. The greater their activity, the more likely we are to feel pain.

If you think back through this discussion, you should be able to recognize the fact that the *relative* amount of activity in the L fibers and the S fibers will ultimately determine the activity level of the T cells. As the proportion of L-fiber activity increases, T-cell activity decreases, and we are unlikely to experience pain. As the proportion of S-fiber activity increases, T-cell activity increases, and we are more likely to experience pain.

How could we increase the proportion of L-fiber activity? Because L fibers have low thresholds and S fibers have high thresholds, any mild stimulation should increase the proportion of L-fiber activity. That makes quite a bit of sense in terms of the ways we react to some kinds of pain: often when people have headaches, they rub or massage their foreheads. This mild stimulation often reduces the pain. I suspect that most people believe that the rubbing relaxes tense muscles, and that the pain reduction is a consequence of muscle relaxation. However, there is no good reason to believe that muscle tension is involved in most headaches. Whether or not it is, the Melzack–Wall Theory provides a fascinating alternative explanation. According to the theory, the mild stimulation provided by rubbing should activate the L fibers but not the high-threshold S fibers. Increasing the L-fiber activity will reduce T-cell activity, and pain will be reduced.

How could we decrease the proportion of L-fiber activity? One way would be to do something that would interfere with the needs of those large-diameter L fibers. Because L fibers are much larger than S fibers, it is probably a safe guess to assume that their metabolic requirements are greater. If we could reduce (but not eliminate) the flow of blood to an area, the L fibers (with their higher metabolic requirements) would probably react to the oxygen deficit first. That is exactly the kind of thing that happens as your foot "falls asleep" when you keep it in an awkward position for awhile. The blood flow to your foot is reduced and usually, before your foot becomes truly numb, there is a period during which stimulation of the foot is rather painful. According to the Melzack–Wall Theory, pain occurs when there is a high proportion of S-fiber activity. Certainly if the L fibers are unable to get the fairly high level of oxygen they need while the S fibers are able to meet their lower oxygen needs, the proportion of S-fiber activity will be high.

The Melzack–Wall Theory does not explain all of our pain perceptions but it is an intriguing theory that points us in the appropriate direction. Its basic assumption is that the language of the nervous system is one in which the overall *pattern of activity* in a variety of neurons is of paramount importance. If you think back to our discussions of vision, audition, and temperature perception, I think you'll discover that the nervous system does indeed emphasize the pattern of activity in groups of neurons and the relationships among the patterns of various groups.

Summary

Be sure you understand and can explain all the italicized terms.

Skin receptors are found within the *dermis*, well below the surface *epidermis*. Most receptors respond to a variety of stimuli. This fact makes a strict interpretation of the *Law of Specific Nerve Energies* inappropriate.

Information from the skin receptors is carried by two different systems. The *lemniscal system* pathway carries information up the spinal cord in the *dorsal tracts*. The dorsal tracts end in *nuclei* in the *medulla*. From the nuclei, information is carried by two crossing bundles, the *medial lemnisci*. The medial lemnisci end in the *ventrobasal complex* of the thalamus. Information from the thalamus arrives at *somatosensory cortex I*.

The other system is sometimes called the *extralemniscal system* and sometimes called the *spinothalamic system*. In this system, information is carried to the opposite side of the spinal cord, where it is carried up by the *spinothalamic tracts*. Axons of the spinothalamic tracts end in the ventrobasal complex and the *posterior nuclear group*, as well as in the *reticular formation* and the *cerebellum*. Eventually the information arrives at *somatosensory cortex II*.

Information from the head and upper neck travels, via the *trigeminal, facial,* and *vagus nerves,* to the thalamus and then to somatosensory cortices I and II.

Both the ventrobasal complex and somatosensory cortex I are well organized. They both have *somatotopic maps,* and they both have their neurons further organized according to the kind of stimulation to which they respond (in the cortex, this additional organization takes the form of *columnar organization*). The thalamic and cortical areas associated with the extralemniscal system are, by contrast, rather disorganized affairs.

In both touch and temperature perception, our sensitivity varies considerably from one body region to another. In both cases, *adaptation* is a prominent feature of our perceptions. In the case of touch, the *Pacinian corpuscle* provides an excellent means of studying neural adaptation—and proves to have a mechanical arrangement that enhances adaptation. In the case of temperature, adaptation involves both a shift in the *physiological zero* and a shift in the *difference threshold.*

Our perceptions of temperature changes involve two different signaling systems: the *"warm spots"* and *warm fibers,* plus the *"cold spots"* and *cold fibers.* The unexpected responses of cold fibers account for the phenomenon of *paradoxical cold.* The perception of "hot" requires the activation of both the warm fibers and the cold fibers.

Our perceptions of pain probably involve patterns of activity in the nervous system, rather than the overstimulation of a single group of neurons. The *Melzack–Wall Theory* provides an excellent scheme for thinking about one possible way in which our nervous system might signal pain.

Recommended Readings

There are two good articles on pain.

Livingston, W. K.   "What is Pain?", *Sci. Amer.,* March 1953 (not available as an Offprint).

Melzack, R.   "The Perception of Pain," *Sci Amer.,* Feb. 1961 (Offprint #457).

There is also a very well-written book that discusses such topics as cultural and situational determinants of pain, kinds of pain, and methods of pain relief (including acupuncture). Take a look at this fascinating book.

Melzack, R.   *The Puzzle of Pain.* Basic Books, 1973.

If acupuncture interests you, also take a look at the following book.

Kurland, H. D.   *Quick Headache Relief Without Drugs.* Morrow, 1977.

For a general discussion of the skin senses, see the following book.

Mueller, C. G.   *Sensory Psychology.* Prentice-Hall, 1965. (Chapter 7.)

For a more advanced discussion, see this book.

Geldard, F. A.   *The Human Senses,* 2nd ed. Wiley, 1972. (Chapters 9–11.)

14

Body Position and Movement

Try a simple experiment on yourself: close your eyes and concentrate on the positions of your head and body. Move your limbs and head and, as you do so, concentrate on the sensations you can feel. Next think about the process of walking. Although we seldom think of it as such, walking is complicated: the contractions and relaxations of muscles in the legs, back, and arms must be carefully coordinated. Usually we don't look at our limbs when we walk—yet, without considerable information about their positions and movements, we would be forever stumbling. How do we know what position we are in and what movements we are making if we don't continually watch our own bodies? Basically, we have two signaling systems available to us. The first system we'll discuss tells us about the angles of our various joints and the degree of contraction of our skeletal muscles. That system is called *kinesthesis* (pronounced, "kin-es-the'-sis"). The second system, called the *vestibular system,* provides information about the position and movements of the head.

Kinesthesis

Kinesthetic information (that is, information arising from joints, muscles, and tendons) is carried primarily via the *lemniscal system.* You may want to return briefly to Chapter 13 and review the lemniscal-system pathway before going any further.

There are several different kinds of receptors associated with kinesthesis. In the joints, two or three different types of dendritic endings can be found in the connective tissues and in the ligaments. In the tendons that form the links between muscles and bones, there is another type of receptor, often called the *Golgi tendon organ.* Finally, in muscles there is yet another type of receptor, the so-called *annulospiral ending.* Most of our ability to detect the position and movements of the body depends upon information arising from the receptors in our joints. The Golgi tendon organs and the annulospiral endings, although providing some information, make a lesser contribution to our kinesthetic abilities.

Joint Positions

Stretch your arm out straight in front of you with your palm up. Now gradually bend your arm, paying attention to the angle formed by your forearm and upper arm, at the elbow. When your arm was out straight, the angle was 180° (that is, the forearm and upper arm formed a straight line). As you brought your forearm up, you gradually reduced this angle, ultimately reaching an angle of about 30° when your forearm was as close to your upper arm as possible. We will refer to this angle, formed by the two sides of a joint, as the *joint angle.* If we are to be aware of the position and movements of our joints, we must have neurons that can signal the joint angle rather precisely.

Neurons of this kind are found arising from the receptors located in joints. The axons of these neurons enter the dorsal side of the spinal cord, along with axons carrying information involved with the skin senses. When recordings are made from the joint-position axons, it soon becomes clear that these neurons do signal joint angle in a very precise way.

Each of the many joint-position axons responds just to a small range of joint angles. For example, one axon may respond whenever the joint angle is between 180° and 165°. Another may respond only when the joint angle is between 70° and 55°. Thus, when you move your arm from a straight-out position to a bent position, first one axon is activated, then a second, then a third, and so on. Each individual axon has a range of approximately 15° over which it responds.

Imagine that we are recording from one axon that responds to joint angles between 100° and 85°. When the joint angle is 100°, the axon produces impulses at a steady rate (the axon has a *maintained discharge*). If the joint angle is suddenly changed to 85° and held there, the axon initially produces impulses at a markedly increased rate, and then the firing rate gradually settles down to a lower, steady rate. We can summarize this in a graph.

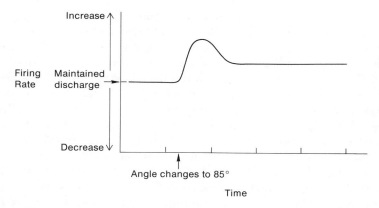

Notice that, when the joint angle is maintained at 85°, the steady rate is higher than it was when the angle was 100°, but it is lower than the activity level that occurred initially when the joint angle was changed.

Imagine now that we suddenly return the joint angle to 100°. The axon responds with an initial firing rate that is markedly reduced. Then it gradually increases its rate until the original rate is again reached.

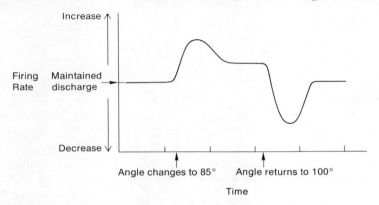

This kind of behavior should seem very familiar to you: it is, of course, an example of *adaptation*. As we've indicated before, adaptation means that the receptors and nervous system react vigorously to a change in stimulation, that they then establish a baseline level as the steady stimulation continues, and that they judge future changes in stimulation against this baseline level. In this particular case, it should be clear to you that we have an additional and very important effect: the axon signals the *direction of change* of stimulation (that is, a decrease or an increase in the joint angle) by the direction of change in its firing rate (an increase or a decrease in the number of impulses per second).

Let's return to our axon. We'll start, again, with a joint angle of 100°. However, now let's consider what happens if the joint angle is suddenly changed to 90°, kept at that position for a while, and then suddenly returned to 100°. As before, the axon markedly increases its firing rate when the angle is first changed, gradually reduces the rate and achieves a steady rate as the angle is maintained, markedly decreases its rate when the angle is returned to 100°, and then achieves its original steady rate. If we compare what happens in this case to what happened when we changed the joint angle from 100° to 85° and back to 100°, we'll find the following.

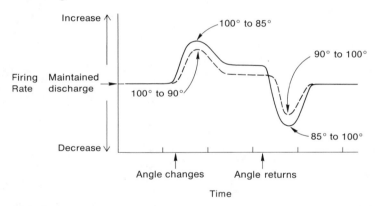

The initial increase in the rate of impulses, the steady rate achieved while the joint angle is maintained, and the decrease that initially occurs when the original joint angle is restored—all will be smaller when the joint angle is changed by 10° rather than by 15°. Thus, the axon signals the *amount of change* in the joint angle by the amount of change in its firing rate.

Finally, let's consider what happens if we repeatedly change the joint angle by 15°, but we vary the speed with which we change that angle. In other words, we will always begin with a joint angle of 100°, move to a joint angle of 85°, hold it there for a while, and then return to a joint angle of 100°. However, we will sometimes change the joint angle very rapidly, and we will sometimes change it slowly. As you look at the next graph, keep the following principle in mind: the more rapidly the change is made, the higher the initial firing rate will be and the sooner the axon will achieve its steady rate.

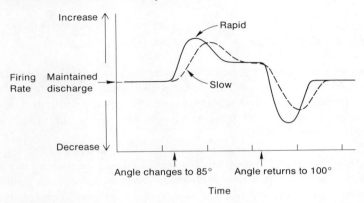

The axon signals the *rate of change* in the joint angle by both the initial firing rate and the time it takes to achieve the steady level.

We can summarize all this as follows.

Quality of Change in Stimulation	*Quality of the Axon's Signal*
Direction of change	Increase vs decrease in firing rate.
Amount of change	Firing rate during the initial period and during the steady period.
Rate of change	Firing rate during the initial period; length of time it takes to achieve the steady rate.

Because the firing rate during the initial period reflects both the amount and the rate of change, the firing rate during the steady period and the length of time it takes to achieve the steady rate are more specific indicators.

Now place your arm straight out in front of you once again. Bend it at the elbow. Think about what you now know is happening in your nervous system as you do so: different neurons are activated as you pass through the various joint angles. All of those neurons signal the direction, amount, and rate of change of the joint angle as you successively pass through the joint angles to which they respond. It is this kind of information that allows you to know where your limbs are without having to look at them.

Golgi Tendon Organs

Skeletal muscles are attached to bones by tendons. Within the tendons, there are numerous dendritic endings that form receptors called the *Golgi tendon organs.* These structures are strategically located: they are activated whenever the muscle changes the amount of "pull" it is exerting on the tendon.

We can, once again, make recordings of the activity of the appropriate axons where they enter the spinal cord. These axons tend to produce impulses at a slow and steady rate when the tension on the tendon is kept constant (that is, they have a *maintained discharge*). If the tension is changed only slightly, the axons do not change their firing rate. It is only when the tension is changed rather markedly and suddenly that the axons react. The easiest way to summarize this is to say that the neurons that make up the Golgi tendon organs have a *high threshold.*

Let's take a look at the results of a typical set of recordings. You should keep in mind that, whenever the muscle contracts, it will increase the tension on the tendon and, whenever the muscle is stretched (by being pulled), it will also increase the tension on the tendon. Both kinds of events can activate the Golgi tendon organs. In the graph, the point marked "contract" means that the muscle briefly contracted and it then returned to its original condition. The point marked "stretch" means that the muscle was briefly stretched and then returned to its original condition.

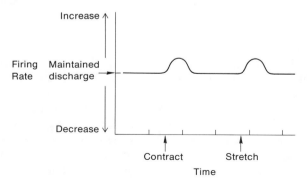

Notice that the axon increases its rate of impulse production whenever any substantial change occurs in the muscle. This is the case because any change in the muscle will produce a change in the tension on the tendon. To understand this, prop your elbow up on a table with your fingers pointing toward the ceiling. Turn your hand so that you are looking at the palm. Now make a fist and alternately bend your fist first toward you and then away from you. When you bend your fist toward you, the muscles running from the inner surface of your wrist to the inner surface of your elbow are contracting. When you bend your fist away from you, the same muscles are being stretched. Let's draw a simplified sketch of these muscles.

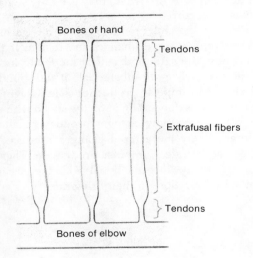

When the muscles contract, they pull on the tendons. Because the tendons are attached to bones, those bones that are free to move (in this case, the bones of your hand) will be pulled into a new position. In those places where the bones cannot be moved (in this case, the bones of your elbow), there will simply be increased tension on the tendons.

When the muscles are stretched (in our example, the muscles are stretched when the muscles on the other side of the forearm contract), movable bones are pulled into a new position. Because of that new position, they, in turn, pull on the tendons and muscles.

Notice that, in both cases, there will be an increase in the tension exerted on the tendons. The Golgi tendon organs, located within the tendons, respond to changes in tension, regardless of the reasons for the changes. Therefore, Golgi tendon organs cannot signal whether muscles contracted or were stretched; they can only signal the fact that a change in tension occurred.

As we said earlier, the Golgi tendon organs have a high threshold. They do not respond to slight changes in tension. If the change in tension is moderate, they respond with a moderate increase in their firing rate. If the change is more substantial, they respond with a larger increase in their rate of impulse production. The Golgi tendon organs also vary their responses depending upon the speed with which tension changes take place. Very slow changes produce no alteration in the firing rate. Progressively more rapid changes produce progressively larger alterations in the rate of impulse production. Therefore, we can say that the Golgi tendon organs signal both the *amount* and *rate of change* in tension by alterations in their firing rate.

Annulospiral Endings

The third source of kinesthetic information we'll consider is a receptor found within the muscle itself. Muscles are made up primarily of contractile fibers that do most of the work of the muscles. These contractile elements are usually called the *extrafusal fibers.* Intermingled with these are a few fibers that can contract only very weakly, but that contain receptors. These fibers are usually called the *intrafusal fibers.* It would be wise for you to stop at this point and figure out a mnemonic that will help you keep these terms straight. The one I use is to remind myself that the *e*xtrafusal fibers form the *e*fferent components of muscles (that is, the *e*xtrafusal fibers are the ones that have a direct *e*ffect on our movements).

The receptors contained in the intrafusal fibers are usually called the *annulospiral endings*. Let's take a look at a simplified sketch of a muscle.

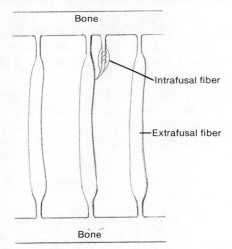

Notice that the extrafusal fibers are attached (by tendons) to bones at each end, but the intrafusal fiber is attached to a bone at one end and to an extrafusal fiber at the other end. This means that the intrafusal fiber will be affected whenever there are changes in the extrafusal fiber.

As you look at the sketch, try to imagine that all the extrafusal fibers have contracted. Contraction of the extrafusal fiber to which the intrafusal fiber is attached is of paramount importance to us. Contraction of that extrafusal fiber will make the intrafusal fiber go slack. If you have trouble picturing why that should occur, think of it this way: as the extrafusal fiber contracts, it carries that portion of the intrafusal fiber that is attached to it in an upward direction. Alternatively, we could say that, when the extrafusal fiber contracts, the bones are brought closer together, and the tension on the intrafusal fiber is therefore reduced.

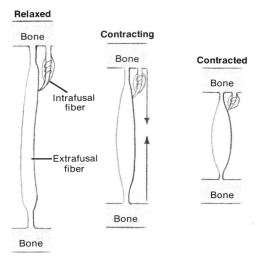

This effectively removes any pull that might have originally been exerted on the intrafusal fiber.

Now imagine what happens when the extrafusal fiber is stretched. The attached portion of the intrafusal fiber will be pulled downward, and the intrafusal fiber will become taut. Alternatively, we could say that, when the bones are moved farther apart, the tension on the intrafusal fiber is increased.

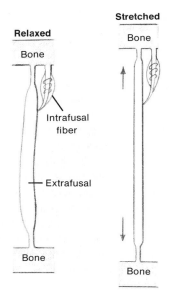

The annulospiral ending is basically the dendritic ending of a neuron, whose axon enters the dorsal spinal cord along with all the other axons bringing skin and kinesthetic information into the spinal cord. If we record from the appropriate axons, we can discover the nature of the information coming from the annulospiral endings.

You will probably not be surprised to discover that the annulospiral ending responds very well and very precisely to changes in the state of the extrafusal fibers. Let's begin by indicating that the axons in this system produce impulses at a rather slow and steady rate whenever the muscle tension is held constant (the axons have a *maintained discharge*). When a muscle contracts, the intrafusal fiber becomes slack, and the axon reduces its firing rate. When a muscle is stretched, the intrafusal fiber becomes taut, and the axon increases its rate of impulse production. The greater the degree of contraction or stretching, the more slack or taut the intrafusal fiber will become, and the greater the change will be in the axon's firing rate. Let's summarize all this in a few graphs. Once again, the points marked "contraction" mean that the extrafusal fiber briefly contracted and it then returned to its original state. The points marked "stretch" mean that the extrafusal fiber was briefly stretched and then returned to its original state.

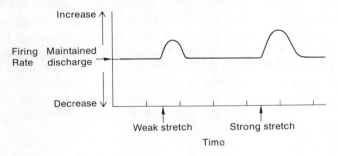

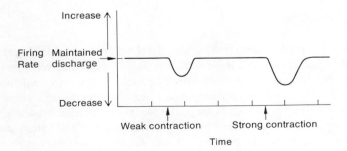

Here we have a system that signals the *direction* of stimulation (a decrease or an increase in tension on the intrafusal fiber) by the direction of change in the firing rate. In addition, it signals the *amount* of stimulation (the degree of contraction or stretching) by the amount of change in its firing rate.

Both the Golgi tendon organ and the annulospiral ending display *adaptation.* They both react initially to a contraction or stretch in a marked way. If the contraction or stretch is maintained, they both respond in a gradually diminished way. In the case of the Golgi tendon organ, the firing rate following the initial response to contraction or stretch will gradually subside to a slower, steady rate. In the case of the annulospiral ending, the firing rate following the initial response to contraction will gradually increase to a higher, steady rate; the firing rate following the initial response to stretch will gradually decrease to a lower, steady rate.

For both the Golgi tendon organ and the annulospiral ending, more rapid or more intense contractions or stretches will result in a longer period before the steady rate is reached. Therefore, both kinds of receptor can signal both the *rate* and the *amount* of change.

So far, it looks as if the annulospiral ending can signal everything the Golgi tendon organ can signal and more besides (remember that the annulospiral ending can indicate whether a muscle has contracted or has been stretched, while the Golgi tendon organ can only indicate that a change has occurred in the muscle). What then is the point of having Golgi tendon organs? To understand the answer, we need to leave our consideration of kinesthesis and discuss one very important reflex activity.

The Stretch Reflex

Before we begin, let me remind you that I said early in this chapter that most of our kinesthetic information is supplied by joint receptors. The Golgi tendon organs and the annulospiral endings do contribute to kinesthesis, but their primary roles are to regulate and coordinate various muscle activities. Perhaps the most well-studied muscle activity has been the *stretch reflex.* This reflex can be described rather simply: whenever a muscle is stretched, it automatically contracts in response to the stretch. Let's see how this works by looking at a simplified sketch of muscle fibers and the spinal cord.

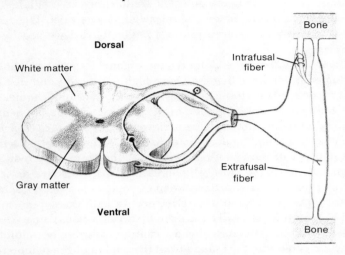

What we have here is one intrafusal fiber with its annulospiral ending. The line running from the annulospiral ending to the spinal cord represents the dendrite, cell body, and axon of one neuron. That neuron synapses, within the spinal cord, on another neuron that runs out of the spinal cord to the extrafusal fiber. Whenever that neuron is activated, it will cause a brief contraction of the extrafusal fiber. There are several ways in which that neuron can be activated, but let's consider just one: if we can increase the firing rate in the neuron associated with the annulospiral ending, we can (via the synapse in the spinal cord) activate the neuron associated with the extrafusal fiber. How can you increase the firing rate in the neuron associated with the annulospiral ending? One sure way is to stretch the muscle. Now you can see that, every time a muscle is stretched, activity in the neuron of the annulospiral ending will increase; this will activate the second neuron, and the muscle will contract. When the muscle contracts, activity in the neuron of the annulospiral ending will decrease and, as a consequence, activity in the neuron of the extrafusal fiber will decrease. The muscle will then relax. If we maintain a continuous pull on the muscle, this cycle (activation of the annulospiral ending→contraction of the muscle→deactivation of the annulospiral ending→relaxation of the muscle) will continue indefinitely. And this is exactly what happens in us most of the time because gravity exerts a continuous pull on certain muscles. When you stand, for example, muscles in the legs and back are stretched by the pull of gravity. Those muscles reflexly contract, relax, contract, relax, and so on, in response to the pull. The contractions are not large, and the period of each contraction and relaxation is very brief. The overall result is a general, low-level response to gravity that we usually call *muscle tone.*

Ah, but what about the Golgi tendon organs? Remember that they are situated in tendons, that they have high thresholds, and that they react to any sudden, strong changes in muscle tension. The neurons associated with the Golgi tendon organs also synapse on the neurons associated with the extrafusal fibers. However, this synapse is *inhibitory.* Thus, when the Golgi tendon organs are active, they suppress activity in the neurons of the extrafusal fibers and, therefore, they reduce or prevent muscle contractions. This inhibition is a protective device: it reduces or prevents contractions when the muscle is already contracting strongly or is being strongly stretched. In both cases, reducing or preventing contractions will reduce the chance of serious damage to the muscle. If the muscle has already contracted strongly, additional contraction could tear the muscle from the tendon or the tendon from the bone. Similarly, contracting a severely stretched muscle could produce the same kind of damage, particularly if the bones are being held firmly in place either by an external object (a weight, for example) or by strong contractions of other muscles.

In order to bring this discussion back to the topic of kinesthesis, you should realize that the neurons associated with the Golgi tendon organs and the annulospiral endings have axons that branch out inside the spinal cord. One branch of each axon joins the *dorsal tract* in the spinal cord and becomes part of the *lemniscal system.*

The Vestibular Apparatus

Associated with the bony wall of each cochlea, there is a complex, bony structure that houses receptors responsible for signaling the position and movements of the head. Contained within each bony structure are three *semicircular canals* and two *otolith organs.* The semicircular canals and otolith organs are collectively known as the *vestibular apparatus.* The vestibular apparatus is closely associated with the cochlea; in fact, the fluids that fill the cochlea (remember the *perilymph* and the *endolymph?*)

also fill the vestibular apparatus. To see just how intimate the relationship is between the cochlea and vestibular apparatus, take a look at the following sketch.

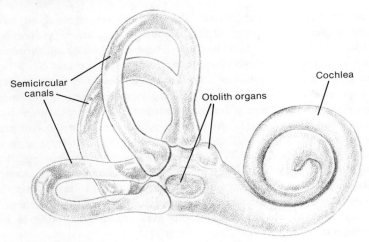

The Semicircular Canals

Notice in the sketch that the three canals lie in different planes. Movements of the head in any direction will affect at least one semicircular canal. In this way, all movements of the head can be detected by the canals.

Each canal is really a bony tube. Notice that at one end of each canal there is an enlarged area. The enlarged area is call the *ampulla* (pronounced, "am'-pew-la"), and it is the location of the receptors.

Each bony canal is lined by a membrane. Between the membrane and the bone, the rather dense fluid called perilymph is found. The space formed by the membrane lining contains endolymph. In a cutaway view of one canal, you can see the membrane and the locations of the fluids:

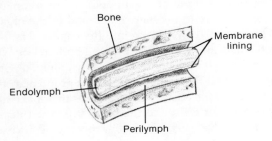

Throughout most of the length of each semicircular canal, we have this arrangement. However, at the ampulla, things are very different. Within each ampulla, there is a large, rather odd-looking structure called the *crista*. The most obvious component of the crista is a big, dome-like mass of gelatinous material called the *cupula* (pronounced, "que'-pew-la"). (You may want to stop here and figure out some mnemonic devices that will help you keep the terms "ampulla," "crista," and "cupula" straight in your mind. For example, you may want to use the following: the *a*mpulla is *a*mply filled by a *c*rest of material called the *c*rista. The *cupula* is the gelatinous material that looks like an inverted *cup*.) The cupula is large enough to fill the interior of the ampulla. In fact, the cupula has such a tight fit that neither the perilymph nor the endolymph can flow around it. This sketch of a cutaway view of the ampulla should give you a good idea of the arrangement.

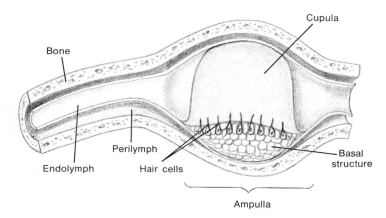

Sticking up from the bottom of the ampulla, there are many *hair cells*, very similar in structure to the hair cells found in the organ of Corti. The tips of the hairs actually jut up into the cupula. The bases of the hairs are embedded in a *basal* (that means "bottom" or "basement") *structure* that is attached to the bony wall of the ampulla.

We can now say that the ampulla contains a group of structures that are collectively called the crista. The structures that make up the crista are the cupula, the hair cells, and the basal structure (please don't go any further until you've worked out your mnemonic devices!).

The dendritic endings of neurons are located very close to the bases of the hair cells, within the basal structure. Hopefully, this reminds you of the situation in the cochlea. The fact that the vestibular apparatus and the cochlea are built along the same general plan reflects the fact that they are evolutionarily and embryologically derived from the same small mass of tissue.

The dendrites lead from the basal structure to a small cavity in the bony wall of the vestibular apparatus. Within the cavity there are cell bodies, and axons lead out of the cavity to join up with the auditory nerve. These axons travel into the brain in conjunction with the axons associated with the cochlea. However, the two sets of axons do not end up going to the same regions in the brain. The axons associated with the vestibular apparatus end up sending information to a variety of locations: the cerebellum, the reticular formation, the nuclei associated with movements of the eyes, nuclei associated with movements of skeletal muscles, nuclei associated with the autonomic nervous system (which controls heart rate, breathing, blood-vessel constrictions and dilations, etc.), and the area of the cortex near the Sylvian fissure.

We said earlier that the semicircular canals are responsible for signaling head movements. Think about what happens to you when you are spun around and around: you make adjustments in your posture and body movements and, although you may not realize it, you make adjustments in your eye movements. If the spinning is rapid and prolonged, your heart may begin to race, you may become sweaty or chilled, and you may eventually become nauseated. All these reactions can be understood if you think about all the different areas of the brain that receive vestibular information.

The Functioning of the Semicircular Canals

When recordings are made from the axons associated with the semicircular canals, we find that they produce impulses at a slow, steady rate when the head is stationary (that is, these axons have a *maintained discharge*). When the head is moved suddenly, some of the axons increase their rate of impulse production, while others decrease their firing rate.

We can arrange to keep the head moving at a steady speed. The easiest way to do this is to strap the organism on a platform and attach a harness that prevents any independent movements of the head. Now we can begin with the platform at rest and then rotate it. We can bring the rotation up to any particular speed and keep it at that speed as long as we wish. And, of course, we can later slow the rotation and finally stop the platform.

Because of all our discussions of *adaptation*, you may be able to predict what will happen to the firing rate in our axons when the platform begins to rotate and then continues to rotate at a constant speed. Following the initial change in the firing rate, the rate of impulse production gradually returns to the original slow, steady rate. Let's put this in graph form:

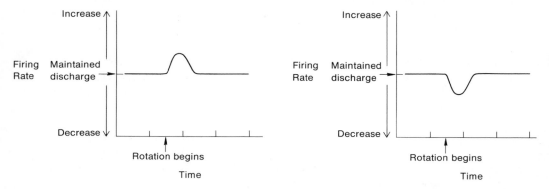

These two graphs indicate that, regardless of whether an axon increases or decreases its firing rate when the platform begins to rotate, adaptation takes place as the speed of rotation is maintained.

When we finally stop the platform, most of the axons respond by doing the opposite of what they did when the platform began to move: axons that originally increased their firing rate now decrease their rate, and those that originally decreased their rate now increase it. A few axons do not respond in this opposite fashion. Instead, they either increase their rate both when the platform begins to move and when it stops, or they decrease their rate in both situations. All the axons gradually return to their original maintained discharge as the platform remains stationary. These axons therefore signal *changes* in movements of the head. We have certainly encountered lots of other examples in which the receptors and nervous system react to changes in stimulation rather than to the actual, steady level of stimulation. As in those other examples, these axons react more vigorously when the change is more sudden or more pronounced. Thus, axons that increase their firing rate when the platform begins rotating will produce a larger increase either if the platform reaches its ultimate rotating speed more rapidly or if the platform reaches a higher ultimate rotating speed. As you may have guessed, it will also take longer for the axon to get back to its original, steady rate under these conditions. You should be able to predict what happens when the platform is stopped suddenly rather than gradually, or when the platform is stopped after rotating at a high rather than a low speed.

Let's continue to focus on those axons that increase their firing rate when the platform begins to move. Suppose that all along we've been rotating the platform in a clockwise direction. What will happen if we once again begin with the platform stationary, but now when we rotate it, we do so in a counterclockwise direction? These axons will now decrease their firing rate when the platform begins to move. Let's use some graphs here:

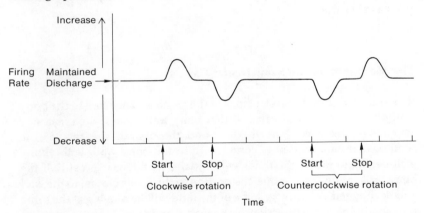

Notice that stopping after moving clockwise produces the same result as starting to move counterclockwise (the axon decreases its firing rate). Starting to move clockwise produces the same result as stopping after moving counterclockwise (the axon increases its firing rate).

This may seem very strange to you until you think about the following: if you've been spinning around in one direction for a while and then you stop, you don't feel stopped. You feel as if you're spinning in the opposite direction. Try it. If you try it once with your eyes closed and once with them open, you'll find that the effect is more pronounced when your eyes are closed. This is because, with your eyes closed, you don't have any visual information to help you decide when you've truly stopped.

The fact that when you stop you feel as if you're spinning in the opposite direction is a direct result of the reactions of those axons associated with the semicircular canals. They signal the end of movement in one direction in precisely the same way as they signal the beginning of movement in the opposite direction. This should bring to mind the afterimages we discussed in Chapter 7. Do you recall that we found that the offset of a red light produces the same change in the firing rate of an LGN opponent cell as the onset of a green light? We have an analogous situation here in the vestibular system.

Now we can say that most of the axons actually signal the *direction* of the change of movement rather than just signaling a change. The minority axons, those that always either increase or decrease their firing rate, can only signal that a change has occurred, without signaling the direction of that change.

What is happening inside the semicircular canals during all this starting, rotating, and stopping? Put another way, why do the axons react as they do?

The Mechanics of the Semicircular Canals

Remember that the basal structure of the crista is connected to the bony wall of the semicircular canal. If that bony wall moves, the crista will also move. However, the fluids found throughout the rest of the semicircular canal are not "connected" to the bony wall. If the bony wall begins to move, the fluids will initially tend to remain still. If the bony wall continues to move, the portion of the fluids closest to the wall will be dragged along. Now some of the fluid will be moving at the same rate and in the same direction as the wall. Gradually, as the movement of the wall continues, more and more of the fluid will move with it.

What's important to understand is what will happen to that gelatinous mass called the cupula during all this. It is rather firmly attached to the basal structure but, because it is gelatinous, it can be compressed and pushed about to some extent. When the bony wall and basal structure begin to move, the cupula will also begin to move. The problem is that it has a mass of fluids in front of it. The fluid cannot stream around it; there just isn't any room between the cupula and the bony wall. Until the fluids are moving at the same rate as the bony wall, they'll push the cupula backwards. The hair cells sticking up into the cupula will be bent, and this shearing (remember "shearing" from our discussion of the organ of Corti?) will affect the nearby dendritic endings.

In case you're having trouble visualizing all this, let's take a look at some sketches. These sketches portray the semicircular canal as being a complete ring; such a conceptualization simplifies the process of understanding what's taking place inside.

(1) Movement begins

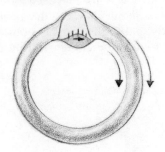

(2) Movement continues

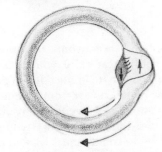

(3) Movement continues and fluids move

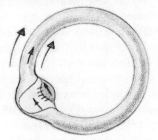

If you look carefully at these sketches, you should be able to predict what will happen when the movement stops. The bony wall and basal organ stop. The cupula begins to stop but it is pushed forward by the fluids. When the fluids finally stop, the cupula will no longer be pushed and the hair cells will no longer be bent. Notice that, when the movement began, the cupula was pushed in a direction opposite to the direction of movement (in our sketches, the movement of the walls and basal organ is clockwise, but the cupula is pushed counterclockwise); when the movement ends, the cupula will be pushed the other way (clockwise).

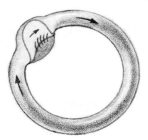

Under what other circumstances would the cupula be pushed clockwise? If you've been reading carefully, you should have a feeling right now of "aha! so that's what's happening." If you don't have that feeling, go back and reread. (The answer to the question is, begin with everything stationary and then move the bony wall in a counterclockwise direction. Now you should recognize why stopping a clockwise motion and beginning a counterclockwise motion, or vice versa, produce the same effects on the cupula. This should allow you to make more sense out of the fact that when you stand still after spinning in one direction, you have the sensation of spinning in the opposite direction.)

Most of the dendrites associated with hair cells produce depolarizations when the hair cells are bent in one direction and produce hyperpolarizations when they are bent in the opposite direction. This accounts for the differences in the responses of the axons when movement begins and ends, and when movement is in one direction or the other. Some of the dendrites always produce either depolarizations or hyperpolarizations, regardless of the direction in which their hair cells are bent. Thus, some axons either always increase or always decrease their rate of impulse production, regardless of whether movement is beginning or ending and regardless of the direction of movement.

The mechanics of the semicircular canals also go a long way toward explaining the adaptation we noted earlier: the axons return to their original, steady firing rate when movement is sustained. This occurs because, when the fluids are finally moving along with the bony wall, the cupula is no longer being pushed, and the hair cells are therefore no longer being bent.

The Otolith Organs

The three semicircular canals on each side of the head are connected to a central structure that contains two additional areas that are part of the vestibular apparatus. These two areas are collectively known as the *otolith organs*. ("Otolith" means "earstone." As you'll soon see, this is a good descriptive name.) The two individual areas are named the *utricle* and the *saccule*.

Like the semicircular canals, the otolith organs contain a membrane lining that separates the perilymph from the endolymph. In addition, within each otolith organ, there is an area that resembles the crista of the semicircular canal: that is, there is a *basal structure* within which the bases of many *hair cells* are found, and there is a *gelatinous mass* into which the tips of the hair cells jut. In the otolith organs, this area is called the *macula* (pronounced, "mack'-u-lah"). There are, however, two very important differences between the crista and the macula. First, the macula does not completely fill the interior of that part of the otolith organ in which it is found. Thus, the fluids are free to move past it and over it. Second, and most crucial, the topmost portion of the gelatinous mass of the macula contains many little crystals of calcium carbonate. These small crystals are rather dense; if we weighed equal volumes of the crystals and the gelatinous material (for example, we might weigh 1 cc of each), we'd find that the crystals are heavier. The crystals are actually suspended in the gelatinous mass, much as small pieces of fruit can be suspended in jello. The crystals are called *otoliths*, and it is because of them that the utricle and saccule are called the otolith organs.

A cutaway view of the macula looks something like this.

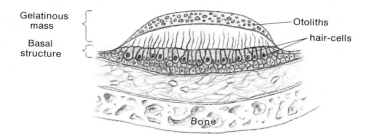

Once again, there are dendritic endings located near the bases of the hair cells. The locations of the cell bodies and axons are the same as the ones we discussed for the semicircular canals. As was the case with the semicircular canals, the axons send information to a wide variety of locations in the brain.

The Functioning of the Otolith Organs

Recordings have been made from axons associated with the utricle and saccule. All the axons produce impulses at a steady rate, no matter in what position the head is held (these axons have a *maintained discharge*). However, each individual axon has a "preferred position." In other words, one particular axon might produce impulses at a steady, high rate whenever the head is held upright and at steady, lower rates whenever the head is held in any other position. Another axon might have its highest firing rate when the head is held in one particular, tilted position (perhaps a position in which the head is tilted 45° to the left). In this way, all the possible head positions can be signaled by the activity of the various axons. As long as a particular head position is held, axons with that position as their "preferred position" continue to produce impulses at a high, steady rate. In other words, the axons do *not* show pronounced adaptation, if indeed they show any adaptation at all. Therefore, the otolith organs do *not* emphasize *changes* in head position. Instead they signal the *actual* head position.

This is quite a departure from the situations we've found before. All the systems we've described earlier clearly display adaptation. In some cases, such as the Pacinian corpuscle, we found that adaptation is due to both neural and mechanical effects. In the case of the semicircular canals, we found that adaptation was due, in large part, to the mechanics of the crista and the fluids. In the otolith organs, perhaps we can understand the apparent absence of adaptation by examining the mechanics of the macula.

The Mechanics of the Otolith Organs

In the semicircular canals, the important point is that changes in movements of the head create unequal changes in movements of the crista and the fluids. In the otolith organs, the important point is that, no matter what position the head is in, gravity will exert more pull on the heavy otoliths than on anything else inside the utricle or saccule. When the otoliths are pulled by gravity, the gelatinous mass in which they're embedded will be shifted in the direction of gravity. This will bend the hair cells and, depending on the direction and degree of bending, the hair cells will produce larger or smaller depolarizations.

Tilt left   **Tilt right**

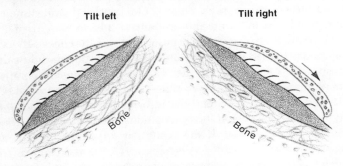

Evidently individual hair cells are situated such that they are subjected to shearing forces most when the gelatinous mass shifts one way or the other, and/or each hair cell is built such that only certain directions of bending increase the depolarizations.

What should be clear to you is that gravity will continue to exert the same pull on the otoliths as long as a particular head position is maintained. Certainly gravity does not weaken when a head position is maintained. And there is nothing inside the otolith organs that gradually counteracts the effects of gravity. Thus, there is no mechanical basis for adaptation. If any adaptation does occur, and there is some disagreement about that, it could only be due to neural changes.

Motion Sickness

There is no doubt that the vestibular apparatus is crucial to our ability to maintain normal erect posture and to adjust our posture when we move. This can be demonstrated in a wide variety of animals. If, for example, just one semicircular canal on one side of a bird's head is damaged, the bird will no longer fly voluntarily. If the bird is forced to fly, its flight will be awkward, and the bird will rapidly descend. If all three canals on one side of the head are destroyed, the bird will be unable to maintain a standing posture. It will repeatedly fall and somersault. In human beings, damage to just one set of semicircular canals creates extreme dizziness, nausea, and vomiting, as well as changes in heartrate, breathing, and blood pressure. Damage to the utricle produces similar symptoms, although they are not as pronounced. (Strangely enough, damage to the saccule does not seem to produce any particular symptoms. There is, understandably, quite a debate going on about the possible reasons for this.)

Notice that damage to the vestibular apparatus on just one side of the head produces very marked effects. Our postural adjustments are based not only on the kind and amount of information arising from each side of the head; they are also based on the differences between the information provided by the vestibular apparatus on the right side and the vestibular apparatus on the left side. Within the brain, the information arising from the two sides of the head is compared. When there is a discrepancy between the information coming from the left and right sides, head and body positions are adjusted so that the discrepancy is minimized. If the vestibular apparatus on one side is damaged, there will always be a discrepancy between the information it provides and the information provided by the intact vestibular apparatus on the other side. In the futile attempt to reduce the discrepancy, head and body positions are continuously altered. Thus the bird with damaged semicircular canals on one side of the head repeatedly falls and somersaults. When the discrepancy cannot be eliminated or substantially reduced, we experience dizziness, nausea, and cardiovascular changes.

If you've had an ear infection, you may well have suffered many of these symptoms. If you recall the intimate relationship between the ear and the vestibular apparatus, it should be clear to you that disturbances of the ear will affect the various vestibular organs. Even sounds can affect the vestibular apparatus; being exposed to very loud sounds for a period of time can produce dizziness and nausea.

Most of us, however, think of dizziness and nausea as components of motion sickness. Motion sickness is most likely to occur when the head is repeatedly jarred. But there are situations in which motion sickness never occurs despite repeated jarrings of the head. For example, walking and running produce repeated jarrings, yet motion sickness does not occur. There are also situations in which motion sickness can be produced despite the fact that the head is kept still. For example, it's possible to become motion sick when the scene at which you're looking is repeatedly jarred but you remain still. Perhaps the best way to view all this is to say that motion sickness is most likely to occur when the information from either the vestibular apparatus or the eyes or both indicates that things are moving about rather erratically, but the information from these two sources is not well correlated.

Individuals seem to differ markedly in their ability to withstand erratic movements. Successful pilots, ballet dancers, and ice skaters are typically far less susceptible to motion sickness than most of us. Part of their ability to withstand erratic motion is based on techniques they acquire. For example, dancers and skaters learn to fix their eyes on one spot as they spin. This reduces the apparent motion of the visual world, and it is a technique often used to combat seasickness. (If you can see a stationary object such as a prominent lighthouse or point on land, you can reduce the feelings of dizziness and nausea by fixing your eyes on that spot.) However, these techniques do not fully account for resistance to motion sickness. Certain individuals are apparently naturally more resistant for reasons that are not well understood.

If you've ever been on a boat for a period of time, you know that, when you return to land, you experience some difficulty moving about. It's as if the rolling motions of the boat became "normal" and, for a time, the absence of those motions feels "abnormal." It's a bit difficult to understand precisely how this phenomenon occurs. Although it bears some resemblance to adaptation, it really is more complicated. Adaptation entails exposure to an unchanging stimulus to which we become adjusted. The rolling motions of a boat are usually erratic, and they certainly do not provide an unchanging stimulus. In fact, quite the opposite occurs: the stimuli keep changing from moment to moment.

Yet, in some sense, we shift our baseline so that the presence of changing stimuli seems "normal." Indeed, judged against this baseline, the absence of changing stimuli seems "abnormal," and it requires a period of readjustment.

Summary

Be sure you understand and can define all the italicized terms.

In this chapter, we've discussed two systems that signal our body position and movements. One system, that of *kinesthesis,* provides information about the positions of our joints and the degree of contraction of our skeletal muscles. The second system, called the *vestibular system,* supplies information about the position and movements of our head.

Kinesthetic information is carried to the brain via the *lemniscal system.* Receptors in our joints signal the *direction of change, amount of change,* and *rate of change* in *joint angles.* Receptors associated with our muscles signal the *direction of change, amount of change,* and *rate of change* in *muscle tension.*

There are two different kinds of receptors associated with muscles. The *Golgi tendon organs* are high-threshold receptors that can only signal the amount and the rate of change in muscle tension. The *annulospiral endings,* located in the *intrafusal fibers,* are able to signal these factors as well as the direction of change. Both of these kinds of receptors are primarily involved in the regulation and coordination of muscle activities. Their roles in events such as the *stretch reflex* have been well studied. Their contribution to kinesthetic information is secondary.

The vestibular system contains a variety of structures that are closely related to the cochlea. The system includes three pairs of *semicircular canals* and two sets of *otolith organs.* Axons associated with these structures form part of the *auditory nerve.* The information from these structures eventually reaches a wide variety of locations in the brain.

The semicircular canals contain a membrane lining that separates the *perilymph* from the *endolymph.* Each canal has an enlarged area, called the *ampulla.* Within the ampulla, there is a large structure called the *crista,* which is composed of a *basal structure, hair cells,* and a gelatinous mass (the *cupula*). Most of the axons associated with the semicircular canals increase their firing rates when the hair cells are bent in one direction and decrease their firing rates when the hair cells are bent in the opposite direction. *Adaptation* occurs primarily because of mechanical changes that take place in the semicircular canals during maintained stimulation.

The otolith organs are individually called the *utricle* and the *saccule.* Like the semicircular canals, these structures contain a membrane lining that separates the *perilymph* from the *endolymph*. The sensory structure inside each otolith organ is called the *macula*. It contains a *basal structure, hair cells,* and a gelatinous mass with *otoliths* embedded in the topmost portion of the mass. The axons associated with the otolith organs typically have a *"preferred position"* to which they react most vigorously by increasing their firing rates. Other positions produce lower firing rates. The axons do not appear to adapt when a head position is maintained. This is probably the case because there is no mechanical adjustment that occurs inside the otolith organs when a position is maintained.

There is no doubt that the vestibular apparatus is important to our ability to maintain posture. Damage to the vestibular apparatus—or intense or erratic stimulation of it—results in dizziness, nausea, and cardiovascular changes.

Recommended Readings

For general information on kinesthesis and the vestibular system, try these books.

Geldard, F. A.   *The Human Senses,* 2nd ed. Wiley, 1972, (Chapters 13 and 14.)

Mueller, C. G.   *Sensory Psychology,* Prentice-Hall, 1965, (Chapter 8.)

For additional information on the activities of muscles, take a look at these two fine books (originally recommended in Chapter 1).

Thompson, R. F.   *Introduction to Physiological Psychology.* Harper & Row, 1975. (Chapter 7.)

Thompson, R. F.   *Foundations of Physiological Psychology.* Harper & Row, 1967. (Chapter 12. A more advanced treatment.)

15

The Chemical Senses

We sense chemical stimulation in two ways: by taste and by smell. Often we think of these as two very different senses. However, if you think about it for a while, you may discover that they are not as different and separate as you supposed. Consider, for example, what happens to your sense of taste when your nose is stuffed up during a cold. Foods taste rather bland, and many foods that normally seem to have distinctively different tastes become indistinguishable from each other. Much of what we think of as taste is actually smell.

Whether we consider taste or smell, we are really talking about the interactions between chemicals (usually in the form of rather complex molecules) and receptors. In large part, we differentiate between taste and smell on the basis of the location of the receptors; chemicals interact with receptors in the mouth and throat to produce taste sensations, while chemicals interact with receptors in the nose to produce smell sensations. The receptors in these locations seem to respond only to certain chemicals, and chemicals that can activate receptors in the mouth and throat are not necessarily those that can activate receptors in the nose. Therefore, we can consider taste to be dependent on one group of receptors and one class or group of chemicals, while smell is dependent upon a different group of receptors and chemicals.

It is necessary for us to discuss taste and smell in a somewhat hesi-
tant way because taste and smell are poorly understood. Many of the
most basic questions about taste and smell have yet to be answered.
As an example of the confusion that exists, try to come to grips with
the following dilemma: no one is certain how many or what kinds
of basic taste or smell sensations there are. During the last three centuries, various individuals have developed lists of the basic taste sensations. Some of the lists included as many as 12 sensations: sweet,
sour, sharp, pungent, harsh, bitter, insipid (I've known insipid people,
but I'm not sure I'd know an insipid taste if it came up and bit me!),
salty, spiritous, aromatic, urinous, and putrid. Most researchers today
believe that there are only four basic tastes: salt, sour, bitter, and sweet.
However, there are some who argue for a fifth, alkaline. Still others note
that some animals seem to detect distilled water as a unique taste.

The situation in smell is even worse. There simply is no agreement.
Some individuals argue that there are just four basic smells: fragrant,
burnt, goaty, and acid. Others list fruity, spicy, flowery, burnt, foul, and
resinous. Still others insist on ethereal (?), camphor, floral, musky,
pungent, putrid, and pepperminty. There are other lists, but I think you
get the point.

We are involved here in a situation that clearly differs from those we
encountered in the other senses. Part of the reason that there is so much
disagreement about the basic sensations of taste and smell is that no
one understands the properties of the stimuli that produce the
sensations. In vision, we had no trouble identifying the properties of
light that produce various visual sensations: the wavelength and
amplitude of light (or if you prefer the quantum view, the energy level
and number of quanta) are responsible for producing sensations of
color and brightness. In audition, we talked about the frequency and
amplitude of a sound wave. But here, in the chemical senses, we do not
know what properties of chemicals are important. When we enter the
realm of the chemical senses, we enter a universe in which little is
certain, much is confusing, and contradictions are everywhere.

Taste Receptors and Pathways

Let's begin on the firmest footing we can find. The taste receptors have
been carefully studied, and a considerable amount is known about their
structure.

If you look at your tongue in a mirror, you can see that it's covered
with small bumps. Each bump is called a *papilla* (pronounced "pa-pill'-
a"; plural, papill*ae*). Each papilla is separated from its neighbors by a

trench. *Taste buds* are located in the walls of the papillae that form the trenches. Every taste bud is actually a collection of between 2 and 12 individual cells called, reasonably enough, *taste cells*. Let's take a look at a cross-section of two papillae and at a blowup view of a taste bud.

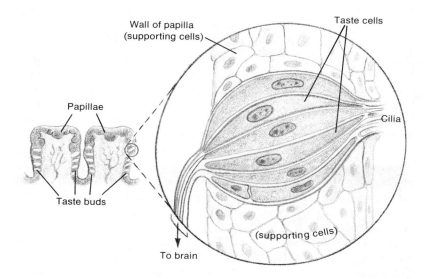

In the blowup, you can see that the wall of the papilla has an opening through which each taste cell sticks a hairlike ending. The opening is called the *taste pore*. The walls of the papillae are covered with taste pores, one for each taste bud. The hair-like endings of the taste cells are called *cilia* (singular, *cilium*). Surrounding and intermingling with the taste cells, there are *supporting cells.*

Individual taste cells do not survive for very long. Their average life span is a matter of days. New taste cells are continuously developed from the supporting cells, and these replace the old taste cells as they degenerate.

The dendritic endings of neurons are found within the papillae, close to the taste cells. The neurons travel as three distinct bundles from the mouth and throat to the brain. The bundle that collects information from the anterior two-thirds of the tongue is called the *facial nerve.* The bundle that collects information from the posterior one-third of the tongue is the *glossopharyngeal nerve* ("glosso-" meaning tongue; "-pharyngeal"-for pharynx). Information from the throat region is carried by the *vagus nerve.* (Do you recall that we met these three cranial nerves in Chapter 13, when we discussed skin information from the head? These three nerves carry a wide variety of information from the head to the CNS and from the CNS to the muscles and glands of the face.) All three of these cranial nerves enter the brain at the *medulla*. They synapse there on neurons that join the *medial lemniscus* and travel, as part of the *lemniscal system*, to the thalamus and then on to the *somatosensory cortex*. Information from both the left and right halves of the tongue and throat goes to both sides of the cortex (you may want to return to Chapter 13 and briefly review the lemniscal system).

There are thousands of papillae, and each one may contain 200 or more taste buds. The total number of papillae and taste buds changes markedly as a function of age. The newborn has relatively few taste buds. During early childhood, there is an increase in the number of taste buds found in papillae. There is also an increase in the number of taste buds found where there are no papillae: on the underside of the tongue, on the insides of the cheeks, and on the throat surfaces. During adulthood, taste buds seem to be confined to the papillae. In later life, the number of papillae and taste buds declines. These differences may partially account for changes in taste preferences. Newborns are relatively insensitive to taste. Children are quite sensitive to (and often intolerant of) bitter and spicy tastes. Adults often enhance taste sensations by adding seasonings and spices.

The fact that individual taste cells are constantly degenerating and being replaced, and the fact that the numbers and locations of taste buds change as we age, should suggest to you that we are dealing with a very changeable system. Its changeable character may be one of the sources of our confusion in understanding taste.

Taste Stimuli

Chemicals that are capable of activating the taste cells all have one property in common: they must be soluble in saliva. Saliva is a mixture of a variety of substances, and its composition varies from one individual to another—and even for one individual, depending upon the time of day, diet, the presence of fever or infection, and so on. For the sake of simplicity, we can consider saliva to be primarily water with a good dose of salt added. Any substance that is not soluble in salty water cannot be tasted.

Let's adopt the most commonly accepted listing of taste sensations: salt, sour, bitter, and sweet. If we can identify substances each of which creates just one of these sensations, we can examine what happens to the substances when they're placed in saliva. Table salt (sodium chloride, NaCl), for example, seems to produce a "pure" salt sensation, while quinine seems to produce a "pure" bitter sensation. When a molecule of sodium chloride is placed in saliva, it ionizes (the molecule splits into atoms that carry positive or negative charges). We end up with a positive sodium ion and a negative chloride ion. Quinine, on the other hand, is not ionized by saliva. A quinine molecule remains in its molecular form in saliva. Let's take a closer look at this kind of examination of substances that produce "pure" taste sensations and see if it provides any information that will reduce some of the confusion about taste stimuli.

As we've said, sodium chloride is ionized by saliva. Therefore, two different stimuli are available to the taste buds: the positive sodium ions and the negative chloride ions. We might ask whether just one or both of these stimuli give rise to the salt sensation. One way to find out is to examine what happens when salts other than sodium chloride are placed in the mouth. We might first try potassium chloride. It is ionized by saliva into the positive potassium ion and the negative chloride ion. And, most importantly, it produces a salt sensation. In fact, potassium chloride is often sold as a "salt substitute" for individuals who must limit their intake of table salt because of high blood pressure.

Because sodium chloride and potassium chloride both produce salt sensations, and because they have in common the negative chloride ion, we might be tempted to say that salt sensations are produced by negative chloride ions. However, it is also the case that sodium bromide produces a salt sensation. It is ionized by saliva into the positive sodium ion and the negative bromide ion. Therefore, it has in common with sodium chloride only the positive sodium ion. Now we have a case in which the salt sensations seem to be produced by positive sodium ions. At this point, it should not surprise you to discover that salt sensations are thought to occur whenever *either* sodium ions or chloride ions are present.

Before we go on to consider substances that produce the sour sensation, let's think carefully about the salt sensation. The three substances we've mentioned (sodium chloride, potassium chloride, and sodium bromide) all produce salt sensations, but they do not taste exactly alike. Individuals can readily discriminate among these three. In addition, the taste sensations produced by these substances change drastically depending upon their concentrations. At very low concentrations, both sodium chloride and potassium chloride tend to taste somewhat sweet. At slightly higher concentrations, sodium chloride tastes salty, but potassium chloride tastes bitter. It is only at very high concentrations that potassium chloride tastes salty. All of this should sound very puzzling to you. Remember that we began by talking about a "pure" salt sensation, and we concluded that either sodium ions or chloride ions can produce that sensation. But now we discover that one so-called "pure" salt sensation is not identical to another, and that a substance that produces the "pure" salt sensation can give rise to other sensations, such as sweet or bitter. Do I need to remind you that a great deal of confusion exists in the universe of the chemical senses?

But on to the sour sensation. All substances that taste sour to us are acids. These acids ionize in saliva, and they all have in common the presence of the positive hydrogen ion.

Now we can say that salt and sour sensations seem to arise in the presence of certain ions. Interestingly, bitter and sweet sensations do not appear to arise in response to ions. Substances that taste bitter or sweet do not ionize in saliva; they remain in their molecular form. Substances that give rise to bitter sensations (e.g., quinine) or sweet sensations (e.g., the sugars) are usually organic compounds (that is, they contain carbon). There is a hint that bitter and sweet sensations may be related to each other. Some substances, such as saccharin, taste sweet in low concentrations, but they taste bitter in high concentrations. In addition, some substances that taste sweet will taste bitter when their chemical constituents are rearranged (this is the process called *isomerization,* which we discussed in Chapter 5 under the topic of the photochemicals of the retina).

Isomers of the same molecule differ from one another only in the geometric arrangement of their chemical constituents. As an analogy, imagine that we have three pieces of water pipe: one short straight piece, one long straight piece, and one curved piece. Let's select just two possible arrangements of these pipes (in all, there are 6 possible arrangements of them).

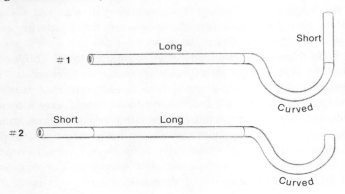

If we were to build forms that would just barely accommodate these two structures, obviously the forms would be very different from each other.

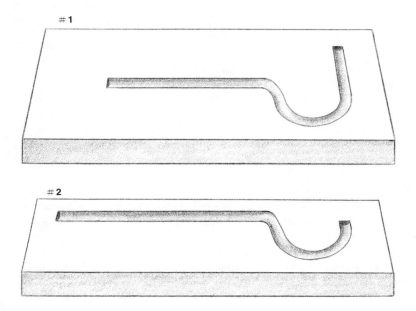

It would only be possible for us to place a given arrangement in just one of these forms. Neither arrangement could be accommodated by both forms.

Interestingly, a different ordering of arrangement #2 would fit into form #2: instead of having first short, then long, then curved, we could have long, then short, then curved. However no other ordering except arrangement #1 would fit into form #1.

What do these pipes and forms have to do with taste? Think of the various arrangements of the pipes as being isomers of a "pipe molecule," and think of the forms as being different cilia projecting from individual taste cells. If individual cilia do indeed have properties that allow them to accommodate only certain isomers, perhaps some of the confusion concerning taste stimuli can be cleared up. Our pipe-and-form analogy indicates that only some isomers should produce identical results (short-long-curved and long-short-curved), while other isomers will produce very different results.

We can go a bit further with this. Imagine that we have the following three forms.

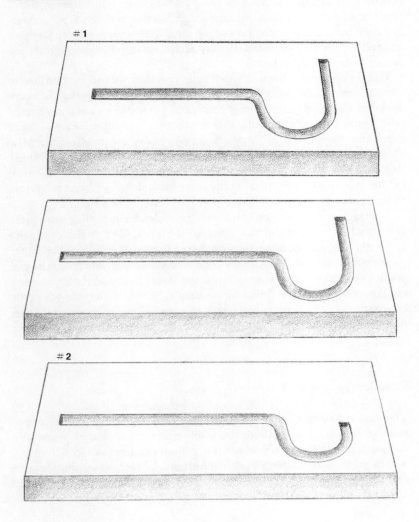

The first form is our original #1. The last form is our original #2. Notice that the middle form can accommodate either of our two different pipe arrangements, although neither arrangement will fit perfectly. The other two forms can each accommodate just one of our two pipe arrangements.

Let's again think of the two pipe arrangements as if they were isomers, and of the three forms as if they were cilia. It should be clear that each isomer may fit two different cilia. Now we can say that these two isomers will produce results that are similar in one respect (they will both be accommodated by the middle cilium), but they will not produce identical results because each isomer will also be accommodated by just one of the remaining cilia. In this way, perhaps we can understand how two substances may each taste bitter or sweet, but they do not taste exactly alike.

The theory we've been discussing is one that should be familiar to you if you've read very much about how enzymes work. Different enzymes have different geometric structures, and the various locations where enzymes can exert influence are thought to contain *receptor sites* of particular shapes. In the "lock-and-key" view of enzyme function, the enzymes are the "keys" and the receptor sites that they precisely fit are the "locks." When the "lock-and-key" view is applied to the chemical senses, it is often referred to as the *stereochemical theory* ("stereo-" refers to shape, form, or spatial arrangement) of taste, or of smell.

Although the stereochemical theory provides an intriguing approach, you should keep in mind that it is only a theory. No one has ever seen variously shaped receptor sites on taste cilia; we don't know whether they really exist. Further, the theory doesn't help our understanding of certain aspects of taste. For example, the stereochemical theory doesn't explain why taste sensations should vary as wildly as they do when the concentration of a taste substance is changed. Despite these problems, the stereochemical theory seems to be the best one we currently have.

Complex Taste Sensations

The vast majority of the substances we taste do not produce "pure" taste sensations. Think about the taste sensations that arise when you eat a dill pickle. Certainly, there is a pronounced sensation of "sour," but there is also a strong "salt" sensation. In fact, most people also detect "bitter" and "sweet" sensations. The taste we associate with dill pickles is a blend of "pure" sensations.

One of the most revealing demonstrations you can perform for yourself is to analyze various substances into their taste components. Start out by producing the four "pure" sensations for yourself: first, taste a little table salt. Remind yourself that the sensation that occurs is the one considered the "ultimate" in saltiness. Rinse your mouth. (This is important! Why?) Then taste some pure lemon juice. Remind yourself that you're now experiencing the "ultimate" in sourness. Rinse your mouth and sample some plain sugar. That will produce the "ultimate" in sweetness. Finally, rinse your mouth, sample some quinine water (this is available in most grocery stores as a mixer for drinks, but be careful to buy quinine water that does not contain sugar or other sweeteners), and experience "ultimate" bitterness. Now that you've experienced the four "pure" sensations, you can assign the value of 100 to each one: table salt produced a value of 100 on the saltiness scale, lemon juice produced a value of 100 on the sourness scale, etc.

Now select a food you want to analyze. You might try an apple or piece of bread or coffee. Whatever you select, try to focus your attention on the component sensations and rank the sensations on four scales. If you chose the apple, as you chew it, try to remember the sensation of 100 on the saltiness scale. Zero on the saltiness scale means the complete absence of any salt sensations. Rank the saltiness of your apple somewhere between zero and 100. Then do the same for the sourness scale, the sweetness scale, and the bitterness scale. When you finish the four rankings, ask yourself whether there is any additional taste sensation produced by the apple. If your answer is "no" (that is, if the sensation produced by the apple is nothing more than the combination of a particular amount of saltiness, of sourness, of sweetness, and of bitterness), you are actually confirming the idea that there are four and only four "pure" tastes. All taste sensations are then nothing more than unique combinations of salt, sour, sweet, and bitter. If you find that the apple produced something more, you are suggesting that there must be something more than the four basic tastes.

Before you come to any firm conclusions, try analyzing several different taste substances. Even better, coerce some friends, relatives, passers-by, or whomever you can find to join you in analyzing taste sensations. The comparisons of the rankings assigned by different individuals are typically fascinating. If you can find someone who has a head-cold, all the better (remember that we said earlier that much of what we normally think of as taste is actually smell).

There are several additional things you should think about as you perform this demonstration. First, consider what happens when you keep the taste substance in one part of your mouth: chew and hold some apple bits in the front of your mouth while you rank them. Then chew and hold them at the sides of your mouth while you assign rankings. Also try chewing and holding them at the back of your mouth. Second, pay attention to what happens to the sensations over time: does the first taste of the substance produce sensations that are different from those produced by the second or third taste? Finally, what happens to the sensations when the temperature of the substance is changed? Does a well-chilled apple receive the same rankings as an apple of room temperature?

We'll discuss what happens to taste sensations as the location or length of exposure or temperature changes. First, however, I'd like you to look at the labels of food items in your home or in a grocery store. Pay particular attention to highly processed foods such as juice-like drinks or prepackaged dessert and snack items. Many of the labels will have lists of ingredients that read like an inventory of a chemistry lab. The point is that many "real" foods produce taste sensations that can be mimicked by the appropriate combinations of chemicals. Insofar as the taste of an apple can be expressed as a particular combination of salt, sour, sweet, and bitter, it ought to be possible to produce an apple taste without any apple at all. In fact, it is not especially difficult to produce a great many different chemical tastes that mimic the tastes of "real" foods. What is difficult is to produce a texture for the chemical combination that closely resembles the texture of a "real" food. As you look at the labels, it should become more than obvious to you that our sense of taste is based on our reactions to particular chemicals.

Electrophysiology of Taste

When you performed your taste analyses, it may have become clear to you that a substance does not taste the same when it is held in different parts of the mouth. Apple bits taste noticeably sweeter when they're held in the front of the mouth, rather than on the sides or in the back. Coffee does not taste especially bitter unless it's held in the back of the mouth. One way to summarize this is to say that the tongue seems to have different regions that are especially sensitive to different taste sensations. The tip of the tongue is more sensitive to sweet than are the sides or back. The back of the tongue is more sensitive to bitter than are the sides or tip. This does not mean that only the tip is sensitive to sweet, or only the back is sensitive to bitter. It does mean that there are *regional variations* in relative sensitivity (just as there are regional variations in skin sensitivity—do you remember coming across that in Chapter 13?). Let's take a look at a graph that summarizes these regional variations.

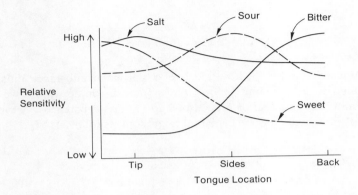

Notice that the graph specifies only three tongue regions: the tip, sides, and back. What about the middle region, that center zone on the top surface of the tongue? Strangely, there are relatively few taste buds found there and, consequently, the middle region of the tongue is rather insensitive to all taste sensations. You can demonstrate this for yourself by sticking out your tongue and placing a small piece of food on the middle region. Unless the food you've chosen has a very strong flavor, you'll experience no sensations (strongly flavored foods actually are likely to produce smell rather than taste sensations in this situation). If you move the piece of food so that it rests on the tip or sides or back of the tongue, you should experience taste sensations. The insensitivity of the middle region of the tongue is not usually a problem. Substances that are taken into the mouth and swallowed pass over the tip, sides (especially if they're chewed), and back of the tongue.

You might expect that, if the tongue has regional variations in sensitivity, the taste buds should also vary in sensitivity depending upon their location. When recordings are made from individual taste buds or from the neurons collecting information from them, it is usually found that there is a bias toward one kind of stimulation. Most of the taste buds at the tip of the tongue are very responsive to sugars. Most of those at the back are very responsive to bitter substances such as quinine. However, individual taste buds inevitably respond to more than one kind of stimulation. Thus, those at the tip that are very responsive to sugars are often also responsive to salts and sometimes to sour substances. The important factor is the *relative* responses to these substances. Perhaps the easiest way to measure the relative responsivity is to ask how much of a particular substance must be applied to a taste bud before it responds. In other words, we can examine the *threshold* of a taste bud to various substances. A typical set of thresholds for one taste bud might look as follows:

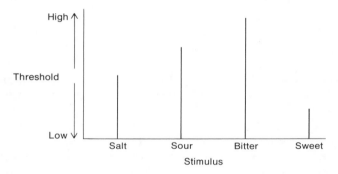

This taste bud is very sensitive to (has a low threshold for) sweet, and it is progressively less sensitive to (has increasing thresholds for) salt, sour, and bitter. Actually, many taste buds are totally insensitive to (have an infinitely high threshold for) one or two kinds of stimulation.

The neurons that collect information from the taste buds respond in a similar manner. They typically react more vigorously to one kind of stimulation and less vigorously to others. Because each neuron collects information from many taste buds (an example of *convergence*—do you remember convergent and divergent arrangements?), it should not surprise you to learn that the neurons are usually a bit less specific in their responses than the taste buds: that is, although most taste buds are totally insensitive to one or two kinds of stimulations, most of the neurons respond to all or most kinds of stimulations.

Many of the neurons produce nerve impulses at a slow and steady rate in the absence of specific taste stimulation (their axons have a *maintained discharge*). This may be a steady response to saliva. When an appropriate taste stimulus is introduced, these neurons markedly increase their firing rate for a brief time. If the stimulus remains, the neurons reduce their rate to a somewhat lower level. When the stimulus is removed, the neuron returns to its original rate of impulse production. We can summarize this in a graph.

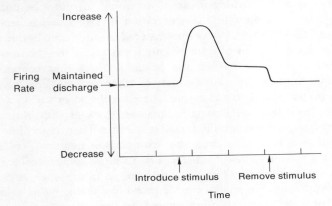

If the neuron has a very low threshold for sweet and progressively higher thresholds for salt, sour, and bitter, it will react to equal concentrations of these substances as follows:

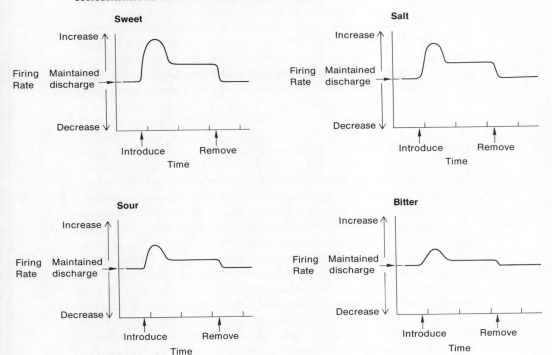

Increasing the concentration of any of these substances will produce a higher initial firing rate and a higher steady rate. In terms of the response of this individual neuron, we would therefore be unable to distinguish between a low concentration of sweet and a very high concentration of bitter. We've encountered this dilemma before (especially in our discussion of color vision). If you recall, the solution to the dilemma is to have, within the brain, neurons that compare the responses they receive from a variety of other neurons. The "comparison neurons" could, for example, compare the information arriving from neurons that are especially sensitive to sweet with information arriving from those especially sensitive to bitter. Then, regardless of the concentration of a substance, the "comparison neurons" could differentiate between a sweet substance and a bitter substance—based on which of the two sets of neurons bringing in information is reacting more vigorously. I hope you are reminded of a theme we've discussed repeatedly: we interpret stimuli based on the *patterns of activity* they create.

Whether such "comparison neurons" in fact exist in the thalamus or in the somatosensory cortex is not known. Research on the appropriate thalamic and cortical areas has been skimpy, in part because most researchers want to sort out the confusions over the nature of taste stimuli and taste sensations before examining the responses in the taste pathway. What is known is that neurons in the thalamus and the cortex react to more than one kind of taste stimulation in a fashion very much like the neurons that collect information from the taste buds.

Taste Adaptation

As you may have already noticed, the responses of taste buds and the neurons associated with them decline rapidly after the initial presentation of taste stimuli. This process is one we've repeatedly encountered: the decline in response represents *adaptation*. In the case of taste, we cannot specify why the decline takes place. There is no obvious mechanical reason for it, and we must assume that the decline occurs because of neural changes within the taste buds and neurons.

You may have also noticed that taste sensations decline markedly when a taste substance is repeatedly sampled. During your taste analyses, you probably realized that the initial sensations produced by the apple were more intense than the later sensations. It is certainly tempting to assume that the reduction in taste sensations is caused by the decline in the responses of the taste buds and their neurons. However, there are some problems here. First, the decline in the responses of taste buds and neurons occurs very soon after the stimulation begins. In most cases, the response level of the neurons has reached its lowered, steady rate within one second following the beginning of stimulation (this can vary, of course, depending on such factors as the intensity and the kind of stimulation that's used). But the reduction in taste sensations usually takes considerably longer before it's complete. Depending upon the intensity and kind of stimulation, the adaptation of taste sensations may take anywhere from several seconds to several minutes. Therefore, we must conclude that the decline in response of the taste buds and their neurons does not fully account for the reduction in taste sensation.

Secondly, the neurons associated with the taste buds continue to produce impulses at a steady rate as long as stimulation continues. Yet if we are exposed to an unchanging level of taste stimulation, we lose all sense of its taste within a few minutes. In other words, the neurons never cease responding to the stimulation, but we cease to detect any taste sensations. Once again, we're forced to conclude that the adaptation of the taste buds and their neurons does not fully account for the adaptation of our sensations.

The suspicion is that additional adaptation events must be taking place in the thalamus and cortex. In fact, such adaptation events probably occur at a variety of locations in the brain in every sensory system. The precise nature of these events is unknown, but you can probably come up with some good notions about the kinds of events that are likely to be occuring.

Let's pause here and consider the now familiar process called adaptation in a slightly different way. We've repeatedly emphasized the idea that our nervous system reacts most to changes in stimulation. Adaptation, or the decline in reaction that occurs when we are presented with ongoing, unchanging stimulation, certainly reflects this. But why have we evolved in such a way that we react most to changes in stimulation? Why are we "prewired" to attend to the first instant of stimulation and then gradually adapt?

To begin suggesting some answers, we need to get away from thinking of taste in terms of the aesthetics of a gourmet meal or a double cheeseburger (depending on your gastronomic bent). We need to think in terms of the biologically important information we derive from taste sensations. Consider, for example, the fact that naturally occurring sweet substances tend to be nontoxic and nutritious. (I'm not thinking of processed or refined substances such as white sugar, but rather of foods such as ripe fruit.) Naturally occurring bitter substances tend to be toxic and nonnutritious (such as unripe fruit, poisonous grasses, etc.).

There is not a perfect correlation between the sweetness or bitterness of a substance and its toxicity or nutritive value, but the relationship is strong. In terms of survival, being able to detect sweetness and bitterness is important. Once you've detected the sweetness or bitterness of a substance, knowing that more of the same substance is equally sweet or bitter is unimportant. Biologically speaking, who cares if the fourth or fifth bite of an apple tastes as sweet as the first? The important piece of information came with the first bite: this apple is sweet, therefore it is safe to eat. If a bite of the apple suddenly tastes bitter, all the important information is provided in that one bite: stop eating this apple, it is unsafe to eat.

Concentrating on changes in stimulation provides us with an economical way of obtaining the information that is of greatest importance. Reducing our reactions to ongoing, unchanging stimulation means doing away with a lot of "clutter" that would otherwise demand our attention. If I stop paying attention to the unchanging sweetness of the apple I'm eating, I'm free to pay attention to something else in my environment.

Although this discussion of the biological significance of our tendency to attend most to changes in stimulation has dealt only with taste, you may want to stop here for a while and consider whether the same kind of discussion could be applied to other senses. Think about the adaptation we described in vision, in audition, in the skin senses, and in the detection of body position and movement before you return to the world of taste adaptation.

We've often described adaptation as a process by which the nervous system resets the baseline against which it will judge future stimulation. In taste, this often leads to some interesting events called *contrast effects*. Suppose, for example, that you sample a bit of quinine. Following this, you eat something sweet for a while. If you then sample the quinine again, it will taste more bitter than it originally did. What has happened is that you became partially adapted to sweet. In fact, sweet began to feel "normal." Judged against this baseline, the quinine seems especially bitter. (I trust that all this reminds you of what happens to temperature sensations when the physiological zero is changed.)

What is interesting is that not all combinations of taste substances produce contrast effects. For example, becoming adapted to salt does not appear to affect our sensations to bitter substances. In addition, adaptation to one substance may enhance our sensations of certain tastes, while reducing our sensations of other tastes; then again, adaptation to one substance may either enhance or reduce our sensations of another, depending on the concentration of the other substance. Thus, adaptation to salt may enhance or reduce our sensations to a sweet substance, depending upon how sweet the substance is.

Needless to say, the contrast effects have attracted a great deal of interest. If we could discover the rules underlying the various contrast effects, we might be in a position to understand better the nature of taste stimuli and the relationships among them. As things now stand, untold numbers of contrast effects have been examined, but no orderly characteristics have emerged.

Temperature Effects

If you analyzed various substances at different temperatures, you probably noticed that a chilled apple received different rankings from those for an apple at room temperature. You may have been aware of this even before you performed your taste analyses. If you season foods while they are hot, you may often discover that the foods taste overseasoned or underseasoned once they've cooled. Or you may have noticed that hot coffee or tea tastes less bitter than iced coffee or iced tea. There is no doubt that our taste sensations vary depending upon temperature. What is perplexing is that the various sensations change in different ways. Our sensitivity to salt seems to increase as the temperature decreases. Thus, a soup may seem correctly salted when it is hot, but oversalted when it cools slightly. In general, our sensitivity to bitter also increases as the temperature decreases. However, our sensitivity to sweet increases as the temperature increases; a moderately sweet chocolate bar may taste overly sweet when it is melted and used as a hot sauce. Finally, our sensitivity to sour remains virtually unchanged by temperature changes. Let's put all this into one graph.

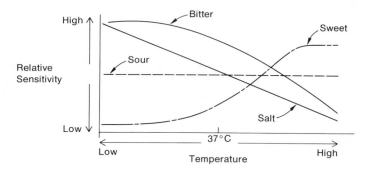

Notice that it is impossible to account for these temperature effects with one simple principle. It is not the case, for example, that increases in temperature merely enhance the various activities of the taste buds and their neurons. If that were the case, all our sensitivities should increase when the temperature is increased. Whatever is going on here is complicated and, once again, we are left with the feeling that, if only we could understand what is going on, we'd probably be a long way along toward understanding taste stimuli and taste sensations.

Olfactory Receptors and Pathways

The sense of smell is technically called *olfaction*. Olfaction is even less understood than taste. Let's again begin with what is relatively well understood: the olfactory receptors and pathways.

The olfactory receptors are located in the topmost portion of the *nasal cavity*. There are two patches of olfactory receptors, those of the left nostril and those of the right nostril, separated from each other by the nasal septum.

The nasal cavity is a complicated structure containing a number of bones and pieces of cartilage. The bones and cartilage channel air downward to the windpipe, and most inhaled air never reaches the olfactory receptors. Sniffing and inhaling deeply produce changes in the movement of air through the nasal cavity such that more air arrives at the receptors. When substances are chewed, some air is carried upward from the back of the throat, through the nasal cavity, to the receptors.

The receptors are actually just the naked dendritic endings of neurons. These endings are called the *olfactory rods*, and they hang down into the nasal cavity. Each olfactory rod bears several tiny hair-like structures, the *cilia*. Let's take a look at some sketches.

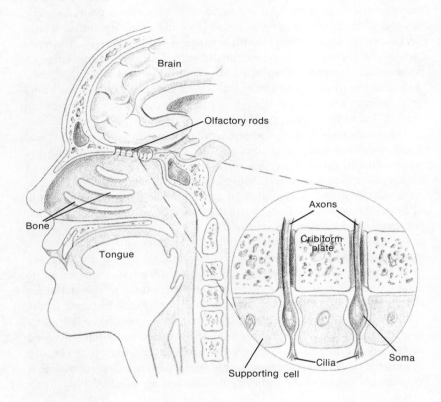

The profile sketch gives you an idea of the location of the olfactory rods within the nasal cavity. The other sketch is a super blowup of two olfactory rods. Notice that their axons pierce the *cribiform plate*, a piece of bone that forms the roof of the nasal cavity.

Each patch of olfactory receptors may contain as many as 30 million olfactory rods, crammed into an area of perhaps only several hundred square millimeters. The information travels from the olfactory rods toward the brain in two bundles of axons called the *olfactory nerves*. The olfactory nerves are short; they extend only to two structures located on the underside of the front portion of the brain. These structures, called the *olfactory bulbs*, are the synaptic relay areas for the olfactory system. From the olfactory bulbs, information may be sent to a wide variety of locations within the brain. Interestingly, olfactory information, unlike any other sensory information, is not ultimately sent to any particular region of the cortex.

Thus, in the olfactory system, the first-order neurons collect information via their dendrites and send it to the olfactory bulbs. The second-order neurons are the neurons of the olfactory bulbs. These second-order neurons fall into three categories: the *mitral cells*, the *tufted cells*, and the *granule cells*. Axons of the *mitral cells* carry information to subcortical structures deep within the brain. The *tufted cells* send their axons to the opposite olfactory bulb. And the *granule cells* send information from one location within an olfactory bulb to another location within that same bulb.

Where an axon of the olfactory nerve terminates within an olfactory bulb, there is usually a little clump of intricate synapses among the axon and the three categories of olfactory bulb cells. The clump of endings is called a *glomerulus* (plural, glomeruli), and you can think of each olfactory bulb as essentially a group of many thousand glomeruli. (I hope it has occurred to you that glomeruli are ideal locations for *convergence* and *divergence* of information.)

In addition to the fact that the olfactory system does not include a particular cortical area, you should notice that there is something else very peculiar about this system. Unlike any other sensory system, the olfactory system does not have a particular area of the thalamus devoted to it. Olfactory information does not appear to travel to the thalamus. These two oddities in the olfactory system have led many researchers to conclude that the olfactory system must have evolved separately from, and probably much earlier than, the other sensory systems. If that conclusion is correct, it seems a bit more reasonable that we should have so much difficulty understanding olfaction.

Olfactory Stimuli

You already know that there is absolutely no agreement concerning so-called "pure" or "basic" smells. Many researchers have tried to identify what properties are common to substances that smell alike. The only approach that has proven at all successful is to focus on the geometric properties of the substances. To a limited extent, substances that smell similar have molecules that are similar in shape. Thus, the *stereochemical theory*, which we discussed under the topic of taste stimuli, is also the most promising theory for olfaction. It suffers from the same problems we mentioned under taste: no one has ever seen a receptor site on an olfactory cilium, and several olfactory phenomena are not well explained by the theory.

The two things that can be said with confidence are that a substance must release some of its molecules into the air (it must be *volatile*) if we are to smell the substance, and that the released molecules must be at least partially soluble in water so that they can combine with the mucus covering the olfactory rods. However, just because a substance is volatile and water-soluble does not guarantee that we can smell it. Distilled water is volatile and its molecules are certainly water-soluble, but we cannot detect any smell associated with distilled water. Thus, we know the conditions that are necessary for olfaction, but these conditions are not always sufficient for olfaction.

We do know that we are able to respond to astoundingly low levels of olfactory stimuli. In terms of the minimum number of molecules required to produce a sensation, we are many thousands of times more sensitive to olfactory stimuli than we are to taste stimuli. We can go further than this, however, in indicating just how sensitive we are to olfactory stimuli. Recall the Hecht, Shlaer, and Pirenne experiment we discussed in detail under the topic of visual thresholds. Their experiment involved determining the minimum number of quanta that must arrive at the cornea if vision is to occur, the losses that occur as the quanta travel to the receptors, the number of quanta required to activate one receptor, and the number of receptors that must be activated if we are to experience a visual sensation.

An attempt has been made to perform the same kind of analysis in olfaction. There is sufficient confusion about which olfactory stimulus to test, whether to allow the individual to sniff it naturally or to literally "blast" the molecules into the nose, the time period during which the stimulus should be presented, and so on, to make us less comfortable about the olfactory analysis than we were about the visual analysis. Yet the results are still interesting.

If we calculate the percentage of molecules that never reach the olfactory rods because they are deflected by obstacles in the nasal cavity or because they adhere to the mucus found at locations other than the olfactory rods or because they pass right by the olfactory rods and end up in the windpipe, we discover that only about 2 percent of the inhaled molecules may ever affect the olfactory rods. Under some conditions, we can detect an odor when only 2,000 molecules are inhaled or, in other words, when only 40 molecules affect the olfactory rods. Considering the sheer number of olfactory rods, it is unlikely that any one receives more than one of those 40 molecules. Thus we can say that an individual olfactory rod can probably be activated by a single molecule.

Of course, our ability to detect odors varies depending upon the time of day (for example, we are far more sensitive to olfactory stimuli before lunch than we are after lunch), what odors are already present, the particular mixture of odors that reaches us at one time, etc. Before we examine some of these factors, let's briefly take a look at what is known of the electrophysiology of olfaction.

Electrophysiology of Olfaction

Recordings have been made from individual axons in the olfactory nerve. These axons tend to maintain a steady but extremely slow firing rate (a *maintained discharge*) when no olfactory stimuli are present. If an appropriate stimulus is continuously presented, the axons initially produce impulses at a very high rate and then rapidly reduce the rate to a lower, steady level. When the stimulus is removed, they return to the original, very slow rate.

Individual axons respond in this way only to a limited number of all the possible olfactory stimuli. In addition, there is some evidence that axons whose dendrites are located in one region of the patch of olfactory receptors all tend to respond to the same olfactory stimuli. It is therefore possible that *regional variations* may exist among the olfactory receptors just as they exist among the taste buds.

Similarly, neurons in the olfactory bulbs may also be regionally organized. For example, in the cat, the anterior portions of the olfactory bulbs seem to be especially sensitive to banana oil (!) while the posterior portions seem to be especially sensitive to the odors of decayed fish or meat.

Research in olfaction has not reached the elegance of work in vision or hearing for several reasons. First, we do not rely heavily on olfactory information in our daily lives; research has tended to focus upon the senses that are of primary importance to us. Second, the important structures, such as the olfactory rods, are situated in rather inaccessible locations. Third, different species of animals have bewilderingly different abilities to detect odors. (Just consider the olfactory reactions of dogs as compared to those of human beings.) Fourth, and most important, no one knows how to begin identifying and classifying all the possible olfactory stimuli. Even if we could record from the olfactory rods with ease, and even if we've agreed upon the appropriate experimental animals to use, we don't know which stimuli to test.

Maybe we should begin with floral odors. But there are an awful lot of different floral odors. Should we try to test every one? Should we select just a few and, if so, on what shall we base our selections? Or maybe we should start with spicy odors or fruity odors or. . . .

It's a problem, to say the least.

Olfactory Adaptation

I don't think anyone is unaware that the intensity of an odor seems to decline the longer you're exposed to that odor. You now also know that the axons of the olfactory nerve reduce their firing rate after the initial exposure to an olfactory stimulus. But just as we found in taste, we cannot conclude that the change in the responses of the axons fully accounts for the change in our sensations. The change in the responses of the axons occurs far more rapidly than the change in our sensations. Further, the axons continue to respond as long as the stimulation is presented, but we stop sensing any odor at all after the stimulation is presented for a while. Again, we must assume that there are additional adaptation mechanisms in the olfactory bulbs or elsewhere within the brain.

Adaptation to one olfactory stimulus may have no effect on our sensitivity to another stimulus, or it may either increase or decrease our sensitivity to other stimuli. Again, this should remind you of the situation in taste. So far, it has not been possible to develop any overall principles or rules that clarify which stimuli produce or do not produce effects on our perceptions of other stimuli.

Olfactory Mixtures

Normally we are confronted with a variety of olfactory stimuli at the same time. These mixtures can produce some interesting results. Sometimes, for example, the mixture of several stimuli produces a sensation that is unique and that is not simply the equivalent of the sum of a set of separate sensations. (This is similar to the situation in vision: when we are presented with a mixture of a particular level of red, a particular level of green, and a particular level of blue, we experience "white.") At other times, a mixture of olfactory stimuli produces a sensation best described as a blend, in which each of the individual stimuli can be identified. (This is similar to the situation in audition:

when we are presented with a mixture of notes, we hear something we call a chord, and all the individual notes can be separately heard.) Sometimes, a mixture of olfactory stimuli can result in the obliteration of some sensations. For example, it is nearly impossible to detect the odor of even a very fragrant rose if you are simultaneously sniffing a freshly cut onion. This situation is called *masking*, and it is one we encountered earlier in our discussion of audition.

As you can see almost any imaginable outcome can result from the mixture of olfactory stimuli. There is no way to deny that olfaction seems to become more complicated and less amenable to analysis, no matter which way we turn.

Summary

Be certain you understand and can explain all the italicized terms.

The chemical senses are the least understood of our sensory systems. In both taste and olfaction, there is considerable confusion over what constitutes the basic sensations and what properties of the stimuli are important.

In taste, we know that the receptors are the *taste buds* found primarily along the walls of *papillae*. A taste bud is actually a cluster of *taste cells*, each of which survives for perhaps a week, to be replaced by a new cell developed from the *supporting cells*. Each taste cell bears a *cilium*, which extends through the *taste pore* into the trench around the papilla.

Information from the taste buds is carried by the *facial, glossopharyngeal,* and *vagus nerves* to the *medulla*. From there, information travels as part of the *lemniscal system* to the *somatosensory cortex*.

In olfaction, we also know a bit about the receptors. The olfactory receptors are actually the dendritic endings of the first-order neurons. These endings, called the *olfactory rods*, enter the top wall of the *nasal cavity* through the *cribiform plate*. Each olfactory rod bears several *cilia* at its tip.

The axons of these first-order neurons form the *olfactory nerves*, which bring information to the *olfactory bulbs*. Where each axon terminates in the olfactory bulb, there is a small region of intricate synapses called a *glomerulus*. It is the location of synapses among the first-order neurons and the *mitral, tufted,* and *granule cells*. Information from the olfactory bulbs travels to various locations within the brain, although there are no regions in the *thalamus* or *cortex* that are devoted solely to olfactory information.

For a substance to be tasted, it must be soluble in saliva. Substances that give rise to salt and sour sensations *ionize* in saliva; substances that produce sweet and bitter sensations remain in *molecular form* in saliva. For a substance to be smelled, it must be *volatile* and water-soluble.

Although no theory exists that completely explains the nature of taste and olfactory stimuli or sensations, the *stereochemical theory* is more promising than most. It provides a way of thinking about how stimuli may interact with *receptor sites* on the cilia.

The axons in the cranial nerves associated with taste and in the olfactory nerves react to appropriate stimuli by briefly increasing their firing rates and then lowering them as the stimulation continues. Although the responses of these axons explain some of the reduction in sensation that occurs during prolonged exposure to a stimulus, they do not fully account for it. Thus, there must be additional *adaptation* mechanisms in the brain.

In the chemical senses, there is evidence for *regional variations* in sensitivity, for complex reactions to multiple stimulation (as in the case of *contrast effects*, for example), and for changes in sensitivity produced by such factors as the time of day or the temperature of the stimulus.

Recommended Readings

There are three good articles dealing with the chemical senses.

Amoore, J. E., J. W. Johnston, Jr., and M. Rubin. "The Stereochemical Theory of Odor," *Sci. Amer.*, Feb. 1964 (not available as an Offprint).

Haagen-Smit, A. J., "Smell and Taste," *Sci. Amer.*, March 1952 (Offprint #404).

Hodgson, E. S. "Taste Receptors," *Sci. Amer.*, May 1961 (not available as an Offprint).

For information on both taste and olfaction, see these books.

Mueller, C. G. *Sensory Psychology.* Prentice-Hall, 1965. (Chapters 5 and 6.)

Geldard, F. A. *The Human Senses,* 2nd ed. Wiley, 1972. (Chapters 15 and 16.)

Finally, there is a remarkable set of essays dealing with a wide variety of topics. The writing is extraordinary; the thoughts are sometimes awesome, sometimes ennobling. I suggest you read all the essays but, with reference to this chapter, I especially recommend the one entitled "Vibes" in the following book.

Thomas, L. *The Lives of a Cell.* Viking, 1974. Paperback edition, Bantam, 1975.

16

Concluding Thoughts

Let's construct an imaginary sensory system that incorporates those attributes most commonly found in our sensory systems. We'd begin, of course, with receptor cells. These are the cells we made such a fuss about in the Introduction. They convert the energy provided by an event in the world into the language of the nervous system. Think about the receptor cells we actually have: rods and cones; hair cells in the cochlea and vestibular apparatus; the receptors found in joints, muscles, and tendons; the array of skin receptors; taste cells; olfactory rods. Of all the sensory systems, olfaction is thought to be evolution-arily the oldest. Notice that of all the sensory systems, only olfaction relies completely on receptor cells that are simply the naked dendritic endings of the first-order neurons. Within the skin senses and the body senses, there are some receptor cells that are just dendritic endings, but there are other receptor cells that bear elaborate nonneural structures. The receptor cells found in the eyes, ears, vestibular apparatus, and taste buds are certainly not naked dendrite endings; they are cells in and of themselves, separate from any neuron.

As you think about these differences, it might occur to you that all receptor cells behave in a neuron-like way. Any neuron will respond by changing its polarization if it is sufficiently poked or squeezed or shocked or otherwise disturbed. In particular, receptor cells behave a lot like dendrites. They produce *graded potentials* that vary in amplitude depending upon the degree of disturbance (for example, rods and cones produce larger responses when the light is made more intense); in some cases, the graded potentials may be either *hyperpolarizations* or *depolarizations* depending upon the nature of the disturbance (for example, hair cells may hyperpolarize when bent in one direction but depolarize when bent in the other direction). But receptor cells do not behave exactly like neurons. The primary difference is to be found in the selectivity of receptor cells. They are typically more responsive to some kinds of disturbances than to others. Their selectivity is the result of two factors. First, receptor cells are strategically located in places where they will be subjected only to certain kinds of disturbances. For example, the olfactory rods are located such that they will rarely, if ever, be subjected to light, sound, heat or cold, touch, pressure, etc. Just about the only events from the outside world that will reach them are olfactory events. The positioning of receptor cells in strategic locations is often associated with the development of nonneural structures that promote the effectiveness of only certain kinds of disturbances. For example, all the elaborate equipment found in the ear is designed to transmit to the receptor cells information about pressure changes created by movements of air molecules. The equipment cannot mechanically react to light or to the ionic or molecular composition of air. These disturbances never reach the receptor cells in the cochlea.

The second factor involved in the selectivity of receptor cells has to do with the design and functioning of the cells themselves. Most receptor cells contain structures that are not found in "true" neurons. Rods and cones, for example, look very different from neurons; no neuron contains the equipment required to manufacture photochemicals or to build disks. Even the olfactory rods bear cilia at their tips; cilia are not part of the standard equipment of neurons.

Perhaps we can summarize all this by saying that receptor cells appear to be derived from neurons. As they developed through evolution, modifications were made in the original neuron plan. Receptor cells that evolved very early (such as the olfactory rods) were modified only slightly. They still show their neuronal heritage very clearly. Receptor cells that evolved later (such as the rods and cones) were substantially modified. They now appear markedly different from their neuronal ancestors.

This view of receptor cells is speculative. No one can be certain that it accurately describes the development of receptor cells, but it does provide one way of thinking about their origins. But let's return now to our imaginary sensory system.

So far, we have stipulated that we need receptor cells that can convert physical events into the language of the nervous system. The next thing we'll need is a series of neurons or neuron-like cells that can carry the information provided by the receptor cells into and through the brain. Each set of neurons in the series will collect information from the previous set. Part of the function of the series is simply to get the information from one place to another. However, there is no reason why these neurons cannot simultaneously modify, compare, and abstract portions of the information while carrying it along. In our sensory systems, each neuron typically performs its modifications, comparisons, and abstractions by collecting information from a partic-ular group of neurons in the previous set (we've described this before as the process of *convergence* of information) and by sending information to a particular group of neurons in the next set (*divergence* of information). The results can be startlingly complex: do you recall our discussion of the way in which simple receptive fields can be developed by combining a group of center–surround receptive fields, and complex receptive fields can be developed from the appropriate grouping of simple receptive fields?

Finally, we need to add the fact that, in us, all this modification, comparison, and abstraction is somehow interpreted, resulting in the personal experience of awareness. I wish I could tell you how the interpretation is performed. However, with all we do know about the workings of the brain, no one is able to explain how the movements of ions across the membranes of neurons finally produce the overwhelm-ingly important, undeniable experience that "yes, I exist"—"yes, I perceive"—"yes, I feel and think and know."

Let's go back to our imaginary sensory system and see what we can specify about the manner in which it should function. You know by now that the first-order neurons of our sensory systems usually have *maintained discharges*. There is a suspicion that maintained discharges may be caused by ongoing activity in the receptor cells, which continues even in the apparent absence of stimulation. For example, it is known that body heat supplies enough energy to isomerize some molecules of the photochemicals found in rods and cones. Therefore, even when no light is physically present, rods and cones are contin-uously activated, albeit at a low level. As a result, cells throughout the visual system are continuously activated. Thus, the source of the maintained discharge may be the receptor cells. Alternatively, it is possible that maintained discharges occur because of a property intrinsic to the cells producing them. Whatever their source, maintained discharges serve as a baseline against which changes can be judged. Whenever the *firing rate* changes from the maintained discharge level, the neuron is signaling the fact that an event occurred.

In our imaginary system, the first-order neurons will have a maintained discharge, and they will change their firing rate whenever the receptor cells from which they receive information are sufficiently disturbed. We already know that the receptor cells are selective. They do not react to all disturbances. The first-order neurons are therefore indirectly selective; the immediate disturbance that affects them is always the same (they are always "set off" by the reactions of the receptor cells), but that disturbance will occur only when the appropriate physical event affects their receptor cells.

Notice the use of the term "their" receptor cells. Each neuron collects its information from a limited set of receptor cells. Another way to say this is to indicate that information from particular receptor cells *converges* on each neuron. As a result, a first-order neuron reacts only when the appropriate physical event impinges on one group of receptor cells. Typically, those receptor cells that send their information to the same first-order neuron are located near each other. This is the basis for the *receptive fields* we described in vision and in the skin senses, and the *response areas* we talked about in audition. (Response areas are usually thought of in terms of the frequencies of sound to which a neuron responds. We can alternatively think of them in terms of the locations along the basilar membrane of those hair cells that must be bent in order to activate particular neurons. Because von Békèsy's findings indicate that particular frequencies of sound have their primary effects on particular locations along the basilar membrane, we are really describing the same thing in these two views of response areas.)

Typically, the first-order neuron rather faithfully reproduces many aspects of the activity and arrangement of its receptor cells. If the receptor cells become intensely disturbed, the first-order neuron alters its firing rate substantially. If the receptor cells are less disturbed, the first-order neuron changes its firing rate less drastically. In some cases, the first-order neuron faithfully records whether the receptor cells hyperpolarize or depolarize, by decreasing or increasing its firing rate. In other cases, the neuron-like cell that collects information from the receptor cells sometimes depolarizes and sometimes hyperpolarizes, even when the receptor cells always hyperpolarize. (I am thinking here of cells in the intermediate layer of the retina.) In the first instance, it is not hard to imagine that hyperpolarizations of the receptor cells inhibit the first-order neuron, while depolarizations of the receptor cells activate it. In the second instance, we have to assume that hyperpolarizations of some receptor cells always inhibit some neuron-like cells, while hyperpolarizations of other receptor cells always excite these neuron-like cells.

A first-order neuron also preserves information about the spatial arrangement of its receptor cells. If its receptor cells are aligned in a row, a first-order neuron will react most vigorously to a physical stimulus that "covers" the row. If the receptor cells are grouped in a circle, the first-order neuron will react most vigorously to a physical stimulus that "covers" the circle. Preservation of information about spatial arrangement becomes most important when we tie it in with the notion that the receptor cells do not all react in the same way to the same physical event. Individual receptor cells have varying sensitivities and responses. If all the receptor cells located in one region of a receptive field react in the same way but those located in a different region react in an opposite fashion, the first-order neuron signals this by increasing its firing rate when the appropriate physical stimulus is located in one position and decreasing its firing rate when the same stimulus is located in another position. (The same principle applies to the ganglion cells of the retina. However, in this case, we need to consider the responses of the intermediate cells rather than the responses of the receptor cells.)

One area in which first-order neurons may not faithfully reproduce the activity of their receptor cells is in the domain of time. Typically, receptor cells continue to signal the presence of a stimulus as long as the stimulus remains. First-order neurons tend to respond less and less the longer a stimulus remains. We know this process well: it is *adaptation.*

The principles that apply to the responses of the first-order neurons also apply to each set of neurons in the series that carries information into and through the brain. The second-order neurons operate on the information brought to them by the first-order neurons, much as the first-order neurons operate on the information brought to them by the receptor cells. A second-order neuron rather faithfully reproduces the level of activity and spatial arrangement of its first-order neurons. The second-order neuron typically displays somewhat more adaptation than its first-order neurons. And so it goes.

We should point out that each set of neurons in the series is arranged in an orderly way. First-order neurons that have neighboring receptive fields (that is, they collect information from groups of receptor cells that lie side-by-side) tend to be located next to each other. Second-order neurons that collect information from adjoining groups of first-order neurons are located next to each other. In this way, information about the overall spatial arrangements of the receptor cells is preserved. Even at the level of the sixth- or seventh-order neurons, the receptive fields (or their equivalents) of neighboring neurons tend to be located next to each other. This orderly arrangement is precisely what we identified as *retinotopic maps*, *tonotopic maps*, and *somatotopic maps*.

Suppose I actually handed you a batch of receptor cells, whatever nonneural structures you desire, and some neurons. Could you arrange these elements so that they would approximate a sensory system? Certainly the most critical decisions you'd have to make would involve the linkages from receptor cells to neurons, and then from each set of neurons to the next in the series. The relationships you established among these elements would determine, to a large extent, the nature of the information analyzed by your sensory system.

If, for example, you arranged the elements such that each neuron received information from just one receptor cell or from just one neuron in the previous set, no broad comparisons could be made anywhere in the system. That is, without convergence and divergence of information, the effects of different stimuli would be very much the same—except to the very limited extent that any individual receptor cell or neuron can react to varying degrees, depending on the nature and intensity of the stimulus, and can perform spatial and temporal summation. Each receptor cell and its associated string of neurons would form a "private line." Information among the private lines would never be shared, and there would be no way to determine the *pattern of activity* within the nervous system. As a result, there would be no basis for abstracting certain features of the stimuli: the size of stimuli could not be known without "comparison neurons" that totalled up the number of private lines that were busy. The location of stimuli, their shapes, their contours or edges, their intensities (an individual receptor cell or neuron can signal only a limited range of intensities; much of the information we have concerning intensity comes about as a result of the threshold differences among receptor cells and among neurons), their quality (just consider the fact that we interpret something as being "hot" when it produces a particular pattern of activity in the nervous system), their very meaning (we apparently understand something as being "painful" because of interactions among neurons)—all would be lost to us. In other words, the information about stimuli that is most important to us requires the presence of neurons that perform comparisons. Exactly which comparisons are performed determine what features or aspects of stimuli we experience.

Notice that without "comparison neurons," the problem of the absolute threshold is partially resolved. If there are no "comparison neurons," we can justifiably talk about an absolute threshold of a receptor cell or any of the neurons in its private line. It is only when we add neurons that compare what occurs before and during a test trial, that contrast the possible consequences of "right" and "wrong" answers, and so on, that we must drop the concept of an absolute threshold in favor of the idea that our sensitivity varies depending upon the situation we're in.

Without "comparison neurons" of any kind, we cannot differentiate among most stimuli. If there are neurons that can "keep track" of the activity in a private line from one moment to the next (that is, neurons that make comparisons over time), we can have very rudimentary *difference thresholds*. But it is only when we have a rich array of "comparison neurons" that we can discriminate well among stimuli.

Without "comparison neurons," *trading ratios* would become extraordinarily limited affairs. The intensity and duration of a stimulus could only be traded off against each other to the extent that a single neuron can increase its firing rate within a limited range either when a stimulus is made more intense or, via temporal summation, when the stimulus lasts longer (or, via spatial summation, when it is simultaneously disturbed at more than one location).

And what about adaptation and the associated idea that we are especially sensitive to changes in stimulation? Certainly an individual neuron can reduce its response to continuous stimulation; if there are neurons that make comparisons of the activity within a private line from one moment to the next, we can have a rudimentary form of *adaptation*. But think about some of the topics we've considered throughout this book that involve our sensitivity to changes in stimulation: afterimages, the Mach Band, sound localization, the perception of temperature, the functioning of the semicircular canals, contrast effects in taste. We could go on and on with this list. The important point is that, without some basis for assessing the pattern of activity in groups of neurons, these phenomena would not occur. Without convergence and divergence of information, without "comparison neurons," we would not be aware of most changes in stimulation.

When we discussed taste adaptation, we described the possible biological significance of our sensitivity to changes. To the extent that our ability to detect changes in the world is important to our survival, convergence and divergence of information is important to our survival.

You may choose to read the previous sentence simply as a comment on the functioning of our sensory systems, or also as a comment on our human need to share what we know.

Recommended Readings

There is a fascinating book that explores the senses from the viewpoint that they are active, information-seeking systems. Please have a look at it.

Gibson, J. J. *The Senses Considered as Perceptual Systems*, Houghton Mifflin Co., 1966.

Appendix:

Measurement
Units

Metric units are based on multiples of ten. Once you get used to thinking in metric terms, it becomes quite easy to convert from one unit of
measurement to another. For example, if I want to change from meters
to centimeters, I simply multiply by 100. If I want to change from
meters to millimeters, I multiply by 1,000. Contrast this with the
situation in the U.S. Customary Units: to go from yards to feet, I must
multiply by 3; to go from yards to inches, I must multiply by 36; and so
on.

The key to understanding metric units is to learn the meaning of
prefixes such as "centi-" and "milli-." Each prefix indicates the multiple
of ten that must be used to convert from one unit to another. The
following table lists the units most commonly used in the study of the

senses, their abbreviations, the meanings of their prefixes, and the equivalent U.S. Customary Units.

Metric Unit	Abbrev.	Meaning of the Prefix	Metric Equivalent	Equivalent in U.S. Customary Units
Meter	m	No prefix	1.0 m	39.37 in
Centimeter	cm	"centi-" $= 0.01$ or 10^{-2}	0.01 m	0.3937 in
Millimeter	mm	"milli-" $= 0.001$ or 10^{-3}	0.001 m	0.03937 in
Micrometer	μm	"micro-" $= 0.000001$ or 10^{-6}	0.000001 m	0.00003937 in
Nanometer	nm	"nano-" $= 0.000000001$ or 10^{-9}	0.000000001 m	0.00000003937 in
Angstrom	Å	No prefix	0.0000000001 m	0.000000003937 in

Sorry about that last unit in the table; it doesn't conform to the metric system of names, although it is a metric unit. (The system of metric prefixes does not cover every possible power of ten.) The angstrom is named after a Swedish physicist, and it is useful in describing the sizes of atoms and molecules. It is equivalent to 10^{-10} meter.

The superscript after the number ten tells you which multiple of ten you must use to convert from any particular unit to meters. One centimeter, for example, is equal to 0.01 m, or 10^{-2} m. To convert from centimeters to meters, you multiply by 0.01, or 10^{-2}. Similarly, to convert from millimeters to meters, you multiply by 0.001, or 10^{-3}. Notice that this actually amounts simply to moving the decimal point to the left by a certain number of spaces; the superscript gives you that number of spaces.

Suppose, for example, that I have something 136.20 millimeters long. I can convert that to meters by moving the decimal point three spaces to the left; the object is 0.13620 meter long. An object 5.3 mm wide is 0.0053 m wide. Something that is 717.35 cm long can also be described as 7.1735 m in length (in this case, the decimal point was moved two spaces to the left to convert from centimeters to meters).

Suppose I want to convert from millimeters to centimeters. A millimeter is one-tenth of a centimeter. I would therefore multiply millimeters by 0.1 to convert them to centimeters. Because $0.1 = 10^{-1}$, this amounts to moving the decimal point one space to the left. For example, something that is 12.0 millimeters long is also 1.20 centimeters in length. Notice that the difference between the *superscripts* for "milli-" (10^{-3}) and "centi-" (10^{-2}) is one; this difference tells you how many spaces the decimal point must be moved to convert from millimeters to centimeters.

Conversion from smaller units to larger units always involves moving the decimal point to the left.

Try the following problems.

1. Something that is 67 angstroms long is also how many nanometers long? (The difference between the superscripts of 10^{-10} and 10^{-9} is one; move the decimal point one space to the left.)

2. Something that is 67 angstroms long is also how many micrometers long? (The difference between the superscripts of 10^{-10} and 10^{-6} is four; move the decimal point four spaces to the left.)

If you want to convert from larger units to smaller units, you move the decimal point the designated number of spaces to the right. Something that is 6.00 meters in length can also be described as being 600.0 centimeters long (moving the decimal point two spaces to the right) or 6,000.0 millimeters long (moving the decimal point three spaces to the right).

Now try these problems.

1. Something that is 9.25 mm long is also how many micrometers long? (The difference between the superscripts of 10^{-3} and 10^{-6} is three; move the decimal point three spaces to the right.)

2. Something that is 1.13 cm long is also how many nanometers long? (The difference between the superscripts of 10^{-2} and 10^{-9} is seven; move the decimal point seven spaces to the right.)

Make up some problems of your own, and practice until you can work readily with the metric units. You will find it very easy to convert from one unit to another, so long as you stay within the metric system. This is why most nations of the world have already switched to the metric system, and the U.S. is in the process of doing so. Confusion arises only when you try to convert back and forth between the metric units and the U.S. Customary Units. For youngsters who learn from the beginning to estimate sizes in metric units, the metric system will seem perfectly natural. For those of us who grew up on inches and pounds, it takes a little practice to develop an intuitive sense of the meaning of a 50 kilometer drive (31.05 miles) or 2 liters of milk (0.53 gallon). But once you get past the need to convert back and forth from the old units, the metric system should seem natural and easy.

One other possible point of confusion should be mentioned. Scientists in the United States (who long ago adopted the metric system) have traditionally used the spellings "meter" and "liter," while European nations have used the spellings "metre" and "litre." It is not yet clear which spellings will be finally adopted for general use when the U.S. has switched over to the metric system for everyday measurements. At the moment, you will probably encounter both spellings, so don't let it confuse you.

Glossary

Numbers in **boldface** represent pages in the text where you will find a full discussion of the term (in many cases, with illustrations). Additional page references for these terms (as well as page references for many other terms) may be found in the index.

absolute threshold   The minimal amount of a stimulus required for us to perceive the presence of the stimulus. **173** (This concept has been abandoned in favor of measures of sensitivity. See also **Signal Detection, Theory of.**)

absorption spectrum   A graph portraying a pigment's ability to absorb various wavelengths of light. **136**

accommodation   The process of changing the shape of the lens in the eye, thus keeping the focal length the same for nearby and distant objects. **67**

acoustic law   See **Ohm's Acoustic Law.**

action potential The temporary electrical equality that occurs between the inside and outside of an axon following a sufficiently intense disturbance to the axon. (Also called nerve impulse, or spike.) **12.**

acuity See **visual acuity.**

adaptation See **dark adaptation; light adaptation.**

additive mixture The result of mixing lights. **146**

afterimages The perceptual effects noted after looking at one stimulus for an extended period of time. **150**

All-or-None Principle An axon reacts to a disturbance either by producing a full-sized action potential or by doing nothing, depending upon the intensity of the disturbance. **18**

amplitude The height from peak to trough of a wave. **92**

ampulla The enlarged portion of each semicircular canal that contains the crista. **323**

annulospiral endings Receptor cells, located in intrafusal fibers, that signal changes in the state of contraction of extrafusal fibers. **316**

auditory cortex The region of cortex, located primarily in the temporal lobes, that is devoted to audition; composed of areas such as AI, AII, and Ep. **230**

auditory nerves The two collections of axons that carry information from the inner ears toward the brain. **193**

aural harmonics The changes in sounds created by the ear. **237**

axon The portion of a neuron that conducts information away from the cell body. **4**

basilar membrane The membrane in the cochlea on which the hair cells are located. **210**

beats When two or more notes that are similar in frequency are played simultaneously, a note midway between the originals appears to wax and wane in loudness (monaural beat) or to rotate within the head (binaural beat). **275**

binocular cues Information about depth, such as stereopsis, that is available to us only when we view the world through both eyes. **183**

blind spot The point in the retina where the ganglion-cell axons leave the eye. (Also called the optic disc.) **83**

bulbs, olfactory See **olfactory bulbs.**

cells See **complex cells; ganglion cells; hair cells; higher-order hypercomplex cells; lower-order hypercomplex cells; nonopponent cells; off cells; on cells; on–off cells; opponent cells; simple cells.**

characteristic frequency   That frequency of sound to which a neuron in the auditory system is most sensitive. **239**

chiasma   See **optic chiasma.**

choroid   The blood-supply layer of the eye, found underneath the sclera. **60**

Chromaticity-units (C-units)   Cells in the intermediate layer of the retina that sometimes depolarize and sometimes hyperpolarize in response to light, depending upon its wavelength. **101**

cilia   Very small, bristle-like endings found at the tips of hair cells, taste cells, and olfactory rods. **213**

cochlea   The coiled structure of the inner ear that is composed of scala vestibuli, Reissner's membrane, scala media, the basilar membrane, and scala tympani. **208**

cochlear duct   Reissner's membrane, scala media, the receptor cells and their associated structures, and the basilar membrane. **212**

cochlear microphonic   The overall electrical response of the cochlea to sound. **234**

cochlear nuclei   Four synaptic areas, located in the brainstem, that are part of the auditory system. **229**

cochlear resting potentials   Electrical differences among various portions of the cochlea that can be recorded when the cochlea is undisturbed; includes the perilymphatic and endolymphatic potentials. **232**

cold, paradoxical   See **paradoxical cold.**

cold fibers   First-order neurons that respond to temperatures below and well above normal skin temperature. **301**

colliculi   See **inferior colliculi; superior colliculi.**

columnar organization   An arrangement of neurons in the cortex whereby neurons that respond to the same stimuli lie in a column extending from the surface inward to the depths of the cortex. **121**

combination tones   The summation tones and difference tones heard when two or more notes are played simultaneously. **274**

complex cells   Neurons in the visual cortex that respond maximally to a bar of light of a particular width and orientation placed anywhere within their receptive fields. **121**

conduction   See **decremental conduction; nondecremental conduction; saltatory conduction.**

conduction deafness   Hearing loss due to malfunctioning of the tympanic membrane or the ossicular chain. **206**

cones   The receptor cells of the eye that are responsive under conditions of bright illumination and that give rise to color vision. **80**

contrast effects   The perceptual effects noted when one substance is tasted following exposure to another substance. **354**

convergent arrangement   Information from several sources is sent to one location. **99**

cornea   The transparent membrane covering the front portion of the eye. **57**

cortex   The deeply folded outer portion of the brain. **47** (See also **auditory cortex; somatosensory cortex; visual cortex.**)

Corti, organ of   See **organ of Corti.**

cranial nerves   Collections of axons (such as the facial nerve, glossopharyngeal nerve, and vagus nerve) that carry information about the head to and from the brain. **289**

crista   The structure contained within an ampulla; it is composed of the cupula, hair cells, and basal structure. **324**

cues   See **binocular cues; monocular cues.**

C-units   See **Chromaticity-units**

d′   A measurement of sensitivity, used in the **Theory of Signal Detection. 262**

dark adaptation   The process of becoming adjusted to dim illumination conditions. **155**

deafness   See **conduction deafness; nerve deafness.**

decibel (db)   A unit of measure of the intensity of a sound wave; one-tenth of a bel. **202**

decremental conduction   A graded potential becomes smaller as it travels along a dendrite or cell body. **23**

dendrite   The portion of a neuron that conducts information toward the cell body. **4**

depolarization   A reduction or removal of the electrical difference normally found between the inside and outside of a neuron. **12**

dermis   The inner layer of skin, within which receptor cells are found. **280**

dichromat   An individual who has only two kinds of cones. **149**

dichromatic theory   See **Hering's dichromatic theory.**

difference threshold   The minimal amount by which stimuli must differ along a particular dimension (such as size or intensity) before we notice that they differ. **159**

diopter   A unit of measurement that describes the bending power of a lens. **66**

discrimination   See **tonal pattern discrimination.**

divergent arrangement   Information from one source is sent to several other locations. **99**

dorsal tracts   Bundles of axons in the spinal cord that form part of the lemniscal system. **284**

ear   See **inner ear; middle ear; outer ear.**

electrical equilibrium   The equal distribution of positive and negative ions inside and outside of a cell. **7**

energies, nerve   See **Specific Nerve Energies, Law of.**

epidermis   The outermost layer of skin. **280**

equilibrium   See **electrical equilibrium; osmotic equilibrium.**

excitatory postsynaptic potential (EPSP)   A depolarization that is recorded postsynaptically. **36**

extralemniscal system   The evolutionarily older, less systematic, and less rapidly conducting pathway by which skin information is sent to the brain. **286**

Fechner's Law   An equation stating that the sensation level associated with a stimulus is proportional to the logarithm of the stimulus. **162**

fibers   See **cold fibers; warm fibers.**

firing rate   The rate at which an axon produces nerve impulses. **113**

first-order neuron   A neuron that collects information from a receptor. **50**

focal length   The distance between a lens and the focal point. **64**

focal point   The point where light rays that have been bent by a lens all converge. **63**

fovea   The area in the center of the retina that contains the highest concentration of cones but no rods. **83**

frequency   The number of cycles per second that occurs in a sound wave; measured in Hertz (Hz). **197** (See also **fundamental frequency.**)

frequency theories of hearing   Theories that propose that the basilar membrane moves up and down in time with the movements of the stapes. **221**

fundamental frequency   The dominant frequency in a complex sound. **274**

ganglion cells   The cells forming the innermost layer of the retina. **103**

geniculate nuclei   See **lateral geniculate nuclei; medial geniculate nuclei.**

glomerulus (plural, **glomeruli**)   An intricate synapse formed by the axons of the olfactory nerve and the granule cells, mitral cells, and tufted cells of the olfactory bulb. **358**

Golgi tendon organs Receptor cells, located in tendons, that signal changes in the tension being placed on the tendons. **314**

graded potential The response of a dendrite or cell body to a disturbance. **22**

gross VIIIth nerve response The overall electrical response of the auditory nerve to sounds played into the ear; composed of the N_1 response, N_2 response, etc. **237**

hair cells The receptor cells found inside the cochlea, the semicircular canals, and the otolith organs. **212**

harmonics Multiples of the fundamental frequency. **274** (See also **aural harmonics.**)

hearing See **frequency theories of hearing; place theories of hearing.**

Hecht, Shlaer, and Pirenne experiment A study of the absolute threshold in vision. **174**

Helmholtz's Resonance Theory A place theory of hearing. **222**

Hering dichromatic theory A theory that postulates that there are two different kinds of elements responsible for color vision. **144**

higher-order hypercomplex cells Neurons in the visual cortex that respond maximally to a bar of light of a particular width and length placed at any orientation in their receptive fields. **122**

hypercomplex cells See **higher-order hypercomplex cells; lower-order hypercomplex cells.**

hyperpolarization An increase in the electrical difference normally found between the inside and outside of a neuron. **36**

impedance matching The process by which the ossicular chain effectively cancels out the difference between the resistances of air and of the cochlear fluids. **205**

inferior colliculi Synaptic areas, located deep within the brain, that are part of the auditory system. **230**

impulse, nerve See **action potential.**

inhibitory postsynaptic potential (IPSP) A hyperpolarization that is recorded postsynaptically. **38**

inner ear The cochlea. **192**

intermediate layer The amacrine cells, bipolar cells, and horizontal cells of the retina. **97**

iris The muscular, pigmented ring in the anterior chamber of the eye that controls the amount of available light entering the eye. **57**

isomerization The process of changing the shape of a molecule without adding or removing atoms. **87**

kinesthesis   Information about the angles of our joints and the degree of contraction of our skeletal muscles. **309**

λ_{max} The particular wavelength of light that is most readily absorbed by a pigment. **136**

lateral geniculate nuclei (LGN)   The portions of the thalamus devoted to vision. **110**

lemniscal system   The evolutionarily newer, more systematic, and more rapidly conducting pathway by which skin information is sent to the brain. **284**

lemnisci   See **medial lemnisci.**

light adaptation   The process of becoming adjusted to bright illumination conditions. **158**

localization   See **sound localization.**

lower-order hypercomplex cells   Neurons in the visual cortex that respond maximally to a bar of light of a particular width, orientation, and length placed in their receptive fields. **122**

Luminosity-units (L-units)   Cells in the intermediate layer of the retina that always depolarize or always hyperpolarize in response to light, regardless of its wavelength. **101**

Mach band   A perceptual effect in which the edge or contour between bright and dim areas is enhanced. **130**

macula   The site of the receptor cells in each otolith organ; it is composed of hair cells, a basal structure, and a gelatinous mass that contains otoliths. **331**

maintained discharge   A slow and steady firing rate that occurs in the apparent absence of stimulation. **113**

map   See **retinotopic map; somatotopic map; tonotopic map.**

masking   The "covering up" of one stimulus by a second, more intense stimulus. **276**

matching   See **impedance matching; metameric match.**

medial geniculate nuclei   The portions of the thalamus devoted to audition. **230**

medial lemnisci   Two broad ribbons of axons that carry information from one side of the medulla to the opposite side of the thalamus; part of the lemniscal system. **285**

Melzack–Wall Theory   See **Pain, Melzack–Wall Theory of.**

membrane   See **basilar membrane; tectorial membrane.**

metameric match   A mixture of monochromatic lights that appears identical to a different monochromatic light. **144**

microphonic   See **cochlear microphonic.**

middle ear   The ossicular chain and the cavity that houses it. **192**

middle-ear muscles   The tensor tympani and stapedius muscles that, when contracted, reduce the movements of the ossicular chain. **216**

mixture   See **additive mixture; subtractive mixture.**

monochromat   An individual who has only one kind of cone. **149**

monocular cues   Information about depth, such as relative size and interposition, that is available to us even when we view the world through only one eye. **182**

moon illusion   The perception that the moon shrinks in size when it is viewed first at the horizon and later overhead. **76**

myelin   An insulating layer, white in color, found along the length of most axons. **20**

nerve   A collection of axons; also called a tract, bundle, or group of fibers. **51** (See also **auditory nerves; cranial nerves; dorsal tracts; medial lemnisci; olfactory nerves; olivocochlear bundles; optic nerves; optic tracts; spinothalamic tracts.**)

nerve deafness   Hearing loss due to damage to the cochlea or auditory nerve. **206**

nerve impulse   See **action potential.**

neuron   A nerve cell. **4** (See also **first-order neurons; second-order neurons.**)

nodes of Ranvier   Breaks in the myelin found at intervals along the length of an axon. **20**

nondecremental conduction   An action potential remains the same size as it travels the length of an axon. **16**

nonopponent cells   Neurons in the LGN that respond in the same way to all wavelengths of light. **142**

nucleus (plural, **nuclei**)   An area containing the dendrites and cell bodies of a collection of neurons. **51** (See also **cochlear nuclei; lateral geniculate nuclei; medial geniculate nuclei; pregeniculate nuclei; superior olivary nuclei.**)

off cells   Ganglion cells that increase their firing rates when light is removed from their receptive fields. **115**

Ohm's Acoustic Law   The ability of the auditory system to analyze a complex tone into its components. **271**

olfactory bulbs   Synaptic relay areas for the olfactory system, located along the underside of the front portion of the brain. **357–358**

olfactory nerves   Two collections of axons that carry information from the nasal cavities to the brain. **357**

olfactory rods   Naked dendritic endings that hang down into the nasal cavity; they are the receptor cells for smell. **357**

olivary nuclei   See **superior olivary nuclei.**

olivocochlear bundles (OCB)   Two collections of axons running from the superior olivary nucleus on one side of the brain to the opposite ear; the axons inhibit the opposite auditory nerve. **248**

ommatidium (plural, **ommatidia**)   A unit of the compound eye, made up of a lens, receptor cells, and a neural cell. **125**

on cells   Ganglion cells that increase their firing rates when light is shined on their receptive fields. **115**

on–off cells   Cells in the visual system that increase their firing rates both when light is shined on and when light is removed from their receptive fields. **117**

opponent cells   Neurons in the LGN that increase their firing rates in response to some wavelengths and decrease their firing rates in response to other wavelengths. **142**

optic chiasma   The crossing point of the optic nerves. **107**

optic disc   See **blind spot.**

optic nerves   The two collections of ganglion-cell axons leaving the eyes. **107**

optic tracts   Two bundles of ganglion-cell axons that run from the optic chiasma into the depths of the brain. **108**

organ of Corti   The supporting cells, inner and outer hair cells, and the tectorial membrane; found within the cochlear duct. **213**

osmotic equilibrium   Equal concentrations of ions inside and outside of a cell. **7**

ossicular chain   The bones of the middle ear: the malleus, incus, and stapes. **192**

otolith organs   The structures called the utricle and saccule, located near the cochlea, which contain receptor cells that signal the position of the head. **331**

otoliths   Small crystals of calcium carbonate that are suspended in the gelatinous masses of the otolith organs. **331**

outer ear   The pinna, external auditory meatus, and tympanic membrane. **191**

outer segments   The portions of rods and cones that point toward the choroid and that contain photochemicals. **80**

oval window   The flexible membrane in the wall of the cochlea against which the stapes pushes. **212**

Pacinian corpuscles   Skin receptors especially sensitive to touch. **297**

Pain, Melzack–Wall Theory of   A theory proposing that our perceptions of pain arise because of particular patterns of activity in the nervous system. **302**

papilla (plural, **papillae**)   The bumps covering the tongue; the taste buds are found in the papillae. **339**

paradoxical cold   The initial perception that a hot stimulus is cold. **302**

photochemicals   Chemicals found in the outer segments of rods and cones that absorb and are changed by light. **86** (See also **rhodopsin.**)

physiological zero   The temperature to which warm fibers and cold fibers have established their baseline firing levels. **300**

place theories of hearing   Theories proposing that different frequencies of sound affect different locations along the length of the basilar membrane. **222**

Poisson probability distributions   Curves that show the probability of reaching or exceeding a particular number of events when the precise number of events cannot be controlled. **180**

polarization   See **depolarization; hyperpolarization.**

posterior nuclear group   The portions of the thalamus devoted to the extralemniscal system. **288**

potential   See **action potential; cochlear resting potentials; excitatory postsynaptic potential; graded potential; inhibitory postsynaptic potential; resting potential; S-potentials.**

Power Law   See **Stevens Power Law.**

pregeniculate nuclei   The areas of the brain that control the muscles of the iris. **58**

probability distributions   See **Poisson probability distributions.**

pupil   The opening in the center of the iris through which light enters the posterior chamber of the eye. **57**

quantum (plural, **quanta**)   The smallest unit of light. **90**

Ranvier, nodes of   See **nodes of Ranvier.**

ratios, trading   See **trading ratios.**

receiver-operating characteristic (ROC)   A graph showing the probability of hits plotted against the probability of false alarms; used in the **Theory of Signal Detection. 261**

receptive field   The area within which a stimulus must fall in order to affect a particular neuron. **114**

reflex   See **stretch reflex.**

Resonance Theory   See **Helmholtz's Resonance Theory.**

response area   The frequencies and intensities of sound to which a neuron in the auditory system responds. **239**

resting potential   The electrical difference between the interior and exterior of an undisturbed neuron. **11** (See also **cochlear resting potentials.**)

retina   The innermost, neural layer of the eye. **79**

retinotopic map   The systematic mapping out of the retina in each area of the visual cortex. **112–113**

rhodopsin   The photochemical found in rods; made up of a vitamin A derivative and a protein. **87**

rods   The receptor cells of the eye that are responsive under conditions of dim illumination. **80**

rods, olfactory   See **olfactory rods.**

Rutherford's Telephone Theory   A frequency theory of hearing. **222**

saltatory conduction   The skipping of an action potential from one node of Ranvier to the next node. **21**

sclera   The outermost, tough membrane of the eye. **57**

second-order neuron   A neuron that collects information from a first-order neuron. **50**

semicircular canals   Structures, located near the cochlea, that contain receptor cells that signal changes in the movements of the head. **323**

shear   The force created when the tectorial membrane slides back and forth over the hair cells, bending their cilia. **214**

Signal Detection, Theory of, (TSD)   An approach to the study of our sensitivity that does not rely on the concept of an absolute threshold. **258**

simple cells   Neurons in the visual cortex that respond maximally to a bar of light of a particular width and orientation placed in one portion of their receptive fields. **121**

sodium pump   The mechanism that actively forces sodium ions outside of neurons. **9**

somatosensory cortex   The region of cortex, located in the parietal lobes, devoted to the skin senses; composed of somatosensory cortex I and somatosensory cortex II. **291**

somatotopic map   The systematic mapping out of the body surface in somatosensory cortex I. **292–293**

sound localization   The ability to determine the direction from which a sound is coming; this ability requires comparisons of the relative intensities, times of arrival, and phases of sounds at the two ears. **245**

spatial summation   The process in which dendrites and cell bodies add together the effects of two or more disturbances that occurred at different locations. **28**

Specific Nerve Energies, Law of   The principle that, no matter how a nerve is stimulated, it always produces the same sensation. **282**

spectrum   See **absorption spectrum; visible spectrum.**

spike   See **action potential.**

spinothalamic tracts   Bundles of axons in the spinal cord that form part of the extralemniscal system. **286**

S-potentials   The graded potentials of cells in the intermediate layer of the retina. **100** (See also **Chromaticity-units** and **Luminosity-units.)**

stereochemical theory   An approach to understanding taste and smell, suggesting that the shape of an ion or molecule determines which receptor cell will be activated. **346**

Stevens Power Law   An equation stating that sensation is proportional to the stimulus raised to a particular power (or exponent). **168–169**

stretch reflex   When a skeletal muscle is stretched, it automatically contracts. **320**

subtractive mixture   The result of mixing pigments. **146**

summation   See **spatial summation; temporal summation.**

superior colliculi   The areas of the brain that control the extraocular muscles. **111**

superior olivary nuclei   Two synaptic areas, located in the brainstem, that are part of the auditory system. **230**

synapse   The point of communication between two neurons or between a neuron and a receptor, a muscle, or a gland. **31**

synaptic cleft   The narrow space between presynaptic and postsynaptic elements. **31**

synaptic transmitters   Chemicals (found within vesicles) that, when released by the presynaptic element, alter the resting potential of the postsynaptic element. **33**

taste buds   Collections of between 2 and 12 individual taste cells. **340**

taste pores   Openings in the wall of a papilla through which the cilia of taste cells project. **340**

tectorial membrane   The membrane in the cochlea that slides back and forth over the hair cells, bending their cilia. **213**

Telephone Theory   See **Rutherford's Telephone Theory.**

temporal summation   The process in which dendrites and cell bodies add together the effects of two or more disturbances that occurred at slightly different times. **26**

thalamus   Two football-shaped groups of nuclei found deep within the brain, through which almost all sensory information passes. **52**

threshold   The minimal amount of disturbance required to change the activity of a receptor cell or neuron. **18** (See also **absolute threshold; difference threshold.**)

tonal gap   A hearing loss limited to a narrow range of sound frequencies. **257**

tonal pattern discrimination   The ability to differentiate between different sequences of the same notes. **250**

tones   See **combination tones; fundamental frequency.**

tonotopic map   The systematic mapping out of the basilar membrane in each area of the auditory cortex. **231**

trading ratios   Equations expressing the idea that we perceive stimuli that produce equal products of intensity, time, and area as being identical stimuli. **170**

transmitters   See **synaptic transmitters.**

Traveling-Wave Theory   See **von Békèsy's Traveling-Wave Theory.**

trichromat   An individual who has three kinds of cones. **149**

trichromatic theory   See **Young–Helmholtz trichromatic theory.**

ventrobasal complex   The portions of the thalamus devoted primarily to the lemniscal system. **286**

vesicles   Small globular structures, found within a presynaptic element, that contain synaptic transmitters. **32**

vestibular system   Provides information about the position and movements of the head; includes the semicircular canals and otolith organs. **322**

visible spectrum   All the colors we can see. **96**

visual acuity   The ability to see clearly the details of objects. **70**

visual angle   The angle formed by light rays as they cross in the eye; measured in degrees, minutes, and seconds. **71**

visual cortex   The region of cortex, located in the occipital lobes, devoted to vision; composed of areas 17, 18, and 19. **112**

Volley Principle   The "platooning" behavior of neurons in the auditory system in response to sounds below 500 Hz. **242**

von Békèsy's Traveling-Wave Theory   A place theory of hearing specifying that sounds of different frequencies set up different wave patterns in the cochlear fluids. **227**

warm fibers   First-order neurons that respond to temperatures above normal skin temperature. **301**

wavelength   The distance from peak to peak of a light wave; measured in nanometers (nm). **91**

Weber's Law   An equation stating that two stimuli must differ by a particular ratio if we are to notice that they differ. **160**

Young–Helmholtz trichromatic theory   A theory postulating that there are three different kinds of receptors responsible for color vision. **143**

Index